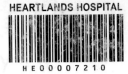
WQ 100

Obstetrics and Gynaecol

THE LIBRARY

Obstetrics and Gynaecology

Lawrence Impey

BA, FRCOG
Consultant in Obstetrics and Fetal Medicine
The John Radcliffe Hospital
Headington, Oxford

and

Tim Child

MA, MD, MRCOG
Senior Fellow in Reproductive Medicine and Surgery
University of Oxford
Honorary Consultant Gynaecologist
The John Radcliffe Hospital
Headington, Oxford

3rd edition

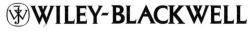

WILEY-BLACKWELL

A John Wiley & Sons, Ltd., Publication

Library of Congress Cataloging-in-Publication Data
Impey, Lawrence.
    Obstetrics & gynaecology / Lawrence Impey and Tim Child. – 3rd ed.
        p. ; cm.
    Includes bibliographical references and index.
    ISBN 978-1-4051-6095-7
    1. Gynecology–Outlines, syllabi, etc.   2. Obstetrics–Outlines, syllabi, etc.   I. Child, Tim.   II. Title.   III. Title: Obstetrics and gynaecology.
    [DNLM: 1. Pregnancy–Outlines.   2. Genital Diseases, Female–Outlines.   3. Pregnancy Complications–Outlines. WQ 18.2 I34o 2008]
    RG101.I47 2008
    618.02′02–dc22

                                                                                    2008012015

ISBN: 978-1-4051-6095-7

A catalogue record for this book is available from the British Library.

Set in 9.5 on 11.5 pt Minion by SNP Best-set Typesetter Ltd., Hong Kong
Printed in Singapore by Fabulous Printers Pte Ltd

3   2010

Contents

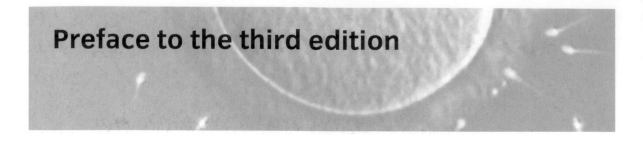

Preface to the third edition

It is over 10 years since, disillusioned with the other texts, I first wrote this book. Many nice things have been written and said about it since the first edition in 1999. One reservation, however, has been that whilst it provides all the information required to pass 'obs and gynae' finals, there was not enough to do really well. This has been rectified for this edition, with Tim Child as co-author. In fact, there was always a huge amount of information here: it is just very tight because we have tried not to waste a single word. Further we have kept out the irrelevant, outdated stuff. We have now expanded the book slightly for this third edition, with more detail; at the same time we have brought the text completely up to date. We hope that this, combined with references and extended further reading, means that the student can do really well and indeed that obstetrician, GP or even midwife in training can get straightforward answers to the essential issues.

LI
TC
Oxford 2008

Preface to the first edition

This book is written for the UK medical student, in line with changes in medical education and the advent of the core curriculum. The level of information is enough to allow a high mark in the final obstetrics and gynaecology examinations. But its strong emphasis on management should also be useful for practising doctors and those about to take postgraduate examinations.

As a student and then a lecturer I was always surprised at the deficiencies of many textbooks: how they failed to emphasize what was common or important, how little emphasis they placed on 'what to do' in a real situation, and how little they allowed understanding of the subject. Problem-based learning is in part a backlash against this. Yet there remains a need for a comprehensive yet straightforward textbook. In this, the space given to

each topic reflects it importance. Subjects are cross-referenced (page cross-references are indicated by superior square brackets). The information is up to date, evidence-based where possible, and referenced, at least for important, new or contentious issues. At the end of each chapter, summaries of all the major topics should aid revision and prevent the need for a separate revision text. At the end of the book, separate management sections describe what to do in all the common clinical situations, from the management of slow progress in labour to the management of the subfertile couple.

Lawrence Impey
1999

Acknowledgements

I am grateful to the many friends and colleagues in the UK and Ireland who have made criticisms in their areas of expertise and have helped with the preparation of this book. These are Mr Mike Bowen, Dr Bill Boyd, Dr Bridgette Byrne, Dr Paul Dewart, Dr Valerie Donnelly, Dr Anne Edwards, Dr Michael Foley, Miss Michelle Fynes, Mr Mike Gillmer, Dr Jonathan Hobson, Mr James Hopkisson, Miss Pauline Hurley, Mr Simon Jackson, Dr Catherine James, Dr Declan Keane, Mr Stephen Kennedy, Dr Peter Lenehan, Dr Graham Lloyd-Jones, Dr Graz Luzzi, Dr Dermott MacDonald, Dr Pamela MacKinnon, Dr Peter McParland, Mr Enda McVeigh, Miss Kathryn MacQuillan, Dr Jane Mellanby, Dr Breda O'Kelly, Miss Meghana Pandit, Dr John Picard, Miss Charlotte Porter, Professor Chris Redman, Miss Margaret Rees, Dr Robin Russell, Miss Susan Sellers, Dr Sarah Sheikh, Dr Orla Sheil, Mr Alexander Smarason, Professor Philip Steer and Dr Mary Wingfield. I am indebted to Blackwell Science, particularly Ms Rebecca Huxley, Dr Andrew Robinson and Dr Michael Stein for their faith, help and encouragement, and to the medical students of The Royal College of Surgeons in Ireland and of Oxford University for their criticisms. And I am particularly grateful to Ms Jane Fallows for her illustrations. Most of all, however, I thank Susan and Cicely Impey for their support and patience during the writing of this book.

Acknowledgements for the third edition

In addition to those who helped with the previous editions, we would like to thank Dr Patricia Boyd, Mrs Jane Child, Ms Jane Fallows, Miss Catherine Greenwood, Ms Rebecca Huxley, Miss Cicely Impey, Mr Simon Jackson, Mr Sean Kehoe, Miss Jane Moore, Miss Jo Morrison, Ms Alice Nelson, Dr Margaret Rees, Mr Alex Slack, Mr Kevin Smith and Mr Alex Swanton for their help, advice or patience.

LI
TC

List of abbreviations

ACE	angiotensin-converting enzyme		DCDA	dichorionic diamniotic
ACT	artemisin combination therapy		DES	diethylstilboestrol
ACTH	adrenocorticotrophic hormone		DEXA	dual X-ray absorptometry
AD	Alzheimer's disease		DI	donor insemination
AFP	alpha fetoprotein		DIC	disseminated intravascular coagulation
AIDS	acquired immune deficiency syndrome		DLE	diathermy loop excision
ALP	alkaline phosphatase		DNA	deoxyribonucleic acid
ALT	alanine aminotransferase		DVT	deep vein thrombosis
AP	antero-posterior		DZ	dizygotic
APH	antepartum haemorrhage		ECG	electrocardiogram
ARDS	adult respiratory distress syndrome		ECV	external cephalic version
ARM	artificial rupture of membranes		EDD	expected day of delivery
ASD	atrial septal defect		EIA	enzyme immunoassay
AST	aspartate aminotransferase		EPAU	early pregnancy assessment unit
BCG	Bacille bilié de Calmette Guérin		EPDS	Edinburgh Postnatal Depression Scale
β-hCG	human chorionic gonadotrophin beta-subunit		ERPC	evacuation of retained products of conception
BMD	bone mineral density		eSET	elective single embryo transfer
BMI	body mass index		ESR	erythrocyte sedimentation rate
BP	blood pressure		EUA	examination under anaesthetic
BSO	bilateral salpingo-oöphorectomy		FBC	full blood count
BV	bacterial vaginosis		FBS	fetal blood sampling
CA	carcinoma		FER	frozen embryo replacement
CA 125	serum carcinoma/cancer antigen 125		FFP	fresh frozen plasma
CEMACH	Confidential Enquiry into Maternal and Child Health		FHR	fetal heart rate
CGIN	cervical glandular intraepithelial neoplasia		FIGO	International Federation of Gynaecology and Obstetrics
CIN	cervical intraepithelial neoplasia		FISH	fluorescence *in situ* hybridization
CMV	cytomegalovirus		FSD	female sexual dysfunction
CNST	Clinical Negligence Scheme for Trusts		FSH	follicle-stimulating hormone
COC	combined oral contraceptive		G&S	group and save
CPP	chronic pelvic pain		GBS	group B streptococcus
CRP	C-reactive protein		GFR	glomerular filtration rate
CSF	cerebrospinal fluid		GnRH	gonadotrophin-releasing hormone
CT	computed tomography		GSI	genuine stress incontinence
CTG	cardiotocography		HAART	highly active antiretroviral therapy
CVA	cerebrovascular accident		Hb	haemoglobin
CVP	central venous pressure		HbF	fetal haemoglobin
CVS	chorionic villus sampling		hCG	human chorionic gonadotrophin
D&C	dilatation and curettage			

HELLP	(syndrome of) haemolysis, elevated liver enzymes and low platelets	NEC	necrotizing enterocolitis
HFEA	Human Fertilization and Embryology Authority	NHS	National Health Service
		NICE	National Institute for Clinical Excellence
HIV	human immunodeficiency virus	NPV	negative predictive value
HMB	heavy menstrual bleeding	NSAID	non-steroidal anti-inflammatory drug
HPV	human papilloma virus	NTD	neural tube defect
HRT	hormone replacement therapy	OA	occipito-anterior
HSG	hysterosalpingogram	OAB	overactive bladder
HSV	herpes simplex virus	OHSS	ovarian hyperstimulation syndrome
HVS	high vaginal swab	OP	occipito-posterior
IA	intermittent auscultation	OT	occipito-transverse
IBS	irritable bowel syndrome	PAPPA	pregnancy-associated plasma protein A
ICAS	Independent Complaints Advocacy Service	PBS	painful bladder syndrome
		PCA	patient-controlled analgesia
ICSI	intracytoplasmic sperm injection	PCB	postcoital bleeding
Ig	immunoglobulin	PCO	polycystic ovary
i.m.	intramuscular	PCOS	polycystic ovary syndrome
IMB	intermenstrual bleeding	PCP	*Pneumocystis carinii* pneumonia
IPT	intermittent preventive treatment	PCR	polymerase chain reaction
IUD	intrauterine device	PDA	patent ductus arteriosus
IUGR	intrauterine growth restriction	PET	positron emission tomography
IUI	intrauterine insemination	PFMT	pelvic floor muscle training
IUS	intrauterine system	PGD	preimplantation genetic diagnosis
i.v.	intravenous	PGE_2	prostaglandin E_2
IVF	*in vitro* fertilization	$PGF_{2\alpha}$	prostaglandin $F_{2\alpha}$
IVP	intravenous pyelogram	PGS	preimplantation genetic screening
KOH	potassium hydroxide	PI	Pearl index
LARC	long-acting reversible contraceptive	PID	pelvic inflammatory disease
LAVH	laparoscopic assisted vaginal hysterectomy	PIGF	placental growth factor
		PMB	postmenopausal bleeding
LDH	lactic dehydrogenase	PMS	premenstrual syndrome
LFT	liver function test	POP	progestogen-only pill
LH	luteinizing hormone	PPH	postpartum haemorrhage
LLETZ	large loop excision of transformation zone	PPV	positive predictive value
LMP	last menstrual period	PSV	peak velocity in systole
LMWH	low-molecular-weight heparin	RCT	randomized controlled trial
LN	lymph node	SBR	serum bilirubin
LSCS	lower segment Caesarean section	SD	standard deviation
LUNA	laparoscopic uterine nerve ablation	SFD	small for dates
MC	monochorionic	SHBG	steroid hormone binding globulin
MCA	middle cerebral artery	SIDS	sudden infant death syndrome
MCDA	monochorionic diamniotic	SLE	systemic lupus erythematosus
MCHC	mean cell haemoglobin concentration	SROM	spontaneous rupture of membranes
MCMA	monochorionic monoamniotic	SSR	surgical sperm retrieval
MCV	mean cell volume	SSRI	selective serotonin reuptake inhibitor
MRI	magnetic resonance imaging	STI	sexually transmitted infection
MSU	mid-stream urine	T3	triiodothyronine
MZ	monozygotic	T4	thyroxine
NAAT	nucleic acid amplification test	TAH	total abdominal hysterectomy

TB	tuberculosis	UAE	uterine artery embolization
TCRE	transcervical resection of endometrium	UDCA	ursodeoxycholic acid
TCRF	transcervical resection of fibroid	USS	ultrasound scan
TEDS	thromboembolic disease stockings	UTI	urinary tract infection
TENS	transcutaneous electrical nerve stimulation	VBAC	vaginal delivery after a previous Caesarean section
TFT	thyroid function test	VDRL	Venereal Disease Research Laboratories
TLH	total laparoscopic hysterectomy	VE	vaginal examination
TOP	termination of pregnancy	VEGF	vascular endothelial growth factor
TOT	trans-obdurator tape	VH	vaginal hysterectomy
TSH	thyroid-stimulating hormone	VIN	vulvar intraepithelial neoplasia
TTN	transient tachypnoea of the newborn	VMA	vanillymandelic acid
TTTS	twin–twin transfusion syndrome	VQ	ventilation/perfusion
TVS	transvaginal sonography	VSD	ventricular septal defect
TVT	tension-free vaginal tape	VTE	venous thromboembolism
U&E	urea and electrolytes	WBC	white blood cell count
UA	umbilical artery	WHO	World Health Organization

List of journal abbreviations

Acta Obstet Gynecol Scand	Acta Obstetricia et Gynecologica Scandinavica
AmJOG	American Journal of Obstetrics and Gynecology
Ann Intern Med	Annals of Internal Medicine
Ann Neurol	Annals of Neurology
BJOG	BJOG: an International Journal of Obstetrics and Gynaecology
BMC Public Health	BMC Public Health
BMJ	British Medical Journal
Br J Cancer	British Journal of Cancer
Cochrane	Cochrane Database System Review
Curr Opin Obstet Gynecol	Current Opinions in Obstetrics and Gynecology
Diabetes Care	Diabetes Care
Diabetes Metab	Diabetes and Metabolism
Epilepsia	Epilepsia
Eur J Obstet Gynecol Reprod Biol	European Journal of Obsterics, Gynecology and Reproductive Biology
Fertil Steril	Fertility and Sterility
Gynecol Oncol	Gynecologic Oncology
Hum Reprod	Human Reproduction
JAMA	Journal of the American Medical Association
JCEM	Journal of Clinical Endocrinology and Metabolism
J Clin Oncol	Journal of Clinical Oncology
J Matern Fetal Neonatal Med	Journal of Maternal–Fetal and Neonatal Medicine
J Med Screen	Journal of Medical Screening
J Natl Cancer Inst	Journal of the National Cancer Institute
J Obstet Gynaecol Res	Journal of Obstetrics and Gynaecology Research
J Periodontol	Journal of Periodontology
Mal J	Malaria Journal
NEJM	New England Journal of Medicine
Neurol	Neurology
Obstet Gynecol	Obsterics and Gynecology
Prenat Diagn	Prenatal Diagnosis
Reprod Biomed Online	Reproductive Biomedicine Online
Soc Sci Med	Social Science and Medicine
Ultrasound Obstet Gynecol	Ultrasound in Obstetrics and Gynecology

Gynaecology section

1 The history and examination in gynaecology

The remit of the doctor is to improve quality of life, not just to treat life-threatening disease: if a symptom is causing distress, treatment should be considered. The type and extent of treatment is determined largely by the patient: the doctor gives information and advice, so the patient can give her *informed* consent. The patient's history should be used not only to help make a diagnosis but also to discover how much her symptom(s) is/are affecting her. Or she may simply be concerned as to the cause of her symptoms (e.g. malignancy) and reassurance is enough.

The gynaecological history

Personal details

Ask her name, age and occupation.

Presenting complaint(s)

How long has the problem been present and how much does it affect her? If it is pain, what alleviates and what exacerbates it, where is it and what is its nature? Allow the patient to elaborate as there may be more than one problem, initially without asking direct questions, perhaps asking her to rate her problems in order of severity. Has she ever consulted a doctor about this problem before and, if so, what has been done? If there are multiple presenting complaints, these should be put in order of severity/effect on her life.

Obstetrics and Gynaecology, 3rd edition. By Lawrence Impey and Tim Child. Published 2008 by Blackwell Publishing, ISBN: 978-1-4051-6095-7.

Specific gynaecological questions

These are asked next, starting with ones that are relevant to this presenting complaint. For example, if it is a menstrual problem, the most appropriate next questions concern menstruation; if it is a urinary problem, one should ask all the appropriate urinary tract questions next.

Menstrual questions. How often does she menstruate (how many days from the first day of bleeding to the next first day?) and how long does menstruation last? (4/28 means bleeding lasts for 4 days and occurs every 28 days.) Is it regular or irregular? Is it heavy? (Number of pads/tampons used or the presence of clots can be useful.) Is it or the days leading up to it painful? Is there ever intermenstrual bleeding (IMB) [→ p.15]? Is there ever postcoital bleeding (PCB) [→ p.17]? Is there ever vaginal discharge and, if so, what is it like? Does she experience premenstrual tension? When was her last menstrual period (LMP)? If postmenopausal, has there been postmenopausal bleeding (PMB)?

Sexual/contraceptive questions. Is she sexually active? If so, is it painful? If so, is it on penetration (superficial dyspareunia) or deep inside (deep dyspareunia) and is it during and/or after (delayed). What contraceptive (if appropriate) does she use and what has she used in the past?

Cervical smear questions. When was her last cervical smear? (This should be done every 3 years between the ages of 25 and 49 years, every 5 years between 50 and 64 years, and not performed thereafter unless never screened or history of recent abnormal tests.) Has she ever had an abnormal smear? If so, what was done [→ p.34]?

Menstrual questions
How often and for how long?
Heavy or painful?
Regularity?
Intermenstrual bleeding (IMB) or postcoital bleeding (PCB)?
When was her last menstrual period (LMP)?

Presenting the history
Start by summing up the important points, including relevant gynaecological questions:
This is . . . , who is a . . . year-old . . . (parity), with a . . . (time) history of . . . , who . . . (most significant findings in history).
Example: This is Mrs X, who is a 38-year-old nulliparous woman, with a 3-month history of postcoital bleeding (PCB), who has a normal menstrual cycle and last had a cervical smear 7 years ago.
N.B. By mentioning the last smear, you have shown understanding that PCB may be a symptom of cervical carcinoma.
Now go through the history in some detail.
Then sum up again, in one sentence.

Urinary/prolapse questions. Does she experience frequency, nocturia, urgency or enuresis? Does she ever leak urine? If so, how severe is it and with what is it associated (e.g. coughing, lifting/straining or urgency)? Is there ever dysuria or haematuria? Does she ever get a dragging sensation or feel a mass in or at the vagina?

Other history

Past obstetric history. This should be brief. Start with 'Have you ever been pregnant'? If the answer is 'No', go on to past medical history. If 'Yes', ask details about previous pregnancies in chronological order. See Chapter 16 for explanation of parity and gravidity. Of deliveries, ask when, what weight, how was the infant born and how the infant is now. Ask about any major complications in the pregnancy or labour.

Past medical history. First ask about any previous, particularly gynaecological, operations, however distant. Then directly ask about venous thrombosis, diabetes, lung and heart disease, hypertension, jaundice, etc. as in any medical history. If you elicit no significant history, ask 'Have you ever been in hospital'?

Systems review. Ask the usual cardiovascular, respiratory and neurological questions. In particular ask about urinary and gastrointestinal symptoms in view of the close pelvic relationship.

Drugs. Does she take any regular medication including prescribed, over-the-counter or complementary? Consider asking about illegal drug use if relevant.

Family history. Is there a family history of breast or ovarian carcinoma, of diabetes, venous thromboembolism, heart disease or hypertension?

Personal/social history. Does she smoke? Does she drink alcohol? If either, how much? Is she in a married or stable relationship and, if not, is there support at home? Where does she live and what sort of accommodation is it?

Allergies. Ask specifically about penicillin and latex.

Gynaecological history: specific essential questions
Presenting complaint, its history
Menstrual questions: last menstrual period (LMP), cycle, flow, intermenstrual bleeding (IMB), postcoital bleeding (PCB)
Urinary/prolapse questions
Sexual/contraceptive questions
Cervical smear history
Past obstetric history

Other questions

Now ask 'Is there anything else you think I ought to know'? This gives her the opportunity to help you if you have not discovered all the important facts.

Summarizing the history

1 Could the symptoms be a manifestation of underlying disease that needs to be treated? (For example, erratic menstrual bleeding may be a sign of malignancy.)

2 Are the symptoms themselves causing physical damage? (For example, erratic menstrual bleeding may lead to severe anaemia.)

3 Are the symptoms themselves causing distress? (For example, erratic menstrual bleeding may disrupt a woman's life such that she may feel unable to leave the home.) Or is she unconcerned?

The gynaecological examination

General examination

This is to:
1 Seek the effects (e.g. secondary spread of malignancy) or, more rarely, the causes (e.g. thyroid abnormalities cause menstrual disturbances) of gynaecological problems.
2 Assess general health and incidental disease, particularly if an anaesthetic may be needed.

General appearance and weight, temperature, blood pressure and pulse, and possible anaemia, jaundice or lymphadenopathy should be noted. More detailed examination of the rest of the body is often perfunctory in the young, fit patient, but is important in the older or more sick patient, or in those about to have an anaesthetic.

Breast and axillary examination

This can be performed as a screening test for breast cancer, although breast examination is not routinely undertaken in UK gynaecological practice unless investigating a potentially malignant pelvic mass (Fig. 1.1). The patient sits back, the breasts are inspected for irregularities and all four breast quadrants are palpated as the patient lies supine with her hands behind her head. The axilla, a principal area for lymph drainage, is then palpated with the patient's arm resting on the examiner's shoulder.

Abdominal examination

The patient lies comfortably on her back with her head on a pillow, discreetly exposed from the xiphisternum to the symphysis pubis. The bladder should be empty.

Inspect

Look for scars, particularly just above the symphysis pubis and in the umbilicus. Look at the distribution of body hair, for irregularities, striae and hernias.

Palpate

Ask about tenderness first, then palpate gently around the abdomen looking for masses or tenderness. Then palpate specifically for masses from above the umbilicus down to the symphysis pubis (Fig. 1.2). If any masses are present, do they arise from the pelvis (i.e. can you get below them)?

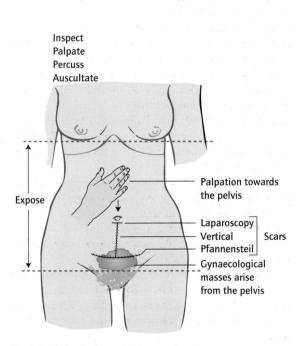

Fig. 1.2 Abdominal examination.

Inspect
Palpate
Percuss
Auscultate

Expose

Palpation towards the pelvis

Laparoscopy
Vertical — Scars
Pfannensteil
Gynaecological masses arise from the pelvis

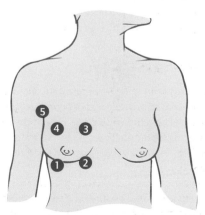

Fig. 1.1 Examination of the breast.

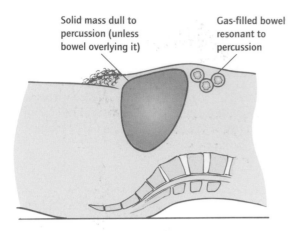

Fig. 1.3 Percussion of the abdomen.

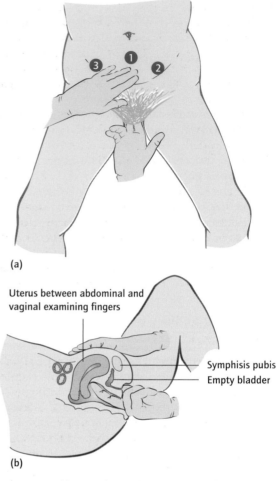

(a)

(b)

Fig. 1.4 Digital bimanual vaginal examination: (a) bimanually palpate areas 1, 2, 3 in order; (b) digital bimanual palpation of the pelvis.

Percuss

Go around the abdomen. The bowel is resonant; fluid-filled and solid cavities (e.g. masses, full bladder) are dull (Fig. 1.3). Look for shifting dullness (free fluid).

Auscultate

Listen to the bowel sounds.

Gynaecological examination
General
(Breast)
Abdomen
Pelvic palpation: digital
Cervical/vaginal inspection: speculum

Vaginal examination

Ensure privacy, explain simply what you intend and ask for the patient's permission. Offer her the opportunity to use the bathroom first. A chaperone must be offered, whether you are male or female. Use lubricating jelly. A metal speculum should be warmed. Internal examination is often uncomfortable, but severe tenderness is abnormal.

Inspect

The vulva and the vaginal orifice are inspected first. Are there any coloured areas, ulcers or lumps on the vulva? Is a prolapse evident at the introitus? Three types of examination have different purposes.

Digital bimanual examination

This assesses the pelvic organs. The patient lies flat, with her ankles together drawn up towards her buttocks and knees apart. Warn the patient before you touch her and ask her to let you know if she finds the examination too uncomfortable. The left hand is placed on the abdomen above the symphysis pubis and is pushed down into the pelvis, so that the organs are palpated between it and two fingers are gently inserted into the vagina (Fig. 1.4a,b).

The uterus is normally the size and shape of a small pear. Size, consistency, regularity, mobility, anteversion or retroversion and tenderness are assessed.

The cervix is normally the first part of the uterus to be felt vaginally and the os is felt as an opening like a toy car tyre. Is the cervix hard or irregular?

The adnexa (lateral to the uterus on either side, containing tube and ovary): tenderness and size and consistency of any mass are assessed. Is it separate from the uterus?

The pouch of Douglas (behind the cervix): the uterosacral ligaments should be palpable. Are these even, irregular or tender, or is there a mass?

Cusco's speculum examination

This allows inspection of the cervix and vaginal walls. The patient lies as for the digital examination. With the blades closed and parallel to the labia and the opening mechanism pointing to the patient's right, gently insert the speculum (Fig. 1.5a). Then rotate it 90° anteriorly and insert it as far as it will go without causing discomfort (Fig. 1.5b). Open it slowly under direct vision and the cervix will come into view (Fig. 1.5c). Common mistakes include not inserting the speculum sufficiently deep and/or posterior with an anterverted uterus. The cervix may be very anterior with a retroverted uterus. Look for ulceration, spontaneous bleeding or irregularities. A cervical smear can be taken. Now slightly withdraw the speculum under direct vision and partly close it without catching the cervix. Slowly withdraw it just open, allowing inspection of the vaginal walls to the introitus, and then close the speculum and remove it, rotating the speculum through 90° on the way out.

Sims' speculum

This allows better inspection of the vaginal walls and, specifically, the prolapse. The patient should be positioned in the left lateral position with the legs partly

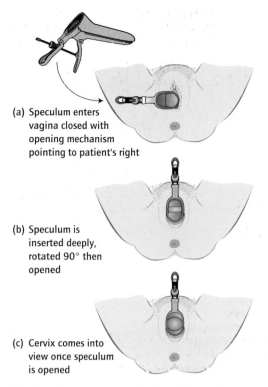

(a) Speculum enters vagina closed with opening mechanism pointing to patient's right

(b) Speculum is inserted deeply, rotated 90° then opened

(c) Cervix comes into view once speculum is opened

Fig. 1.5 Cusco's speculum examination of the cervix and vaginal walls. (a) Speculum enters vagina closed with opening mechanism pointing to patient's right. (b) Speculum is inserted deep, rotated 90°, then opened. (c) The cervix comes into view once the speculum is opened.

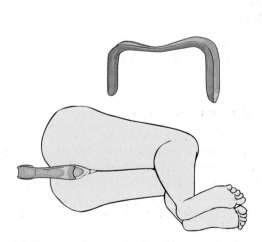

Fig. 1.6 Sims' speculum examination of the vaginal walls.

curled up. Insert the curved speculum into the vagina from behind, with one end pressing against the posterior wall to allow inspection of the anterior wall. Then reverse the speculum, pressing back the anterior wall so that the posterior wall can be seen (Fig. 1.6). If the patient is asked to bear down, the prolapse of either wall and the cervix or vaginal vault can be assessed.

Rectal examination

This is occasionally appropriate if there is posterior wall prolapse, to distinguish between an enterocoele and a rectocoele, and in assessing malignant cervical disease.

Presenting the examination

Present the examination findings, including relevant positive or negative findings:

Mrs X is . . . (describe general appearance sensitively), her blood pressure, temperature and pulse are . . . and abdominal and pelvic examination reveals. . . . There is . . . (mention important positive and negative findings).

Example: Mrs X looks thin and clinically anaemic, her blood pressure is 120/60 mmHg, temperature is normal and pulse is 90 beats/min; abdominal examination reveals a mass arising from the pelvis up to the level of the umbilicus, with no obvious ascites. There is no lymphadenopathy or breast abnormality.

N.B. By mentioning ascites, lymphadenopathy and the breasts, you demonstrated your understanding of the possible aetiology and effects of a pelvic mass.

Management plan. Now decide on a course of action. Plan what investigations (if any) are needed and what course of action (if any) is most appropriate.

Gynaecological History at a Glance

Personal details	Name, age, occupation
Presenting complaint	Details, time-scale, any previous treatment. Prioritize
Gynaecological questions	(Start with most relevant to complaint)

	Menstrual:	Last menstrual period (LMP), cycle, heaviness, intermenstrual bleeding (IMB), postcoital bleeding (PCB)
	Sex/contraceptive:	Sexually active, dyspareunia, contraception?
	Cervical smear:	Last smear, ever abnormal?
	Urinary/prolapse	Frequency, incontinence, lump at introitus

Other history	Past obstetric history:	Ever pregnant? If so, details
	Past medical history:	Operations, major illnesses. Ever in hospital?
	Systems review, drugs, personal (smoking, alcohol), social, family history (particularly breast/ovarian/heart disease), allergies	

Summarize	Presenting complaint and relevant history findings

Gynaecological Examination at a Glance

General	Appearance, anaemia, lymph nodes, blood pressure, pulse
(Breasts/axillae)	Inspect, palpate
Abdomen	Inspect, palpate (particularly suprapubically), percuss, auscultate
Vaginal	Inspect vulva; digital examination; Cusco's speculum, Sims' speculum if prolapse
Summarize	Positive and important negative findings; consider management

2 The menstrual cycle and its disorders

Physiology of puberty

Puberty is the onset of sexual maturity. It is marked by the development of secondary sex characteristics. The *menarche*, or onset of menstruation, is normally the last manifestation of puberty in the female, and in the West occurs on average at 13 years of age. Normal puberty is controlled centrally. The hypothalamic–pituitary axis can be considered as 'waking' and then 'waking up' the ovaries. After the age of 8 years, hypothalamic gonadotrophin-releasing hormone (GnRH) pulses increase in amplitude and frequency, such that pituitary follicle-stimulating hormone (FSH) and then luteinizing hormone (LH) release increases. These stimulate oestrogen release from the ovary (Figs 2.1, 2.2).

Oestrogen is responsible for the development of secondary sexual characteristics: the *thelarche*, or beginning of breast development, occurs first at 9–11 years; the *adrenarche*, or growth of pubic hair (also dependent on adrenal activity), starts at 11–12 years; the final stage is the *menarche* (Fig. 2.2). Menstruation may be irregular at first; as oestrogen secretion rises, it will become regular. Pregnancy is now possible. These changes are accompanied by the growth spurt, due to increased growth hormone release. By the age of 16 years, most growth has finished and the epiphyses fuse. The average age of the menarche is reducing.

Physiology of the menstrual cycle

The hormonal changes of the menstrual cycle cause

Obstetrics and Gynaecology, 3rd edition. By Lawrence Impey and Tim Child. Published 2008 by Blackwell Publishing, ISBN: 978-1-4051-6095-7.

ovulation and induce changes in the endometrium that prepare it for implantation should fertilization occur.

Days 1–4: menstruation

At the start of the menstrual cycle (designated as the first day of menstruation) the endometrium is shed as its hormonal support is withdrawn. Myometrial contraction, which can be painful, also occurs.

Days 5–13: proliferative phase

Pulses of GnRH from the hypothalamus stimulate LH and FSH release which induce follicular growth. The follicles produce oestradiol and inhibin which suppress FSH secretion in a 'negative feedback', such that (normally) only one follicle and oocyte matures. As oestradiol levels continue to rise and reach their maximum, however, a 'positive-feedback' effect on the hypothalamus and pituitary causes LH levels to rise sharply: ovulation follows 36 hours after the LH surge. The oestradiol also causes the endometrium to re-form and become 'proliferative': it thickens as the stromal cells proliferate and the glands elongate.

Days 14–28: luteal/secretory phase

The follicle from which the egg was released becomes the corpus luteum. This again produces oestradiol, but relatively more progesterone, levels of which peak around a week later (day 21 of a 28-day cycle). This induces 'secretory' changes in the endometrium, whereby the stromal cells enlarge, the glands swell and the blood supply increases. Towards the end of the luteal phase, the corpus luteum starts to fail if the egg is not fertilized, causing progesterone and oestrogen levels to fall. As its hormonal support is withdrawn, the endometrium breaks down, menstruation follows and the cycle restarts (Fig. 2.3). Continuous administration of exogenous progestogens maintains a secretory endometrium. This can be used to delay menstruation.

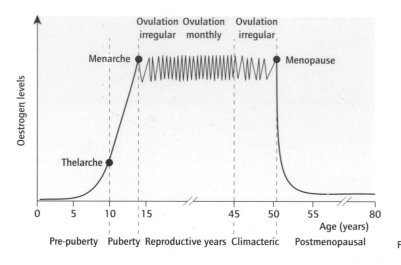

Fig. 2.1 Oestrogen levels in a lifetime.

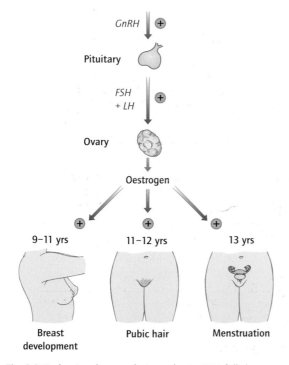

Fig. 2.2 Endocrine changes during puberty. FSH, follicle-stimulating hormone; GnRH, gonadotrophin-releasing hormone; LH, luteinizing hormone.

Normal menstruation
Menarche <16 years Menopause >40 years Menstruation <8 days in length Blood loss <80 mL Cycle length 23–35 days No intermenstrual bleeding (IMB)

Abnormal menstruation and definitions of terms	
Menorrhagia	Heavy menstrual bleeding
Intermenstrual bleeding	Bleeding between periods
Irregular periods	Periods outside the range of 23–35 days with a variability of >7 days between the shortest and longest cycle
Postcoital bleeding	Bleeding after intercourse
Primary amenorrhoea	Periods never start
Secondary amenorrhoea	Periods stop for 6 months or more
Oligomenorrhoea	Infrequent periods (> every 35 days–6 months)
Postmenopausal bleeding	Bleeding 1 year after the menopause
Dysmenorrhoea	Painful periods
Premenstrual syndrome	Psychological and physical symptoms worse in the luteal phase

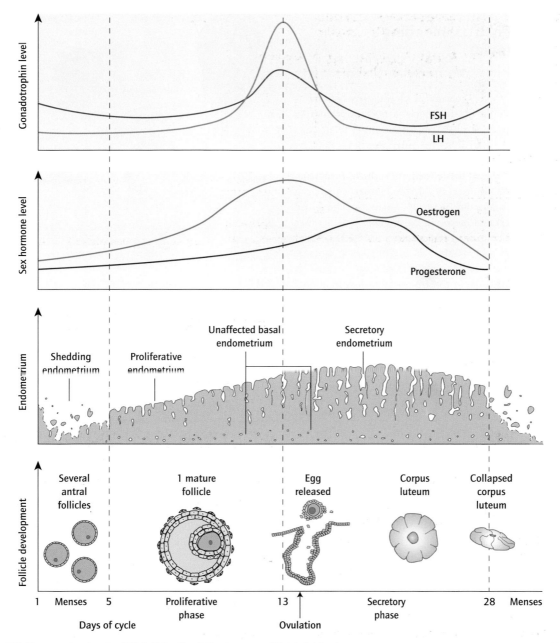

Fig. 2.3 The menstrual cycle. FSH, follicle-stimulating hormone; LH, luteinizing hormone.

Heavy menstrual bleeding (menorrhagia)

Menorrhagia (heavy menstrual bleeding) is defined as excessive bleeding in an otherwise normal menstrual cycle. It is largely a subjective definition, as what constitutes heavy bleeding to one woman may be quite normal for another. Clinically heavy menstrual bleeding (HMB) can be defined as excessive menstrual blood loss that interferes with the woman's physical, emotional, social and material quality of life, and which can occur alone or in combination with other symptoms. Objectively, menorrhagia has been defined as blood loss of >80 mL in an otherwise normal menstrual cycle. This value was chosen because it appears to be the maximum amount that a woman on a normal diet can lose per cycle without becoming iron deficient. In practice, actual blood loss is rarely measured.

Epidemiology

One-third of women complain of heavy periods although most do not seek medical help (*Soc Sci Med* 2007; **65**).

Causes

The majority of women with menorrhagia have no histological abnormality that can be implicated in its causation. The term dysfunctional uterine bleeding is seldom used nowadays. Mechanisms vary. Most women with regular cycles are ovulatory and menorrhagia may result from subtle abnormalities of the endometrial fibrinolytic system or uterine prostaglandin levels. Uterine fibroids (approximately 30% of women) and polyps (approximately 10% of women) are the most common form of pathology found. Chronic pelvic infection, ovarian tumours, and endometrial and cervical malignancy (Fig. 2.4) are rare and are likely to cause irregular bleeding.

Thyroid disease, haemostatic disorders, such as von Willebrand's disease, and anticoagulant therapy are rare causes of menorrhagia. A coagulopathy may be suggested by a history of excessive bleeding after surgery/trauma or easy bruising.

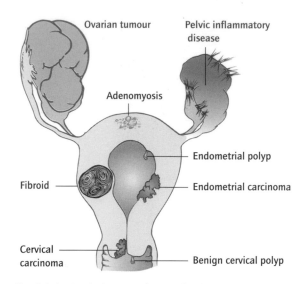

Fig. 2.4 Anatomical causes of menorrhagia.

Clinical features

History: This should assess both the amount and timing of the bleeding. A menstrual calendar is helpful. 'Flooding' and the passage of large clots indicate excessive loss. Any method of contraception should be ascertained.

Examination: Anaemia is common. Pelvic signs are often absent. Irregular enlargement of the uterus suggests fibroids; tenderness with or without enlargement suggests adenomyosis. An ovarian mass may be felt; tenderness and immobile pelvic organs are common with infection and endometriosis (which is not a cause of menorrhagia but which often coexists).

Investigations

To assess the effect of blood loss and fitness, the patient's haemoglobin is checked.

To exclude systemic causes, coagulation and thyroid function are checked only if the history is suggestive of a problem.

To exclude local organic causes, a *transvaginal ultrasound* of the pelvis is performed. This will assess endometrial thickness, exclude a uterine fibroid or ovarian mass and detect larger intrauterine polyps. If the endometrial thickness is >10 mm or a polyp is suspected, or if the woman is over 40 years old with recent onset menorrha-

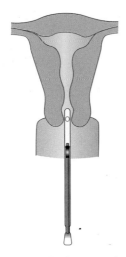

Fig. 2.5 Pipelle endometrial biopsy going through the cervix.

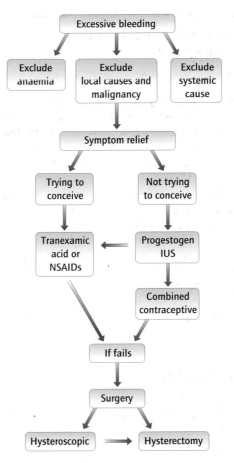

Fig. 2.6 Management of heavy menstruation. IUS, intrauterine system; NSAIDs, non-steroidal anti-inflammatory drugs.

gia, also has IMB, or has not responded to treatment, an *endometrial biopsy* (at hysteroscopy or with a Pipelle; Fig. 2.5) should be performed to exclude endometrial malignancy or premalignancy [→ p.20]. Hysteroscopy allows, in addition to biopsy, an inspection of the uterine cavity, and therefore detection of polyps and submucous fibroids that could be resected. A dilatation and curettage (D&C) is not a treatment for menorrhagia.

Treatment

Treatment can be instigated once pathology has been excluded and depends on the woman's contraceptive needs (Fig. 2.6). Thus, while intrauterine progestogens are very effective and recommended as a first line by the National Institute for Clinical Excellence (NICE), this is not an option for a woman who wishes to conceive (http://guidance.nice.org.uk/CG44/niceguidance/pdf/English).

Medical treatment

First line

Intrauterine system (IUS): This progestogen-impregnated intrauterine device (IUD; Fig. 2.7) is a 'coil' [→ p.99] that reduces menstrual flow by >90% with considerably fewer side effects than systemic progestogens. It is a highly effective alternative to both medical and surgical treatment of menorrhagia (*Cochrane* 2005: CD002126).

It is a contraceptive and also provides the progestogen component of hormone replacement. It should be distinguished from copper IUDs which may increase menstrual loss.

Second line

Antifibrinolytics (tranexamic acid) are taken during menstruation only. By reducing fibrinolytic activity they can reduce blood loss by about 50%. There are few side effects (*Cochrane* 2000: CD000249).

Non-steroidal anti-inflammatory drugs (NSAIDs; e.g. mefanamic acid) inhibit prostaglandin synthesis, reducing blood loss in most women by about 30% (*Cochrane* 2007: CD000400). They are also useful for dysmenorrhoea. Side effects are similar to those of aspirin.

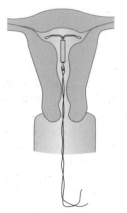

Fig. 2.7 Progestogen impregnated intrauterine system (IUS) *in situ* in the uterus.

The combined oral contraceptive usually induces lighter menstruation, but is less effective if pelvic pathology is present. Its role is more limited because its complications [→ p.96] are more common in older patients and it is these patients who have the most menstrual problems (*Cochrane* 2000: CD000154).

Third line

Progestogens [→ p.98] taken in high doses orally or by intramuscular injection will cause amenorrhoea, but bleeding will follow withdrawal (*Cochrane* 2000: CD001016).

Gonadotrophin-releasing hormone [→ p.68] agonists produce amenorrhoea. Unless add-back hormone replacement therapy (HRT) is used, duration is limited to 6 months. Bleeding will follow withdrawal.

Pharmalogical treatments for menorrhagia

First line
Intrauterine system (IUS)

Second line
Antifibrinolytics (tranexamic acid)
Non-steroidal anti-inflammatory drugs (NSAIDs)
Combined oral contraceptive

Third line
Progestogens (high dose oral or intramuscular)
Gonadotrophin-releasing hormone (GnRH) analogues

Surgical treatment

Hysteroscopic

Polyp removal: If localized abnormalities such as polyps are seen they can be resected. This can be performed under general or local anaesthesia.

Endometrial ablation techniques involve removal or destruction of endometrium. Amenorrhoea or lighter periods usually follow. Long-term patient satisfaction with endometrial destructive techniques is less than with hysterectomy, although surgical complications and hospital stay are less (*Cochrane* 2006: CD003855). Such techniques are most effective in older women with pure menorrhagia.

The first generation techniques include transcervical resection of endometrium (TCRE) and transcervical rollerball ablation [→ p.125]. These use monopolar diathermy with electric current passing down the hysteroscope into either a cutting loop (TCRE) or a rollerball to excise or ablate the endometrium. The current then passes from the patient back to the generator via a pad on the thigh. Second generation techniques include a microwave probe or thermal balloons passed into the uterine cavity which heat and destroy the endometrium. The potentially serious complication of uterine perforation is less common with second than first generation techniques. Endometrial ablation is most appropriate when the uterus is <10 weeks' size with any fibroids <3 cm diameter. The procedures reduce fertility but are non-sterilizing and so effective contraception should be advised.

Transcervical resection of fibroid (TCRF) uses the same hysteroscopic equipment as for a TCRE. Submucosal fibroids up to 3 cm diameter are resected to reduce menstrual flow and improve fertility. If fertility is not desired then a TCRE can be performed at the same time as the TCRF.

Myomectomy is the removal of fibroids from the myometrium. It can be open or laparoscopic (if <4 fibroids of <8 cm diameter, depending on surgeon's experience) [→ p.125] and is used if fibroids are causing symptoms but fertility is still required. GnRH agonists are often used to reduce the size of fibroids first.

Hysterectomy [→ p.126] should be the last resort in the treatment of abnormal uterine bleeding and the numbers of women undergoing this procedure are falling in the UK (*BMJ* 2005; **330**: 938). The operation can be vaginal, abdominal or laparoscopic. The uterus is found to be normal in about half of women having hysterectomy for menorrhagia.

Uterine artery embolization (UAE) treats menorrhagia due to fibroids and is suitable for women who want to retain their uterus and avoid surgery. The effects of UAE on fertility are not clear and such women should consider other options first (*Cochrane* 2006: CD005073).

When to do an endometrial biopsy (Pipelle or hysteroscopy)
If endometrial thickness >10 mm in premenopausal; >4 mm in postmenopausal Age >40 years Menorrhagia with intermenstrual bleeding (IMB) If ultrasound suggests a polyp (perform hysteroscopy) Before insertion of intrauterine system (IUS) if cycle not regular Prior to endometrial ablation/diathermy as tissue will not be available for pathology If abnormal uterine bleeding has resulted in acute admission

Irregular menstruation and intermenstrual bleeding

Epidemiology

This may coexist with heavy menstrual bleeding and is more common at extremes of reproductive age.

Causes

Anovulatory cycles are common in the early and late reproductive years (i.e. just after the menarche and before the menopause).
Pelvic pathology: Non-malignant causes include fibroids, uterine and cervical polyps, adenomyosis, ovarian cysts and chronic pelvic infection. However, with older women, particularly if there has been a recent change, the chances of malignancy, ovarian and cervical, and most particularly endometrial, are slightly increased.

Clinical features

Women should be assessed as for menorrhagia. Speculum examination may reveal a cervical polyp.

Investigations

To assess the effect of blood loss and fitness, the patient's haemoglobin is checked.
Investigations should exclude malignancy, except in young women where malignancy is rare, and exclude local treatable pathology. A cervical smear is taken if required. An *ultrasound* examination of the cavity is performed for women over the age of 35 years with irregular or intermenstrual bleeding, and in younger women if medical treatment has failed, and will also detect a uterine fibroid or ovarian mass. *Endometrial biopsy*, with a Pipelle, preferably at hysteroscopy, is then used if the endometrium is thickened, a polyp is suspected, the woman is over 40 years, or if ablative surgery or the IUS are to be used.

Treatment

Medical treatment

This is appropriate where no anatomical cause is detected: cycles are considered anovulatory. *The IUS* or the *combined oral contraceptive* are first line treatment options. The contraceptive pill usually induces regular and lighter menstruation. Its role is limited because its complications are more common in older patients (although it can be used until the menopause in suitable women). *Progestogens* in high doses will cause amenorrhoea, but bleeding will follow withdrawal. They induce secretory changes in the endometrium and so, when given on a cyclical basis, can mimic normal menstruation. HRT may regulate erratic uterine bleeding during the perimenopause. *Other treatments* that are second line treatments for menorrhagia may also be used.

Surgical treatment

A cervical polyp can be avulsed and sent for histological examination. Surgery is as for women with menorrhagia, except that ablative techniques tend to be less helpful as some endometrium often remains and so irregular but light bleeding may continue.

Amenorrhoea and oligomenorrhoea

Definitions

Amenorrhoea is the absence of menstruation. *Primary*

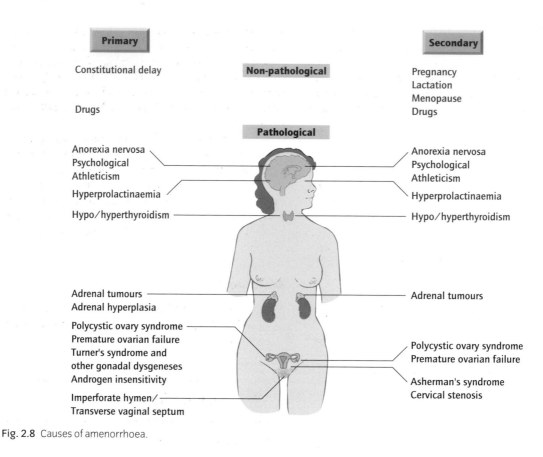

Fig. 2.8 Causes of amenorrhoea.

amenorrhoea is when menstruation has not started by the age of 16 years. It may be a manifestation of *delayed puberty*, which is when secondary sex characteristics are not present by the age of 14 years. Amenorrhoea may also occur in girls with otherwise normal secondary sexual characteristics, when a problem of menstrual outflow is likely. *Secondary amenorrhoea* is when previously normal menstruation ceases for 6 months or more (Fig. 2.8). *Oligomenorrhoea* is when menstruation occurs every 35 days to 6 months.

Classification of causes

Physiological amenorrhoea occurs during pregnancy, after the menopause and, usually, during lactation. Constitutional delay is common and often familial.

Pathological causes may lie in the hypothalamus, the pituitary, the thyroid, the adrenals, the ovary or the uterus and 'outflow tract'. Drugs such as progestogens, GnRH

analogues and, sometimes, antipsychotics (through increasing prolactin levels) cause amenorrhoea.

Where pathological, primary amenorrhoea is due either to rare congenital abnormalities or acquired disorders that arise before the normal time of puberty. Secondary amenorrhoea or oligomenorrhoea is due to acquired disorders that arise later. The most common causes of secondary amenorrhoea or oligomenorrhoea are the premature menopause [→ p.105], polycystic ovary syndrome (PCOS) [→ p.82] and hyperprolactinaemia [→ p.84].

Hypothalamus

Hypothalamic hypogonadism [→ p.84] is common and is usually due to psychological factors, low weight/anorexia nervosa or excessive exercise. Tumours are an uncommon cause and are excluded by brain magnetic resonance imaging (MRI). GnRH and therefore FSH, LH and oestradiol are reduced. Treatment is supportive; bone density is reduced if there has been prolonged hypo-oestrogenism and requires monitoring. Oestrogen replacement is required (plus progesterone for endometrial protection) using either the combined oral contraceptive or HRT. Anorexia nervosa is life-threatening and requires psychiatric treatment.

Pituitary

Hyperprolactinaemia is usually caused by pituitary hyperplasia or benign adenomas. Treatment is with bromocriptine, cabergoline or, occasionally, surgery. Rare pituitary causes include other pituitary tumours and Sheehan's syndrome [→ p.84], in which severe postpartum haemorrhage causes pituitary necrosis and varying degrees of hypopituitarism.

Adrenal or thyroid gland

Over-activity or under-activity of the thyroid can cause amenorrhoea. Hyothyroidism leads to raised prolactin levels and amenorrhoea. Congenital adrenal hyperplasia or virilizing tumours are rare.

Ovary

Acquired disorders: The most common is *polycystic ovary syndrome* [→ p.82]. This can cause primary or secondary amenorrhoea, although oligomenorrhoea is more common. It is extremely important as it is common, is also associated with subfertility and has long-term health consequences. *Premature menopause* occurs in 1 in 100 women [→ p.105]. Rare *virilizing tumours* can arise in the ovary.

Congenital causes: The most common is *Turner's syndrome*, in which one X chromosome is absent, producing the 45 XO genotype. These women have short stature and poor secondary sexual characteristics, but normal intelligence. In other forms of *gonadal dysgenesis* the ovary is imperfectly formed due to mosaic abnormalities of the X chromosomes. Gonadal agenesis and androgen insensitivity [→ p.19] are extremely rare.

Outflow tract problems: menstrual flow is obstructed or absent

Congenital problems cause primary amenorrhoea with normal secondary sexual characteristics. The *imperfo-*

rate hymen and the *transverse vaginal septum* obstruct menstrual flow, which therefore accumulates over the months in the vagina (haematocolpos) or uterus (haematometra), which may be palpable abdominally. Treatment is surgical. Rarer causes include absence of the vagina with or without (Rokitansky's syndrome) a functioning uterus.

Acquired problems usually cause secondary amenorrhoea. *Cervical stenosis* prevents release of blood from the uterus, causing a haematometra [→ p.26]. *Asherman's syndrome* is an uncommon consequence of excessive curettage at evacuation of retained products of conception (ERPC) [→ p.127]; *endometrial resection* or *ablation* [→ p.125] produces this effect intentionally.

Management

The important conditions of premature menopause [→ p.112], PCOS [→ p.83] and hyperprolactinaemia [→ p.84], are discussed elsewhere.

Postcoital bleeding

Definition

Vaginal bleeding following intercourse that is not menstrual loss. Except for first intercourse, this is always abnormal and cervical carcinoma must be excluded.

Causes

When the cervix is not covered in healthy squamous epithelium it is more likely to bleed after mild trauma. Cervical ectropions [→ p.31], benign polyps [→ p.31] and invasive cervical cancer [→ p.35] account for most cases. The bleeding occasionally comes from the vaginal wall, usually if it is atrophic.

Causes of postcoital bleeding
Cervical carcinoma (Fig. 2.9)
Cervical ectropion
Cervical polyps
Cervicitis, vaginitis

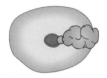

Fig. 2.9 Cervical carcinoma.

Management

The cervix is carefully inspected and a smear is taken. If a polyp is evident, it is avulsed and sent for histology: this is normally possible without anaesthesia. If the smear is normal, an ectropion can be frozen with cryotherapy. If not, colposcopy [→ p.34] is undertaken to exclude a malignant cause.

Dysmenorrhoea

This is painful menstruation. It is associated with high prostaglandin levels in the endometrium and is due to contraction and uterine ischaemia.

Causes and their management

Primary dysmenorrhoea is when no organic cause is found. It usually coincides with the start of menstruation and is very common (50% of women, 10% severe), particularly in adolescents. Pain usually responds to NSAIDs or ovulation suppression (e.g. the combined oral contraceptive) (*Cochrane* 2001: CD002120). Reassurance in the young adolescent is important. Pelvic pathology is more likely if medical treatment fails.
Secondary dysmenorrhoea is when pain is due to pelvic pathology. Pain often precedes and is relieved by the onset of menstruation. Deep dyspareunia and menorrhagia or irregular menstruation are common. Pelvic ultrasound and laparoscopy are useful. The most significant causes are fibroids, adenomyosis, endometriosis, pelvic inflammatory disease and ovarian tumours, which

should be treated appropriately. *Laparoscopic uterine nerve ablation* (LUNA) is not beneficial (*Cochrane* 2005: CD001896).

Precocious puberty

This is when menstruation occurs before the age of 10 years *or* other secondary sexual characteristics are evident before the age of 8 years. It is very rare. The growth spurt occurs early, but final height is reduced due to early fusion of the epiphyses. Investigation is essential, as it may be a manifestation of other disorders. Treatment is essential to arrest sexual development and allow normal growth.

Causes and their management

In 80% of cases, no pathological cause is found. GnRH agonists [→ p.68] are used to inhibit sex hormone secretion, causing regression of secondary sex characteristics and cessation of menstruation.
Central causes: increased GnRH secretion: Meningitis, encephalitis, central nervous system tumours, hydrocephaly and hypothyroidism may prevent normal prepubertal inhibition of hypothalamic GnRH release.
Ovarian/adrenal causes: increased oestrogen secretion: Hormone-producing tumours of the ovary or adrenal glands will also cause premature sexual maturation. Regression occurs after removal. The McCune–Albright syndrome consists of bone and ovarian cysts, *café au lait* spots and precocious puberty. Treatment is with cyproterone acetate (an anti-androgenic progestogen).

Ambiguous development and intersex

There are many causes and degrees of ambiguous genitalia. Psychological support is important and gender assignation should be consistent.

Increased androgen function in a genetic female

Congenital adrenal hyperplasia is recessively inherited. Cortisol production is defective, usually as a result of 21-hydroxylase deficiency: adrenocorticotrophic hormone (ACTH) excess causes increased androgen production. The condition normally presents at birth with ambiguous genitalia; glucocorticoid deficiency may cause Addisonian crises. Occasionally, it presents at puberty with an enlarged clitoris and amenorrhoea. Treatment involves cortisol and mineralocorticoid replacement: lack of these can be fatal. Androgen-secreting tumours and other causes of Cushing's syndrome are rare.

Reduced androgen function in a genetic male

Androgen insensitivity syndrome (AIS) occurs when a male has cell receptor insensitivity to androgens, which are converted peripherally to oestrogens. The individual appears to be female: the diagnosis is only discovered when 'she' presents with amenorrhoea. The uterus is absent and rudimentary testes are present. These are removed because of possible malignant change and oestrogen replacement therapy is started.

Premenstrual syndrome

Premenstrual syndrome (PMS) encompasses psychological, behavioural and physical symptoms that are experienced on a regular basis during the luteal phase of the menstrual cycle and often resolve by the end of menstruation.

Epidemiology

Ninety-five per cent of women experience some premenstrual symptoms; in about 5% they are severely debilitating (Fig. 2.10).

Aetiology

This is unknown, but is dependent on normal ovarian function and the hormone progesterone. Exogenous

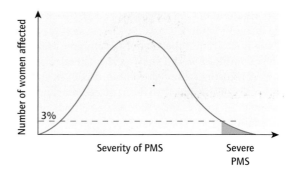

Fig. 2.10 Distribution of premenstrual syndrome (PMS) in the population.

progestogens are known to cause PMS-like symptoms. Differing neurochemical responses to ovarian function (certain neurotransmitter levels may be altered during the luteal phase in severely affected women) may account for the differing severities of the syndrome.

Clinical features

History: These vary and it is the cyclical nature rather than the symptoms themselves that enable diagnosis. Behavioural changes include 'tension', irritability, aggression, depression and loss of control. In addition, a sensation of bloatedness, minor gastrointestinal upset and breast pain can occur.

Examination: Psychological evaluation may be helpful as depression and neurosis can present as PMS. There are no biochemical markers for PMS. Women should be asked to complete menstrual charts, recording their moods and other symptoms for at least two cycles.

Management

Drug treatments

Selective serotonin uptake inhibitors (SSRIs) are effective, given either continuously or intermittently in the second half of the cycle. Because true PMS is in some way caused by the fluctuation of hormones in the second half of the cycle, ablating the cycle may be effective. If the woman needs contraception, continuous oral contraception should help; 100 μg oestrogen HRT patches are often effective. If this is unsuccessful and symptoms are extreme a trial of GnRH agonists and add-back oestrogen therapy to induce a pseudomenopause may be tried. If this is successful, then agonists with add-back HRT can be continued or, as a final resort, bilateral oophorectomy considered (although combined HRT or the contraceptive pill would then be required for bone and endometrial protection). The role of progesterone is uncertain.

Supplements

Oil of evening primrose oil is good for breast tenderness. Pyridoxine (vitamin B$_6$) 50 mg twice daily helps in mild PMS, but can cause a neuropathy in excessive doses. Vitex agnus-castus extract helps PMS.

Cognitive–behavioural therapy

This changes the way a woman copes with her life.

Further reading

Duckitt K, Collins S. Menorrhagia. *BMJ Clinical Evidence* [online web publication May 2006].

Kwan I, Onwude JL. Premenstrual syndrome. *BMJ Clinical Evidence* [online web publication Nov 2006].

Lethaby A, Cooke I, Rees M. Progesterone/progestogen-releasing intrauterine systems for heavy menstrual bleeding. *Cochrane Database of Systematic Reviews (Online: Update Software)* 2005: CD002126.

Lethaby A, Hickey M, Garry R. Endometrial destruction techniques for heavy menstrual bleeding. *Cochrane Database of Systematic Reviews (Online: Update Software)* 2005: CD001501.

Slap GB. Menstrual disorders in adolescence. *Best Practice & Research Clinical Obstetrics & Gynaecology* 2003; **17**: 75–92.

Menstrual Cycle Disorders at a Glance

Types	Menorrhagia, irregular menstruation, intermenstrual bleeding (IMB)
Epidemiology	One-third of women describe heavy periods (not age-related), most do not seek help
Aetiology	*Menorrhagia:* usually ovulatory cycles. Cause not usually found. May be anatomical *Irregular bleeding:* often anovulatory, polycystic ovary syndrome (PCOS) most common cause. Sometimes anatomical *Local anatomical problem:* e.g. endometrial or cervical carcinoma (usually irregular or intermenstrual bleeding, also postcoital bleeding), fibroids, endometrial/cervical polyps; also pelvic inflammatory disease, ovarian tumours, adenomyosis *Systemic problem* (unusual): e.g. disorders of thyroid or coagulation
Investigations	Full blood count (FBC), pelvic ultrasound, ±endometrial biopsy (sometimes combined with hysteroscopy) if thickened or irregular endometrium, or age >40 years
Treatment	Treat systemic disease appropriately. Then symptom relief *Medical:* To reduce volume: intrauterine system (IUS), tranexamic acid, mefanamic acid, combined contraceptive To regulate timing: IUS (amenorrhoea in most), combined contraceptive or cyclical/continuous progestogens *Surgical:* Hysteroscopic surgery: resection or ablation, hysterectomy occasionally, myomectomy/embolization if fibroids

3 The uterus and its abnormalities

Anatomy and physiology of the uterus

Anatomy and function

The uterus nourishes, protects and, ultimately, expels the fetus. Inferiorly it is continuous with the cervix, which acts as its neck and communication with the vagina. The superior part is the fundus; on either side of this the uterus communicates with the fallopian tubes at the cornu. It is supported predominantly at the inferior end, at the cervix, by the uterosacral and cardinal ligaments. In 80% of women it tilts up towards the abdominal wall—anteversion. In 20% of women it is retroverted, tilting back into the pelvis. The wall is made of smooth muscle (the tissue of origin of the benign tumours *fibroids*) that encloses the uterine cavity. This is lined by glandular epithelium—the endometrium (the tissue of origin of *endometrial carcinoma*). The outside coat of the uterus, or serosa, is the peritoneum posteriorly. This also covers the uterus anteriorly down to the bladder, which is on the anterior surface of the lower uterus, the cervix and the vagina. (The proximity of the bladder to the lower uterus and vagina explains the ease with which it can be damaged at surgery or in childbirth.) Laterally this peritoneum is continuous with the broad ligaments that run between the uterus and pelvic side wall. These have little function as supports, but are continuous with the fallopian tubes and round ligaments superiorly, and inferiorly contain the uterine blood supply, ureters and parametrium (Fig. 3.1).

Blood and lymph

The uterine blood supply (Fig. 3.1) is from the uterine

Obstetrics and Gynaecology, 3rd edition. By Lawrence Impey and Tim Child. Published 2008 by Blackwell Publishing, ISBN: 978-1-4051-6095-7.

arteries, which cross over the ureters lateral to the cervix and pass inferiorly and superiorly supplying the myometrium and endometrium. At the cornu there is an arterial anastomosis with the ovarian blood supply. Inferiorly, there is an anastomosis with the vessels of the upper vagina. Lymph drainage of the uterus (Fig. 3.1) is mostly via the internal and external iliac arteries.

The endometrium

The endometrium is supplied by the spiral and basal arterioles. The former are important in menstruation and in nourishment of the growing fetus. The endometrium is responsive to oestrogen and progesterone. In the first 14 days of the menstrual cycle, it proliferates: the glands elongate and it thickens largely under the influence of oestrogens (proliferative phase). After ovulation, under the influence of progesterone, the glands swell and the blood supply increases (luteal or secretory phase; see Fig. 2.3). Towards the end of this phase, progesterone levels drop and the secretory endometrium disintegrates as its blood supply can no longer support it: menstruation occurs. Poor hormonal control commonly causes erratic bleeding patterns.

Fibroids

Definition and epidemiology

Also known as leiomyomata, these are benign tumours of the myometrium. They are present in at least 25% of women and are more common approaching the menopause, in Afro-Caribbean women and those with a family history. They are less common in parous women and those who have taken the combined oral contraceptive or injectable progestagens.

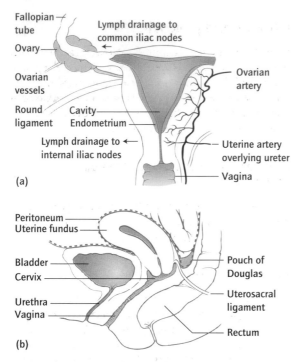

(a)

Fallopian tube
Ovary
Ovarian vessels
Round ligament
Lymph drainage to common iliac nodes
Ovarian artery
Cavity
Endometrium
Lymph drainage to internal iliac nodes
Uterine artery overlying ureter
Vagina

Peritoneum
Uterine fundus
Bladder
Cervix
Urethra
Vagina
Pouch of Douglas
Uterosacral ligament
Rectum

(b)

Fig. 3.1 The uterus. (a) Blood supply and lymph drainage. (b) Relations of the pelvic organs.

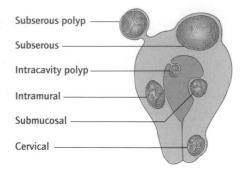

Subserous polyp
Subserous
Intracavity polyp
Intramural
Submucosal
Cervical

Fig. 3.2 Sites of fibroids showing intramural, subserosal and submucosal.

Pathology and sites of fibroids

The sizes vary from a few millimetres to massive tumours filling the abdomen. The fibroid may be intramural, subserosal or submucosal (Fig. 3.2). Submucosal fibroids occasionally form intracavity polyps. Smooth muscle and fibrous elements are present, and in transverse section the fibroid has a 'whorled' appearance.

Aetiology

Fibroid growth is oestrogen and probably progesterone dependent. During pregnancy, fibroids are equally likely to grow, shrink or show no change. Fibroids regress after the menopause due to the reduction in circulating oestrogen. Each fibroid is of monoclonal origin.

Clinical features

History: Fifty per cent are asymptomatic and discovered only at pelvic or abdominal examination. Symptoms are related more to the site than the size.

● Menstrual problems: menorrhagia occurs in 30%, although the timing of menses is usually unchanged. Intermenstrual loss may occur if the fibroid is submucosal or polypoid. Fibroids are common in the perimenopausal woman and may be incidental: menstrual problems may also be the result of hormonal irregularities or malignancy.

● Pain: fibroids can cause dysmenorrhoea. They seldom cause pain, unless torsion, red degeneration or, rarely, sarcomatous change occur.

● Other symptoms: large fibroids pressing on the bladder can cause frequency and occasionally urinary retention, those pressing on the ureters can cause hydronephrosis; other pressure effects may also be felt. Fertility can be impaired if the tubal ostia are blocked or submucous fibroids prevent implantation. Intramural fibroids not distorting the cavity also reduce fertility though the mechanism is unclear.

Examination: A solid mass may be palpable on pelvic or even abdominal examination. It will arise from the pelvis and be continuous with the uterus. Multiple small fibroids cause irregular 'knobbly' enlargement of the uterus.

Symptoms of fibroids
None (50%)
Menorrhagia (30%)
Erratic/intermenstrual bleeding (IMB)
Pressure effects
Subfertility

Natural history/complications of fibroids

Enlargement can be very slow. Fibroids stop growing and often calcify after the menopause, although the oestrogen in hormone replacement therapy (HRT) may stimulate further growth. In mid-pregnancy they may enlarge. Pedunculated fibroids occasionally undergo torsion, causing pain.

'Degenerations' are normally the result of an inadequate blood supply: 'red degeneration' is characterized by pain and uterine tenderness; haemorrhage and necrosis occur. In 'hyaline degeneration' and 'cystic degeneration' the fibroid is soft and partly liquefied.

Malignancy: Around 0.1% of fibroids are leiomyosarcomata [→ p.29]. This may be the result of malignant change or *de novo* malignant transformation of normal smooth muscle.

Complications of fibroids	
Torsion of pedunculated fibroid	
Degenerations:	Red (partic. in pregnancy)
	Hyaline/cystic
	Calcification (postmenopausal and asymptomatic)
Malignancy:	Leiomyosarcoma

Fibroids and pregnancy

Premature labour, malpresentations, transverse lie, obstructed labour and postpartum haemorrhage can occur. Red degeneration is common in pregnancy and can cause severe pain. Fibroids should not be removed at Caesarean section as bleeding can be heavy. Pedunculated fibroids may tort postpartum.

Hormone replacement therapy and fibroids

HRT [→ p.109] can cause continued fibroid growth after the menopause. Treatment is as for premenopausal women or the HRT is withdrawn.

Investigations

To establish diagnosis: Ultrasound is helpful (Fig. 3.3) but magnetic resonance imaging (MRI) or laparoscopy may be required to distinguish the fibroid from an ovarian mass. Adenomyosis can exist as a fibroid-like mass, differentiated by MRI. Hysteroscopy or hysterosalpingogram (HSG) is used to assess distortion of the uterine cavity, particularly if fertility is an issue.

To establish fitness: The haemoglobin concentration may be low as a result of vaginal bleeding, but also high as fibroids can secrete erythropoetin.

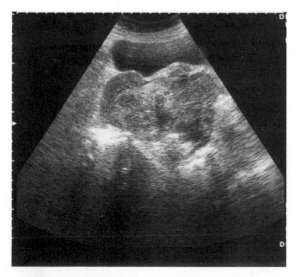

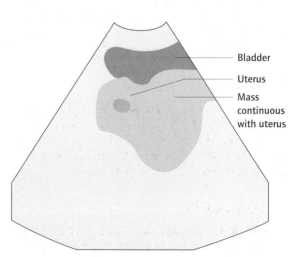

Bladder

Uterus

Mass continuous with uterus

Fig. 3.3 Ultrasound of fibroids on the uterus.

Treatment

Asymptomatic patients with small or slow-growing fibroids need no treatment. The risk of malignancy is small enough not to warrant routine removal or monitoring. Larger fibroids that are not removed should be serially measured by examination or ultrasound because of the remote possibility of malignancy.

Medical treatment

Tranexamic acid, *non-steroidal anti-inflammatory drugs* or *progestogens* are often ineffective when menorrhagia [→ p.12] is due to fibroids but may be worth trying as a simple first line treatment. Gonadotrophin-releasing hormone (GnRH) agonists cause temporary amenorrhoea and fibroid shrinkage by inducing a temporary menopausal state. Side effects and bone density loss restrict their use to only 6 months, usually near the menopause or to make surgery easier and safer. However, concomitant use of ('add-back') HRT may prevent such effects without causing enlargement, allowing longer administration. Once the GnRH agonist is stopped and oestrogen levels return to normal then fibroids will return to their previous size. GnRH agonist treatment is not appropriate for women trying to conceive due to the anovulation induced and return of the fibroids with drug cessation. Consequently, surgery is usually used to manage fibroids under these circumstances.

Is the fibroid malignant?
Uncommon, but more likely if: Pain and rapid growth Growth in postmenopausal woman not on hormone replacement therapy (HRT) Poor response to gonadotrophin-releasing hormone (GnRH) agonists

Surgical treatment

Hysteroscopic: The fibroid polyp or small (up to 3–4 cm) submucous fibroid that is causing menstrual problems or subfertility can be resected at hysteroscopy [→ p.125]. Pretreatment with GnRH agonist for 2 months will shrink the fibroid, reduce vascularity and thin the endometrium so making resection easier and safer.
Radical: Fibroids are a common indication for hysterectomy. The hysterectomy can be performed laparoscopically, vaginally (if fibroids not so large to prevent

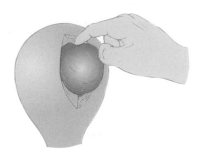

Fig. 3.4 Myomectomy.

removal of the uterus through the vagina) or abdominally. Fibroids can also be removed from the uterus: open or laparoscopic myomectomy (see Chapter 2; Fig. 3.4). Blood loss may be heavy (risk of hysterectomy to save life) and small fibroids can be missed, causing problems to recur. Myomectomy is performed if medical treatment has failed but preservation of reproductive function is required. Hysteroscopic or open (but not laparoscopic as conversely the fibroid excision becomes more difficult) operations are usually preceded by 2–3 months' treatment with GnRH analogues (*Cochrane* 2001: CD000547). If the endometrial cavity is opened during myomectomy then Caesarean section is usually used to deliver future babies because of an increased risk of uterine rupture during labour.
Embolization: Uterine artery embolization (UAE) by radiologists has an 80% success rate and is an alternative to hysterectomy or myomectomy. The volume of embolized fibroids reduces by around 50%. The hospital stay is shorter with a quicker return to normal activities. Symptoms such as pain may get worse, however, and readmission rates are higher with UAE. As the effects of UAE on fertility are unclear it should not be offered to women desiring future pregnancy. Hysterectomy may still be required (*Cochrane* 2006: CD005073).

Adenomyosis

Definition and epidemiology

Previously called 'endometriosis interna', this is the presence of endometrium and its underlying stroma

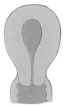

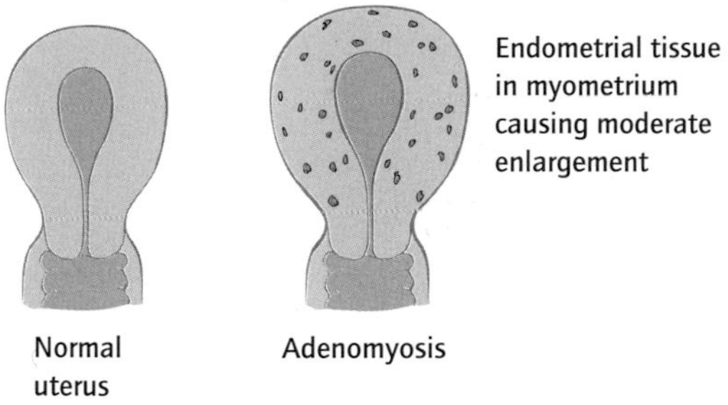

Endometrial tissue
in myometrium
causing moderate
enlargement

Normal
uterus

Adenomyosis

Fig. 3.5 Adenomyosis.

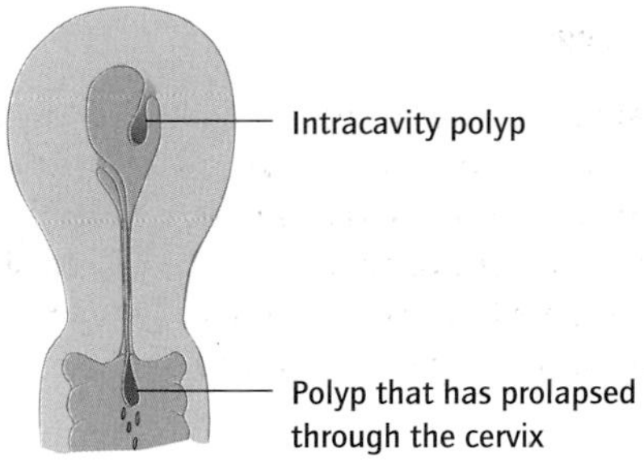

Intracavity polyp

Polyp that has prolapsed
through the cervix

Fig. 3.6 Endometrial polyps.

within the myometrium (Fig. 3.5). Its true incidence is unknown, but it occurs in up to 40% of hysterectomy specimens. It is most common around the age of 40 years and is associated with endometriosis and fibroids. Symptoms subside after the menopause.

Pathology and aetiology

The endometrium appears to grow into the myometrium to form adenomyosis. The extent is variable, but in severe cases pockets of menstrual blood can be seen in the myometrium of hysterectomy specimens. Occasionally, endometrial stromal tissue in the myometrium displays varying degrees of atypia or even invasion [→ p.26].

Clinical features

History. Symptoms may be absent, but painful, regular, heavy menstruation is common.
Examination. The uterus is mildly enlarged and tender.

Investigations

Adenomyosis is not easily diagnosed by ultrasound but can be seen on MRI.

Treatment

Medical treatment with the progesterone intrauterine system (IUS) or the combined oral contraceptive pill with or without NSAIDs may control the menorrhagia and dysmenorrhoea, but hysterectomy is often required. For some women the trial of GnRH analogue

therapy may determine if symptoms attributed to adenomyosis are likely to improve with hysterectomy. The condition is oestrogen dependent, but why it occurs is unknown. The effects on fertility are unclear.

Other benign conditions of the uterus

Endometritis [→ p.74]

This is often secondary to sexually transmitted infections, as a complication of surgery, particularly Caesarean section and intrauterine procedure (e.g. surgical termination) [→ p.117], or because of foreign tissue, particularly intrauterine devices (IUDs) [→ p.99] and retained products of conception. Infection in the postmenopausal uterus is commonly due to malignancy. The uterus is tender and pelvic and systemic infection may be evident. A pyometra is when pus accumulates and is unable to escape. Antibiotics and occasionally evacuation of retained products of conception (ERPC) [→ p.127] are required.

Intrauterine polyps

These are small, usually benign tumours that grow into the uterine cavity. Most are endometrial in origin (Fig. 3.6), but some are derived from submucous fibroids. They are common in women aged 40–50 years and when oestrogen levels are high. In the postmenopausal woman, they are often found in patients on tamoxifen for breast carcinoma. Occasionally they contain endometrial

hyperplasia or carcinoma. Although sometimes asymptomatic, they often cause menorrhagia and intermenstrual bleeding and very occasionally prolapse through
the cervix. They are normally diagnosed at ultrasound
or when a hysteroscopy is performed because of
abnormal bleeding. Resection of the polyp with cutting diathermy or avulsion normally cures bleeding
problems.

Haematometra

This is menstrual blood accumulating in the uterus
because of outflow obstruction. It is uncommon. The
cervical canal is usually occluded by fibrosis after endometrial resection, cone biopsy or by a carcinoma. Congenital abnormalities, for example imperforate hymen
or blind rudimentary uterine horn, present in
adolescence.

Congenital uterine malformations

Abnormalities result from differing degrees of failure
of fusion of the two müellerian ducts at about 9
weeks (Fig. 3.7). These are common but are seldom
clinically significant. Total failure of fusion leads
to two uterine cavities and cervices (didelphys) with
sometimes a longitudinal vaginal septum; or one duct
may fail, causing a 'unicornuate' uterus. If one duct
develops better than the other one, a smaller 'rudimentary horn' is formed. Its cavity can be blind or continuous with the dominant horn. At the other end of the
spectrum, there may simply be a small septum at the
fundus.

About 25% cause pregnancy-related problems that
lead to their discovery. These include malpresentations
or transverse lie, premature labour, recurrent miscarriage (<5% of these) or retained placenta. Treatment
for pregnancy-related problems, however, should not
be undertaken lightly as congenital abnormalities
may be incidental. Simple septa can be resected
hysteroscopically; rudimentary horns need removal
at either open or laparoscopic surgery. Bicornuate
uteri are no longer treated surgically by resecting
the medial walls and forming a single uterus, as the
complication rates were too high. Women with a congenital uterine anomaly have an increased incidence
of renal anomalies and should undergo renal tract
imaging.

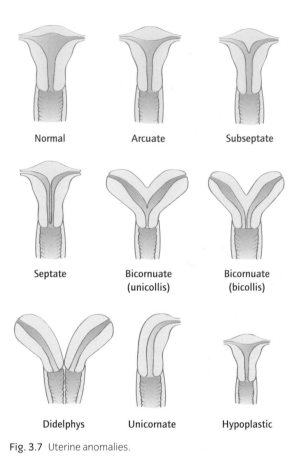

Normal Arcuate Subseptate

Septate Bicornuate (unicollis) Bicornuate (bicollis)

Didelphys Unicornate Hypoplastic

Fig. 3.7 Uterine anomalies.

Endometrial carcinoma

Epidemiology

This is now the most common genital tract cancer (Fig.
3.8). Prevalence is highest at the age of 60 years, with
only 15% of cases occurring premenopausally and <1%
in women under 35 years of age. Because it usually presents early, it is often incorrectly considered to be relatively benign, but stage for stage the prognosis is similar
to ovarian malignancy.

Pathology

Adenocarcinoma of columnar endometrial gland cells
accounts for >90%. Of the rest, the most common is

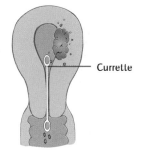

Fig. 3.8 Endometrial carcinoma.

adenosquamous carcinoma, which contains malignant squamous and glandular tissue and has a poorer prognosis.

Aetiology

The principal risk is a high ratio of oestrogen to progestogen. Malignancy therefore is most common when oestrogen production is high or when oestrogen therapy is used 'unopposed' by progestogens.

Risk factors

Exogenous oestrogens without a progestogen increase the rate sixfold. Obesity (through peripheral conversion of androgens to oestrogen), polycystic ovary syndrome (PCOS) associated with prolonged amenorrhoea, nulliparity and a late menopause, and ovarian granulosa cell (oestrogen-secreting) tumours are all risk factors. Tamoxifen increases the risk of endometrial carcinoma (*Lancet* 1994; **343**: 448): although an oestrogen antagonist in the breast and used in the treatment of breast carcinoma, it is mainly an agonist in the postmenopausal uterus. Hypertension and diabetes are common, but probably not independent risk factors. A history of combined oral contraceptive or pregnancy is protective.

Premalignant disease: endometrial hyperplasia with atypia

Oestrogen acting unopposed or erratically can cause 'cystic hyperplasia' of the endometrium. Further stimulation predisposes to abnormalities of cellular and glandular architecture or 'atypical hyperplasia'. This may cause menstrual abnormalities or postmenopausal bleeding and is premalignant. Hyperplasia with atypia often coexists (40%) with carcinoma elsewhere in the uterine cavity but is seldom recognized prior to the diagnosis of malignancy. The discovery of atypia is unusual in women of reproductive age, but if the uterus must be preserved, progestogens in combination with 6-monthly endometrial biopsy are used. Otherwise hysterectomy is indicated.

Risk factors for endometrial carcinoma	
Endogenous oestrogen excess:	Polycystic ovary syndrome (PCOS) (due to unopposed oestrogen) and obesity Oestrogen-secreting tumours Nulliparity and late menopause
Exogenous oestrogens:	Unopposed oestrogen therapy Tamoxifen therapy
Miscellaneous:	Diabetes; hypertension (not independent) Lynch type II syndrome (familial non-polyposis colonic, ovarian and endometrial carcinoma)

Clinical features

History: Postmenopausal bleeding (PMB; 10% risk of carcinoma) [→ p.105] is the most common presentation. The likelihood that PMB is due to endometrial cancer rather than benign or unknown causes increases with age. Premenopausal patients have irregular or intermenstrual bleeding (IMB), or, occasionally, only recent-onset menorrhagia. A cervical smear may contain abnormal columnar cells (cervical glandular intraepithelial neoplasia [CGIN]; [→ p.34]).

Examination: The pelvis often appears normal and atrophic vaginitis may coexist.

Spread and staging

The tumour spreads directly through the myometrium to the cervix and upper vagina (Fig. 3.9). The ovaries may be involved. Lymphatic spread is to pelvic and then para-aortic lymph nodes. Blood-borne spread occurs late. Staging is surgical and histological and, in contrast to cervical carcinoma, includes lymph node involvement.

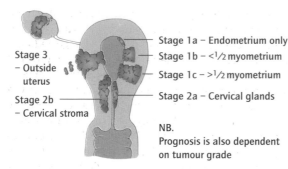

Stage 3 – Outside uterus

Stage 2b – Cervical stroma

Stage 1a – Endometrium only
Stage 1b – <½ myometrium
Stage 1c – >½ myometrium
Stage 2a – Cervical glands

NB.
Prognosis is also dependent on tumour grade

Fig. 3.9 Stages of endometrial carcinoma.

Spread and staging for endometrial carcinoma	
Stage 1	*Lesions confined to uterus:*
1a	In endometrium only
1b	Deepest invasion <½ of myometrial thickness
1c	Deepest invasion >½ of myometrial thickness
Stage 2	*As above but in cervix also:*
2a	In endocervical glands only
2b	In cervical stroma
Stage 3	*Tumour invades through the uterus:*
3a	Invades serosa and/or adnexae and/or positive cytology
3b	Vaginal metastases
3c	Metastases to pelvic/para-aortic lymph nodes
Stage 4	*Further spread:*
4a	In bowel or bladder
4b	Distant metastases

Histological grade: G1–3 is also included for each stage, G1 being a well-differentiated tumour.

Investigations

Abnormal vaginal bleeding is investigated as discussed in Chapter 2 for premenopausal patients and in Chapter 13 for postmenopausal women. Depending on age, menopausal status and symptoms (i.e. likelihood of underlying cancer), an ultrasound scan and/or endometrial biopsy with a Pipelle or hysteroscopy is performed. Endometrial biopsy is required to make the diagnosis. Staging is only possible following hysterectomy. Either an MRI is performed in all patients or only in those where spread is suspected due to symptoms or higher

risk endometrial histology. A chest X-ray is required to exclude rare pulmonary spread.

To assess the patient's fitness, full blood count (FBC), renal function, glucose testing and an electrocardiogram (ECG) are normally required as most patients are elderly.

Treatment

Surgery: Seventy-five per cent of patients present with Stage 1 disease. Unless the patient is unfit or has disseminated disease, a hysterectomy and bilateral salpingo-oöphorectomy (BSO) is performed either abdominally or laparoscopically.

As staging is surgico-pathological, disease that appears to be Stage 1 at surgery may subsequently turn out to be Stage 3 if lymph nodes are involved. However, routine lymphadenectomy is not beneficial in early stage disease based on findings from the recent UK-based ASTEC trial (www.ctu.mrc.ac.uk/studies/ASTEC.asp) and so is not routinely done, but if lymphadenectomy is not performed, an estimate of stage and risk should be made to determine further management including radiotherapy. Management protocols are complicated and controversial as there are more prognostic factors than can be incorporated into a usable treatment algorithm.

General indications for radiotherapy
High risk for extrauterine disease: deep myometrial or cervical stromal spread, poor grade
Proven extrauterine disease
Inoperable and recurrent disease
Palliation for symptoms, e.g. bleeding

Prognosis of endometrial carcinoma	
Stage	*5-year survival rate (%)*
1	85
2	70
3–4	50
4	25
Overall	75

External beam radiotherapy is then used following hysterectomy in patients with, or considered 'high risk' for, lymph node involvement. Risk factors from pathological examination of the uterus are deep myometrial spread, poor tumour histology or grade, or cervical stromal involvement (i.e. Stage 2b).

The ASTEC, and other trials, showed that radiotherapy does not improve long-term survival following surgery for early stage disease (*Cochrane* 2007: CD003916; www.ctu.mrc.ac.uk/studies/ASTEC.asp). Radiotherapy is used for pelvic recurrence and is most beneficial if it has not been given previously. *Vaginal vault radiotherapy* is also used where the above risk factors are present. Its usage reduces local recurrence but does not prolong survival. *Progestogens* are seldom used nowadays. *Chemotherapy* may have a limited role, in advanced disease, and is under investigation in a large randomized controlled trial (RCT).

Prognosis

Recurrence is most common at the vaginal vault, normally in the first 3 years. Poor prognostic features are older age, advanced clinical stage, deep myometrial invasion in Stage 1 and 2 patients, high tumour grade and adenosquamous histology.

Uterine sarcomas

These are rare tumours, accounting for only 150 cases per year in the UK. There are three categories. *Leiomyosarcomas* are 'malignant fibroids'. *Endometrial stromal tumours* are tumours of the stroma beneath the endometrium. Histological types vary from the benign endometrial stromal nodule to the highly malignant endometrial stromal sarcoma. These are most common in the perimenopausal woman. *Mixed müllerian tumours*, derived from the embryological elements of the uterus, are more common in old age. They usually present with irregular or postmenopausal bleeding or, in the case of leiomyosarcomas, rapid painful enlargement of a fibroid. Treatment is with hysterectomy. Radiotherapy or chemotherapy can be used subsequently, but overall survival is only 30% at 5 years.

Further reading

Farquhar C, Brosens I. Medical and surgical management of adenomyosis. *Best Practice & Research Clinical Obstetrics and Gynaecology* 2006; **20**: 603–16.

Kehoe S. Treatments for gynaecological cancers. *Best Practice & Research Clinical Obstetrics and Gynaecology* 2006; **20**: 985–1000.

http://info.cancerresearchuk.org/cancerstats/types/uterus/symptomsandtreatment/

Lethaby A, Vollenhoven B. Fibroids (uterine myomatosis, leiomyomas). *BMJ Clinical Evidence* [online web publication May 2007].

Fibroids at a Glance	
Epidemiology	25% of women, older, nulliparous, Afro-Caribbean
Pathology	Benign tumours of myometrium
Aetiology	Monoclonal, oestrogen dependent
Clinical features	None (50%). Menstrual problems, dysmenorrhoea, pressure effects, subfertility and pain
Complications	Torsion of pedunculated fibroid. Degenerations: red or hyaline degeneration. Sarcomatous change. Complicates pregnancy
Investigations	Full blood count (FBC), hysteroscopy, ultrasound. Magnetic resonance imaging (MRI) or laparoscopy if diagnosis unsure
Treatment	Observation or . . . *Conservative*: Symptomatic relief *Surgical*: Hysteroscopic resection if intrauterine. Myomectomy (fertility preserving), embolization or hysterectomy

Endometrial Carcinoma at a Glance

Epidemiology   Most common gynaecological carcinoma, usually over 60 years of age

Pathology   >90% adenocarcinomas; also adenosquamous

Aetiology   High oestrogen: progesterone ratio. Nulliparity, late menopause, polycystic ovary syndrome (PCOS) if long-term amenorrhoea, obesity. Unopposed oestrogens and tamoxifen
Combined pill and pregnancy protective

Clinical features   Postmenopausal bleeding (PMB) (10% risk of endometrial cancer). Premenopausal get a 'change': irregular, intermenstrual or heavier bleeding

Screening   Not routine. Presents early. Probably worthwhile if taking tamoxifen

Investigations   If PMB then ultrasound scan plus, if endometrium > 4 mm thick or multiple episodes, biopsy by Pipelle or during hysteroscopy
If premenopausal do ultrasound scan then biopsy if abnormal or change in periods and > 40 years. Consider magnetic resonance imaging (MRI). Full blood count (FBC), urea and electrolytes (U&E), chest X-ray, glucose, electrocardiogram (ECG)

Staging   Staging is surgico-pathological
1 Uterus only. 1a: endometrium; 1b: $<\frac{1}{2}$ myometrial invasion; 1c: $>\frac{1}{2}$ myometrial invasion
2 Cervix also
3 Outside uterus, not outside pelvis
4 Bowel and bladder or distant spread

Treatment   Usually total abdominal or laparoscopic hysterectomy and bilateral salpingo-oöphorectomy (BSO)
Radiotherapy if lymph nodes positive/likely to be positive

Prognosis   Dependent on clinical stage, histology, grade, patient's fitness
Overall 75% 5-year survival

The cervix and its disorders

Anatomy and function of the cervix

Anatomy

The cervix is a tubular structure, continuous with the uterus, 2–3 cm long and made up predominantly of elastic connective tissue. It connects the uterus and vagina, allowing sperm in and menstrual flow out. In pregnancy it holds the fetus in the uterus and then dilates in labour to allow delivery. It is attached posteriorly to the sacrum by the uterosacral ligaments and laterally to the pelvic side wall by the cardinal ligaments. Lateral to the cervix is the parametrium, containing connective tissue, uterine vessels and the ureters.

Histology and the transformation zone

The endocervix (canal) is lined by columnar (glandular) epithelium. The ectocervix, continuous with the vagina, is covered in squamous epithelium. The two types of cell meet at the 'squamocolumnar junction' (Fig. 4.1). During puberty and pregnancy, partial eversion of the cervix occurs. The lower pH of the vagina causes the now exposed area of columnar epithelium to undergo metaplasia to squamous epithelium, producing a 'transformation zone' at the squamocolumnar junction (Fig. 4.1). Cells undergoing metaplasia are vulnerable to agents that induce neoplastic change, and it is from this area that cervical carcinoma commonly originates.

Blood supply and lymph drainage

The blood supply is from upper vaginal branches and the uterine artery. Lymph drains to the obturator and internal and external iliac nodes, and thence to the common iliac and para-aortic nodes. Cervical carcinoma characteristically spreads in the lymph and locally by direct invasion into the uterus, vagina, bladder and rectum.

Benign conditions of the cervix

Cervical ectropion (previously called erosion) is when the columnar epithelium of the endocervix is visible as a red area around the os on the surface of the cervix (Fig. 4.2a). This is due to eversion and is a normal finding in younger women, particularly those who are pregnant or taking the 'pill'. Normally asymptomatic, ectropions occasionally cause vaginal discharge or postcoital bleeding (PCB). This can be treated by freezing (cryotherapy) without anaesthetic, but only after a smear and, ideally, colposcopy has excluded a carcinoma. Exposed columnar epithelium is also prone to infection.

Acute cervicitis is rare but often results from sexually transmitted disease [→ p.72]. Ulceration and infection are occasionally found in severe degrees of prolapse when the cervix protrudes or is held back with a pessary [→ p.56].

Chronic cervicitis is chronic inflammation or infection, often of an ectropion. It is a common cause of vaginal discharge and may cause 'inflammatory' smears. Cryotherapy is used, with or without antibiotics, depending upon bacterial culture.

Cervical polyps are benign tumours of the endocervical epithelium (Fig. 4.2b). They are most common in women above the age of 40 years and are seldom larger than 1 cm. They may be asymptomatic or cause intermenstrual bleeding (IMB) or PCB. Small polyps are avulsed without anaesthetic and examined histologically, but bleeding abnormalities must still be investigated [→ p.15].

Nabothian follicles occur where squamous epithelium has formed by metaplasia over endocervical cells. The

Obstetrics and Gynaecology, 3rd edition. By Lawrence Impey and Tim Child. Published 2008 by Blackwell Publishing, ISBN: 978-1-4051-6095-7.

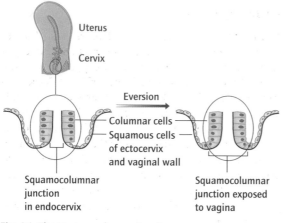

Fig. 4.1 The squamocolumnar junction.

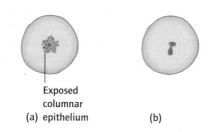

Fig. 4.2 (a) Cervical ectropion; (b) cervical polyp.

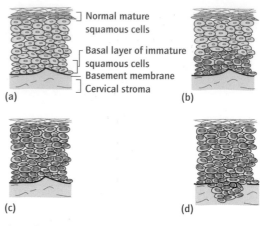

Fig. 4.3 The cervical epithelium and cervical intraepithelial neoplasia (CIN). (a) Normal cervical epithelium; proliferation in basal layer only with small nuclei. (b) CIN I–II: abnormal cells with larger nuclei proliferating in the lower one-third to two-thirds of the epithelium. (c) CIN III: abnormal cells occupying the entire epithelium. (d) Microinvasion: abnormal cells have penetrated the basement membrane.

columnar cell secretions are trapped and form retention cysts, which appear as white or opaque swellings on the ectocervix. Treatment is not required unless symptomatic (rare).

In *congenital malformations* the uterus and cervix may be absent or varying degrees of duplication may occur [→ p.26].

Premalignant conditions of the cervix: cervical intraepithelial neoplasia

Definitions

Cervical intraepithelial neoplasia (CIN), or cervical dys-

plasia, is the presence of atypical cells within the squamous epithelium. These atypical cells are dyskaryotic, exhibiting larger nuclei with frequent mitoses. The severity of CIN is graded I–III and is dependent on the extent to which these cells are found in the epithelium (Fig. 4.3). CIN is therefore a *histological* diagnosis.

CIN I (mild dysplasia): Atypical cells are found only in the lower third of the epithelium.

CIN II (moderate dysplasia): Atypical cells are found in the lower two-thirds of the epithelium.

CIN III (severe dysplasia): Atypical cells occupy the full thickness of the epithelium. This is carcinoma *in situ*: the cells are similar in appearance to those in malignant lesions, but there is no invasion. Malignancy ensues if these abnormal cells invade through the basement membrane.

Natural history

If untreated, about one-third of women with CIN II/III will develop cervical cancer over the next 10 years. CIN I has the least malignant potential: it can progress to CIN II/III, but commonly regresses spontaneously (Fig. 4.4).

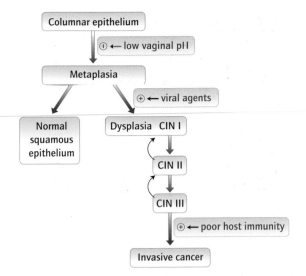

Fig. 4.4 Natural history of cervical intraepithelial neoplasia (CIN).

Epidemiology

CIN is becoming more common. Ninety per cent of cases of CIN III are in women under 45 years, with peak incidence in those 25–29 years of age.

Aetiology

Human papilloma virus (HPV): The most important factor is the number of sexual contacts, particularly at an early age: CIN is almost unknown in virgins. This is because infection with a HPV (particularly types 16, 18, 31, 33) is sexually transmitted. Vaccination against individual viruses reduces the incidence of precancerous cervical lesions, and therefore, potentially, cervical cancer. The vaccine should be administered before first sexual contact as it has a prophylactic effect, and does not help to treat established CIN (i.e. to children/young adolescents) (*Br J Cancer* 2006; **95**: 1459). A UK national vaccination programme for adolescent girls is in progress.

Other factors: Oral contraceptive usage (*Lancet* 2002; **359**: 1085) and smoking are associated with a slightly increased risk of CIN. Immunocompromised patients (e.g. human immunodeficiency virus [HIV], those on long-term steroids) are also at increased risk and of early progression to malignancy.

Pathology

As the columnar epithelium undergoes metaplasia to squamous epithelium in the transformation zone, exposure to certain HPV results in incorporation of viral deoxyribonucleic acid (DNA) into cell DNA. Viral proteins inactivate key cell tumour suppressor gene products and push the cell into a cell cycle. Over time other mutations accumulate and can lead to carcinoma. Viruses also cause changes to hide the infected cell from the immune system. Failure of the immune system to detect and destroy such cells, either because of these cell changes or because of immunosuppression (transplant patient or acquired immunodeficiency syndrome [AIDS]), can result in malignancy.

Diagnosis: screening for cervical cancer

CIN causes no symptoms and is not visible on the cervix. However, the diagnosis identifies women at high risk of developing carcinoma of the cervix who could be treated before the disease develops. Identification of CIN is therefore the principal step in screening for cervical cancer.

Cervical smears

Screening is performed with cervical smears. These should be performed on all women from the age of 25 years, or after first intercourse if later, and then repeated every 3 years until the age of 49. Between 50 and 64 years of age smears are performed 5-yearly. From the age of 65 only those who have not been screened since age 50 or have had recent abnormal tests are screened. The abnormal smear identifies women likely to have CIN and therefore at risk of subsequent development of invasive cancer. Women younger than 25 years often have abnormal cervical changes but the risk of cervical cancer is very low. Commencing screening at 25 reduces the number of unnecessary recalls and colposcopies.

Method
Using a Cusco's speculum [→ p.7] a spatula (or brush) is gently scraped around the external os of the cervix to pick up loose cells over the transformation zone (Fig. 4.5). The spatula is then smeared over a slide and the sample is fixed instantly and then stained and examined with a microscope. If a brush is used the tip can be broken into preservative fluid, transported to the laboratory

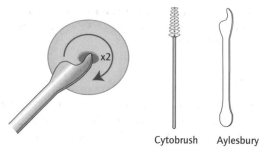

Fig. 4.5 Taking a cervical smear.

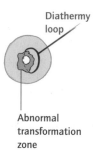

Fig. 4.6 Large loop excision of transformation zone (LLETZ).

then the fluid centrifuged and spread on a slide for microscopy ('liquid-based cytology'). The combination of smear testing with HPV tests may improve screening (*NEJM* 2007; **357**: 1650).

Results

Smears identify cellular, not histological, abnormalities as only superficial cells are sampled. Cellular abnormalities are called *dyskaryosis* and graded mild, moderate and severe. Dyskaryosis suggests the presence of CIN, and the grade partly reflects the severity of CIN. Smears are therefore often reported in histological terms: if severe dyskaryosis is seen, for instance, the report may read 'CIN III'. This does not mean that CIN III is present, merely that a biopsy would be likely to find it. Colposcopy is used to investigate the abnormal smear (see box). Occasionally, abnormal columnar cells are visible (cervical glandular intraepithelial neoplasia [CGIN]). Adenocarcinoma of the cervix or endometrium should then be excluded, using both colposcopy and endocervical curettage (sampling cells within the cervical canal) or with cone biopsy [→ p.36]. Hysteroscopy is used if the cause of the abnormal cells is still unclear.

Colposcopy

If a cervical smear is severely or persistently abnormal, a colposcopy is performed to detect the presence and grade of CIN. The cervix is inspected via a speculum using an operating microscope with magnification 10- to 20-fold. Grades of CIN have characteristic appearances when stained with 5% acetic acid, although the diagnosis is only confirmed histologically and therefore biopsy is usual.

Management of the abnormal smear	
Smear result	*Action*
Normal	Repeat every 3 years
Mild dyskaryosis	Repeat in 6 months. If still present: colposcopy
Borderline changes	Repeat in 6 months. If still present: colposcopy
Moderate dyskaryosis	Colposcopy
Severe dyskaryosis	Urgent colposcopy
Cervical glandular	Colposcopy, if abnormality not found then hysteroscopy intraepithelial neoplasia (CGIN) (any grade)

Prevention of cervical cancer
Human papilloma virus (HPV) vaccination
Prevention of cervical intraepithelial neoplasia (CIN): sexual and (barrier) contraceptive education
Identification and treatment of CIN: cervical smear programmes

Treatment: prevention of invasive cervical cancer

If CIN II or III are present, the transformation zone is excised with cutting diathermy under local anaesthetic. This is called 'large loop excision of transformation zone' (LLETZ; Fig. 4.6), also sometimes called diathermy loop excision (DLE). The specimen is examined histologically. Occasionally an unsuspected malignancy is detected. LLETZ enables diagnosis and treatment to be achieved at the same time ('see and treat') and has replaced laser or diathermy treatment. Alternatively, a small biopsy of the abnormal area can be taken colposcopically and confirmatory results awaited before performing LLETZ. The only major complication of LLETZ, postoperative haemorrhage, is uncommon, but the risk of subsequent preterm delivery is slightly increased (*Obstet Gynecol* 2007; **109**: 309).

Results and problems with screening for cervical cancer

Cervical screening by 3-yearly smear reduces the cumulative incidence of cervical cancer by 91%: most women with cervical carcinoma have never had a smear, and those who have tend to be identified at an earlier stage. Nevertheless, there is a significant false negative rate with cervical smears, dependent on both sampling and interpretation techniques. Furthermore, the distinctions between grades of dyskaryosis and CIN are blurred and spontaneous regression of CIN can occur. Some women do not have cervical smears through fear or ignorance.

Psychological aspects of cervical screening

The woman with an abnormal smear must be handled sensitively. Many will assume they have cancer so an explanation of the 'early warning cells' found will allay fears. Discussion of sexual history and the papilloma virus is usually inappropriate because of feelings of guilt and recrimination. If CIN III is found then the woman can be advised that *without treatment* she has around a 30% chance of developing cancer over 8–15 years. However, colposcopic treatment is straightforward and successful and the national smear programme has reduced the number of cervical cancers in the UK by 75% over the last 20 years.

Malignant disease of the cervix

Epidemiology

The incidence of cervical carcinoma (8.0 per 100 000 women) is falling in the UK, largely due to the success of screening programmes. The disease can occur at any age after first intercourse, but has two peaks of incidence: during a woman's 30s and her 80s. The increased incidence in older women is due to a 'cohort effect' of higher cervical cancer rates in women born during the 1920s who first became sexually active during or after the Second World War.

Pathology

Ninety per cent of cervical malignancies are squamous cell carcinomas. Ten per cent are adenocarcinomas originating from the columnar epithelium: these have a worse prognosis and are increasing in proportion as the smear programme prevents proportionally more squamous carcinomas.

Aetiology

Cervical intraepithelial neoplasia is the preinvasive stage: causative factors are therefore the same. HPV is found in all cervical cancers; vaccination is likely to prevent many cases in the future. Cervical cancer is more common when screening has been inadequate. Immunosuppression (e.g. HIV or steroids) accelerates the process of invasion from CIN. Cervical cancer is not familial.

Clinical features

Occult carcinoma

This is when there are no symptoms, but the diagnosis is made by biopsy or LLETZ.

Clinical carcinoma

History: Postcoital bleeding, an offensive vaginal discharge and IMB or postmenopausal bleeding (PMB) are common. Pain is not an early feature. In the later stages of the disease, involvement of ureters, bladder, rectum and nerves causes uraemia, haematuria, rectal bleeding and pain, respectively. Smears have usually been missed.

Examination: An ulcer or mass may be visible (Fig. 4.7) or palpable on the cervix. With early disease, the cervix may appear normal to the naked eye.

Spread and staging

The tumour spreads locally to the parametrium and vagina and then to the pelvic side wall. Lymphatic spread to the pelvic nodes is an early feature. Ovarian spread is

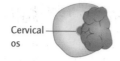

Fig. 4.7 Cervical carcinoma.

rare with squamous carcinomas. Blood-borne spread occurs late. The International Federation of Gynaecology and Obstetrics (FIGO) classification is clinical (from examination), although divisions of Stage 1 are histological (from local excision). It is limited as a predictor of survival because it does not include whether or not there is lymph node (LN) involvement. LN involvement is, however, more likely with advanced stages.

Spread and staging for cervical carcinoma	
Stage 1	*Lesions confined to the cervix:*
1a(i)	Microinvasion <3 mm from the basement membrane, <7 mm across, with no lymph/vascular space invasion
1a(ii)	Invasion >3 mm, <5 mm deep, <7 mm across
1b(i)	Tumour size <4 cm
1b(ii)	Tumour size >4 cm
Stage 2	*Invasion is into vagina, but not the pelvic side wall:*
2a	Invasion of upper two-thirds vagina but not parametrium
2b	Invasion of parametrium
Stage 3	*Invasion of lower vagina or pelvic wall, or causing ureteric obstruction*
Stage 4	*Invasion of bladder or rectal mucosa, or beyond the true pelvis*

Investigations

To confirm the diagnosis, the tumour is biopsied.

To stage the disease, vaginal and rectal examination are used to assess the size of the lesion and parametrial or rectal invasion. Unless it is clearly small, examination under anaesthetic (EUA) is performed. Cystoscopy detects bladder involvement and magnetic resonance

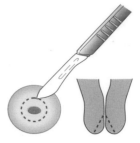

Fig. 4.8 Cone biopsy.

imaging (MRI) detects tumour size, spread and LN involvement.

To assess the patient's fitness for surgery, a chest X-ray, full blood count (FBC) and urea and electrolytes (U&E) are checked. These may be abnormal with advanced disease. Blood is cross-matched before surgery.

Treatment of cervical malignancies

Microinvasive disease

Stage 1a(i) can be treated with cone biopsy (Fig. 4.8), as the risk of LN spread is only 0.5%. Postoperative haemorrhage and preterm labour in subsequent pregnancies are the main complications. Simple hysterectomy is preferred in older women.

All other stage 1 and stage 2a

The choice is between surgery and chemo-radiotherapy. If the LNs are involved, the latter is preferred: treatment is as for beyond stage 2a. LN involvement can be established at MRI, but LN sampling is still required if apparently negative, as MRI is not sensitive enough.

The *lymph nodes are dissected*, frequently laparoscopically, and if negative (either at 'frozen section' or as a second procedure), *radical abdominal hysterectomy* is performed. This Wertheim's hysterectomy involves pelvic node clearance, hysterectomy and removal of the parametrium and upper third of the vagina (Fig. 4.9). The ovaries are left only in the young woman with squamous carcinoma. Specific complications include haemorrhage, ureteric and bladder damage and fistulae, voiding problems and accumulation of lymph (lymphocyst).

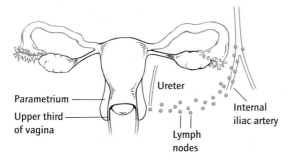

Fig. 4.9 Wertheim's hysterectomy.

Radical trachelectomy is a less invasive procedure for women who wish to conserve fertility. Laparoscopic pelvic lymphadenectomy is first performed. If nodes are positive then chemo-radiotherapy is used instead of surgery. If nodes are negative then radical trachelectomy is an option and involves removal of 80% of the cervix and the upper vagina (*Gynecol Oncol* 2006; **105**: 807). It is appropriate within Stage 1a(ii)–1b(i) provided the tumour is <20 mm in diameter. A cervical suture is inserted to help prevent preterm delivery [→ p.192]. If the incision margins are incomplete then chemo radiotherapy is required.

Proceeding straight to chemo-radiotherapy, particularly in older or medically unfit women, remains an alternative even if the nodes are negative, and survival rates are actually similar to surgery.

Stage 2b and worse *or* positive lymph nodes

These should be treated with radiotherapy and chemotherapy, e.g. platinum agents, the use of which reduces recurrence and increases survival. Palliative radiotherapy is used for bone pain or haemorrhage.

Recurrent tumours

Chemo-radiotherapy is given if it has not been used before. If the patient has received previous chemoradiotherapy, then pelvic exenteration can be considered if the disease is central. Preoperative MRI and positron emission tomography (PET) scans are used to look for metastases. Pelvic exenteration involves removal of the vagina (the uterus and cervix if not already removed), the bladder and/or rectum, and is tried in the young, fit woman, with a central recurrence. There is about a 50% cure rate in carefully selected patients.

Stages of cervical carcinoma and treatment	
Stage	*Treatment*
1a(i)	Cone biopsy or simple hysterectomy
1a(ii)–1b(i)	Laparoscopic lymphadenectomy and radical trachelectomy
1a(ii)–2a	Radical hysterectomy (if lymph nodes [LNs] negative) or chemo-radiotherapy
2b and above or LNs positive	Chemo-radiotherapy alone

Indications for chemo-radiotherapy for cervical carcinoma
Lymph nodes positive on magnetic resonance imaging (MRI) or after lymphadenectomy
If lymph nodes negative as an alternative to hysterectomy
Surgical resection margins not clear
Palliation for bone pain or haemorrhage (radiotherapy)

Prognosis of cervical carcinoma	
Indicator	*5-year survival (%)*
Stage 1a	95
Stage 1b	80
Stage 2	60
Stage 3–4	10–30
Lymph nodes (LNs) involved	40
LNs clear	80
Overall	65

Prognosis

Patients are reviewed at 3 and 6 months and then every 6 months for 5 years. Recurrent disease is commonly central. Poor prognostic indicators are LN involvement, advanced clinical stage, large primary tumour, a poorly differentiated tumour and early recurrence. Death is commonly from uraemia due to ureteric obstruction.

Further reading

Green J, Kirwan J, Tierney J, *et al.* Concomitant chemotherapy and radiation therapy for cancer of the uterine cervix. *Cochrane Database of Systematic Reviews (Online: Update Software)* 2005; Issue 3: CD002225.

Kehoe S. Treatments for gynaecological cancers. *Best Practice & Research Clinical Obstetrics and Gynaecology* 2006; **20**: 985–1000.

NHS Cervical Screening Programme online (http://www.cancerscreening.nhs.uk/cervical/)

Proietto A. Gynaecological cancer surgery. *Best Practice & Research Clinical Obstetrics and Gynaecology* 2006; **20**: 157–72.

Schiffman M, Castle PE, Jeronimo J, *et al*. Human papillomavirus and cervical cancer. *Lancet* 2007; **370**: 890–907.

Carcinoma of the Cervix at a Glance

Epidemiology	Becoming less common in the UK, deaths reducing
Pathology	90% squamous, also adenocarcinomas
Aetiology	Human papilloma virus (HPV), which is sexually transmitted, causing cervical intraepithelial neoplasia (CIN). HPV vaccine now available. Smoking, combined oral contraceptive, immunosuppression
Clinical features	None if occult. Postcoital (PCB) or intermenstrual bleeding (IMB), offensive discharge. Cervix initially appears normal, then ulcerated, then replaced by irregular mass
Screening	Routine use. Three-yearly cervical smears age 25–49; 5-yearly ages 50–64, colposcopy if abnormal
Investigations	Biopsy. Unless early, examination under anaesthetic (EUA), + cystoscopy and magnetic resonance imaging (MRI) to stage. Chest X-ray, urea and electrolytes (U&E), full blood count (FBC)
Staging	**1** Cervix and uterus: 1a(i) <3 mm depth, <7 mm across; 1a(ii) <5 mm depth, <7 mm across; 1b rest **2** Upper vagina also: 2a not parametrium; 2b in parametrium **3** Lower vagina or pelvic wall, or ureteric obstruction **4** Into bladder or rectum, or beyond pelvis
Treatment	Depends on clinical stage: Microinvasion: Cone biopsy or simple hysterectomy 1a(ii)–1b(i) Laparoscopic lymphadenectomy (to confirm negative LNs) and radical trachelectomy to preserve fertility Stage 1a(ii)–2a: LNs negative: Wertheim's hysterectomy or chemo-radiotherapy LNs positive: Chemo-radiotherapy without surgery Stage 2b–4: Chemo-radiotherapy without surgery
Prognosis	Depends on LN involvement, clinical stage and histological grade Overall 65% 5-year survival

Cervical Intraepithelial Neoplasia (CIN) at a Glance

Definitions	Histological abnormality of the cervix in which abnormal epithelial cells occupy varying degrees of the squamous epithelium
	CIN I/mild dysplasia: Atypical cells in lower third
	CIN II/moderate dysplasia: Atypical cells in lower two-thirds
	CIN III/severe dysplasia: Atypical cells in full thickness (carcinoma *in situ*)
	Dyskaryosis: Describes cellular (nuclear) abnormality only from cervical smear. Suggests presence of CIN
Epidemiology	Becoming more common
Aetiology	As for cervical carcinoma
Diagnosis	No clinical features. Cervical smear abnormality and colposcopic abnormality suggests presence. Diagnosis confirmed histologically
Treatment	Rationale: to prevent progression to invasion
	CIN I usually observed; CIN II and III removed with large loop excision of transformation zone (LLETZ)
	This treats, and also identifies, hitherto unexpected invasion

5 The ovary and its disorders

Anatomy and function of the ovaries

The normal ovaries occupy the ovarian fossa on the lateral pelvic wall overlying the ureter, but are attached to the broad ligament by the mesovarium, to the pelvic side wall by the infundibulopelvic ligament and to the uterus by the ovarian ligament. Blood supply is from the ovarian artery, but there is an anastomosis with branches of the uterine artery in the broad ligament (Fig. 5.1).

The ovaries have an outer cortex covered by 'germinal' epithelium (*the most common carcinoma derives from this layer*). The inner medulla contains connective tissue and blood vessels. The cortex contains the follicles and theca cells. Oestrogen is secreted by granulosa cells in the growing follicles and also by theca cells. The rare tumours of these cells secrete oestrogens. A few follicles start to enlarge every month [→ p.11] under the influence of pituitary follicle-stimulating hormone (FSH), but only one will reach about 20 mm in size and rupture in response to the mid-cycle surge of pituitary luteinizing hormone (LH) to release its oocyte (see Fig. 2.3). After ovulation, the collapsed follicle becomes a corpus luteum, which continues to produce oestrogen and progesterone to support the endometrium whilst awaiting fertilization and implantation. If none occurs then the corpus luteum involutes, hormone levels decline and menstruation begins. If fertilization and implantation occur then human chorionic gonadotrophin (hCG) produced from trophoblast maintains corpus luteum function and hormone production until 7–9 weeks' gestation when the fetoplacental unit takes over. Follicular and lutein cysts result from persistence of these structures in non-pregnant women.

Ovarian symptoms

Ovarian masses are often silent and detected either when they are very large and cause abdominal distension, or on ultrasound scan. Acute presentation is associated with 'accidents'.

Ovarian cyst 'accidents'

Rupture of the contents of an ovarian cyst into the peritoneal cavity causes intense pain, particularly with an endometrioma or dermoid cyst (Fig. 5.2a). *Haemorrhage* into a cyst (Fig. 5.2b) or the peritoneal cavity often causes pain. Peritoneal cavity haemorrhage is occasionally so severe as to cause hypovolaemic shock. *Torsion* of the pedicle (bulky due to the cyst) causes infarction of the ovary +/– tube and severe pain (Fig. 5.2c). Urgent surgery and detorsion is required if the ovary is to be saved.

Disorders of ovarian function

Polycystic ovary syndrome (PCOS) is a common disorder that causes oligomenorrhoea, hirsutism and subfertility [→ p.82]. The 'cysts' are actually small, multiple, poorly developed follicles.

Premature menopause is when the last period is reached before the age of 40 years [→ p.105].

Problems of gonadal development include the gonadal dysgeneses, the most common of which is Turner's syndrome [→ p.17].

Obstetrics and Gynaecology, 3rd edition. By Lawrence Impey and Tim Child. Published 2008 by Blackwell Publishing, ISBN: 978-1-4051-6095-7.

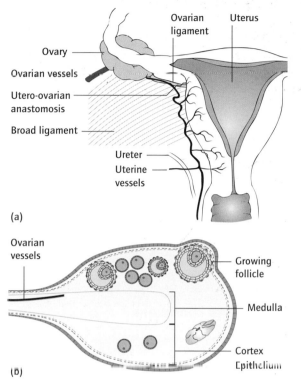

Fig. 5.1 Anatomy of the normal ovary. (a) Relations of the ovary. (b) Transverse section of the normal ovary.

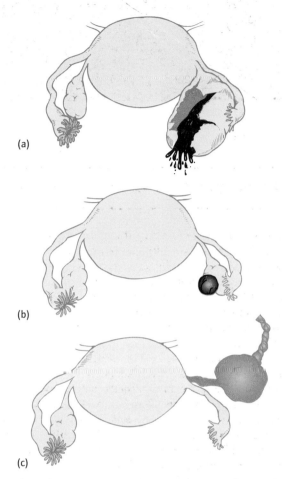

Fig. 5.2 (a) Rupture of an ovarian cyst. (b) Haemorrhage into an ovarian cyst (view from the abdomen). (c) Cyst twisting on its blood supply.

Classification of ovarian tumours

Primary neoplasms

These can be benign or malignant. They are classified together because a benign cyst may undergo malignant change. They fall into three main groups.

Epithelial tumours

Derived from the epithelium covering the ovary, these are most common in postmenopausal women. Uniquely, histology may demonstrate 'borderline' malignancy, when malignant histological features are present but invasion is not. Such tumours may become frankly malignant: surgery is advised but their optimum management is disputed. In younger women with a borderline cyst, close observation may be offered following

removal only of the cyst or affected ovary to retain fertility. Recurrence, as a borderline or invasive tumour, can occur up to 20 years later.

Serous cystadenoma or adenocarcinoma: The malignant variety is the most common malignant ovarian neoplasm (50% of malignancies). Benign and 'borderline' forms also exist.

Mucinous cystadenoma or adenocarcinoma can become very large and are less frequently malignant (10% of ovarian malignancies). A rare 'borderline' variant is pseudomyxoma peritonei, in which the abdominal cavity fills with gelatinous mucin secretions. An appendiceal primary tumour should be excluded.

Endometrioid carcinoma: This malignant variant accounts for 25% of ovarian malignancies. It is similar histologically to endometrial carcinoma, with which it is associated in 20% of cases.

Clear cell carcinoma is a malignant variant that accounts for less than 10% of ovarian malignancies but has a particularly poor prognosis.

Brenner tumours are rare and usually small and benign.

Germ cell tumours

These originate from the undifferentiated primordial germ cells of the gonad.

Teratoma or dermoid cyst is a common benign tumour usually arising in young premenopausal women. It may contain fully differentiated tissue of all cell lines, commonly hair and teeth. They are commonly bilateral, seldom large and often asymptomatic. However, rupture is very painful. A malignant form, the solid teratoma, also occurs in this age group but is very rare.

Dysgerminoma is the female equivalent of the seminoma. Although rare, it is the most common ovarian malignancy in younger women. It is sensitive to radiotherapy.

Sex cord tumours

These originate from the stroma of the gonad.

Granulosa cell tumours are usually malignant but slow growing. They are rare and are usually found in postmenopausal women. They secrete high levels of oestrogens and inhibin: stimulation of the endometrium can cause bleeding, endometrial hyperplasia, endometrial malignancy and, rarely, in young girls, precocious puberty. Serum inhibin levels are used as tumour markers to monitor for recurrence.

Thecomas are very rare, usually benign, and can secrete both oestrogens or androgens.

Fibromas are rare and benign. They can cause Meigs' syndrome, whereby ascites and a (usually) right pleural effusion are found in conjunction with the small ovarian mass. The effusion is benign and cured by removal of the mass.

Common ovarian masses	
Premenopausal:	Follicular/lutein cysts
	Dermoid cysts
	Endometriomas
	Benign epithelial tumour
Postmenopausal:	Benign epithelial tumour
	Malignancy

Secondary malignancies

The ovary is a common site for metastatic spread, particularly from the breast and gastrointestinal tract. Secondaries account for up to 10% of malignant ovarian masses. A few contain 'signet-ring' cells and are called Krukenberg tumours. The primary malignancy may be difficult to detect and the prognosis is very poor.

Tumour-like conditions

The word 'cyst' can include anything from the malignant to the physiological, but is often interpreted as cancer by patients.

Endometriotic cysts: Endometriosis commonly causes altered blood to accumulate in 'chocolate cysts'. In the ovary, such cysts are called endometriomas. Rupture is very painful.

Functional cysts: Follicular cysts and lutein cysts are persistently enlarged follicles and corpora lutea, respectively. They are therefore only found in premenopausal women. The combined pill protects against functional cysts by inhibiting ovulation. Lutein cysts tend to cause more symptoms. If symptoms are absent, treatment is not required and the cyst is observed using serial ultrasound scans. However, because of the remote possibility of malignancy, if an apparently functional cyst >5 cm persists beyond 2 months, the serum carcinoma/cancer antigen 125 (CA 125) level is measured and a laparoscopy considered to remove or drain the cyst.

Carcinoma of the ovary

The silent nature of this malignancy causes it to present late. The overall prognosis is therefore poor.

Epidemiology

There are over 6600 new cases per year in the UK, causing 4400 deaths (more deaths than cervical and endometrial cancer combined). Rates increase with age and over 85% of cases occur in women over 50 years of age. There is marked geographical variation and is getting more common in the West. The lifetime risk of developing ovarian cancer in the UK is 1 in 48.

Histological types of primary ovarian malignancy	
Serous cystadenocarcinoma	50%
Endometrioid carcinoma	20%
Mucinous cystadenocarcinoma	10%
Clear cell carcinoma	10%
Other (non-epithelial)	10%

Pathology

Ninety per cent overall are epithelial carcinomas and the management outlined applies largely to this group. Germ cell tumours are the most common in the rare event of a woman under the age of 30 years being affected.

Aetiology

Benign cysts can undergo malignant change, but a pre-malignant phase is not normally recognized. The risk factors relate to the number of ovulations. Therefore, an early menarche, late menopause and nulliparity are risk factors, whilst pregnancy, lactation and use of the pill are protective. Ovarian carcinoma may also be familial (5%) via the *BRCA1*, *BRCA2* or hereditary non-polyposis colorectal cancer gene (*HNPCC*) gene mutations. If two relatives are affected, the lifetime risk is 13%: if the *BRCA1* mutation is present, the risk approaches 50%. *BRCA1* and *BRCA2* gene mutations are also associated with breast cancer whilst *HNPCC* (also called Lynch's syndrome) is also associated with an increased risk of bowel (80% lifetime risk) and endometrial cancer.

Screening for ovarian carcinoma

There is currently no UK national screening programme for ovarian cancer. Ovarian carcinoma presents late and the prognosis is much better for early disease, so such screening is under investigation (www.ukctocs.org.uk). Unlike cervical cancer, screening is generally for early

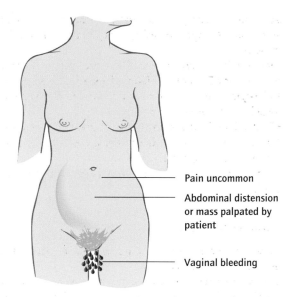

Fig. 5.3 Ovarian cancer presents late as it is commonly asymptomatic.

Pain uncommon

Abdominal distension or mass palpated by patient

Vaginal bleeding

malignant, rather than premalignant disease. Combinations of CA 125 with transvaginal ultrasound are most promising. Screening is currently risk-directed rather than of the general population although the value of screening in women with a high risk of developing ovarian cancer is unknown (trial outcomes awaited). Those with a family history can be referred to regional centres and offered testing for genetic mutations in *BRCA1* and *BRCA2* genes, counselling and prophylactic oöphorectomy (*J Clin Oncol* 2007; **25**: 2921), or yearly transvaginal ultrasound and CA 125 screening.

Clinical features

History: Symptoms are usually initially absent and 70% of patients present with Stage 3–4 disease. Then, abdominal distension is most common or the patient may palpate a mass, or occasionally experience pain or abnormal bleeding (Fig. 5.3). It is important to ask about breast and gastrointestinal symptoms because a mass may be metastatic from these sites.

Examination: Examination may reveal cachexia, an abdominal or pelvical mass and ascites. Very large masses are less likely to be malignant. The breasts should be palpated.

Is the ovarian mass malignant?

More likely if:
    Rapid growth, >5 cm
    Ascites
    Advanced age
    Bilateral masses
    Solid or septate nature on ultrasound scan
    Increased vascularity

Spread and staging for ovarian carcinoma

Stage 1   *Disease macroscopically confined to the ovaries:*
1a   One ovary is affected, capsule is intact
1b   Both ovaries are affected, capsule is intact
1c   One/both ovaries are affected, and capsule is
           not intact, or malignant cells in the abdominal
           cavity (e.g. ascites)

Stage 2   *Disease is beyond the ovaries but confined to the*
           pelvis

Stage 3   *Disease is beyond the pelvis but confined to the*
           abdomen:
           The omentum, small bowel and peritoneum are
           frequently involved

Stage 4   *Disease is beyond the abdomen, e.g. in the lungs*
           or liver parenchyma

The degree of differentiation or 'grade' is also reported

Spread and staging

Ovarian adenocarcinoma spreads directly within the pelvis and abdomen (called transcoelomic spread). Lymphatic and, more rarely, blood-borne spread also occur. Staging is surgical and histological.

Investigations

To help establish the diagnosis and stage, ultrasound is used (Fig. 5.4). Features suggestive of malignancy are solid or septate tumours, high vascularity and ascites. Laparoscopy also helps differentiate malignancy from other pelvic masses. Blood levels of the tumour marker CA 125 are often (80%) raised, but this glycoprotein is neither totally specific nor sensitive for ovarian carcinoma. Liver function tests and a chest X-ray are performed. Paracentesis of ascites may be used to make diagnosis (if malignant cells are found the disease is at least Stage 1c and the patient will require chemotherapy) and to treat pressure symptoms. Drainage of large volumes will worsen intravascular dehydration so an intravenous infusion is required, with monitoring of renal function.

To establish fitness for surgery, blood is taken for full blood count (FBC), urea and electrolytes (U&E) and cross-match.

Management of suspected ovarian carcinoma

The diagnosis and histological type is only established with certainty after surgery, as prior biopsy is seldom practical. This disease is best managed in a cancer centre.

If malignancy is likely

Surgery: Postmenopausal patients and premenopausal patients with almost certain malignancy undergo a *laparotomy* through a vertical incision (Fig. 5.5). The aim is to assess the stage and, if the disease is advanced, to remove as much tumour as possible (debulking). Total abdominal hysterectomy (TAH) with bilateral salpingo-oöphorectomy (BSO) and removal of the omentum should be performed. Bowel preparation is required. Ascites is sent for cytology, and peritoneal washings taken if none present. With very early stage or borderline disease in the woman who wants more children, the uterus and the unaffected ovary are preserved. This may be achieved *laparoscopically*. Meticulous follow-up is required.

Chemotherapy is then normally given to all patients with epithelial carcinoma apart from those with low risk Stage 1a tumours. In early stage disease, this increases survival from 74% to 82% at 5 years (*J Natl Cancer Inst* 2003; **95**: 125). Carboplatin is used (fewer side effects than cisplatin); Taxol increases toxicity without clear benefits. Pegylated liposomal doxorubicin hydrochloride (Caelyx) has a second-line role. A number of trials are currently assessing the value of different treatment options. If initially elevated, CA 125 levels can be used to monitor the response. The best results are seen when as little as possible of the tumour is left after surgery.

Radiotherapy is only used for dysgerminomas.

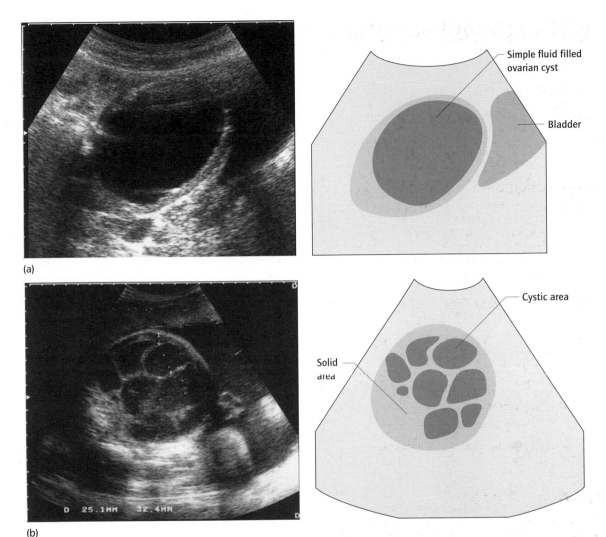

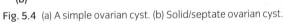

(b)

Fig. 5.4 (a) A simple ovarian cyst. (b) Solid/septate ovarian cyst.

If malignancy is possible

This applies to premenopausal patients with a mass that warrants investigation because it is >5 cm or is persistent or growing. Laparoscopy is used. A simple functional cyst can be biopsied and drained laparoscopically; a dermoid cyst can be removed from the ovary (cystectomy). If the appearances prompt suspicions of malignancy a full laparotomy (as above) is needed.

Follow-up and prognosis

Levels of CA 125 are useful after, as well as during chemotherapy. Computed tomography (CT) scanning aids detection of residual disease or relapse. Interval debulking of residual tissue if not all could be removed at first surgery may be beneficial. Routine 'second look' laparoscopy or laparotomy to monitor the response is not beneficial. Chemotherapy prolongs short-term survival and improves quality of life. Poor prognostic indicators

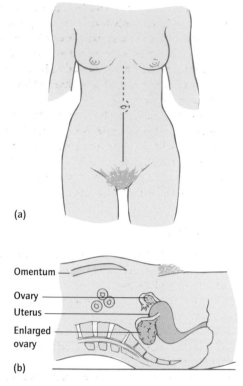

(a)

Omentum

Ovary

Uterus

Enlarged
ovary

(b)

Fig. 5.5 (a) Site of incision for suspected ovarian carcinoma (dotted line is potential extension if abdominal disease). (b) Laparotomy for ovarian carcinoma. The uterus, ovaries, omentum and as much of the affected tissue as possible are removed.

are advanced stage, poorly differentiated tumours, clear cell tumours and poor response to chemotherapy. Death is commonly from bowel obstruction or perforation. The prognosis of ovarian cancer prognosis is improving, but largely for the minority of women with early stage disease.

Prognosis of ovarian cancer	
Stage	*5-year survival (%)*
1a	80
1c	55
2	40
3 (most patients)	15
4	5
Overall	25

Palliative care

Only 30% of women are cured of their gynaecological carcinoma. Ovarian carcinoma causes the most deaths, but the principles outlined are applicable to all terminal disease.

Definition and aims

Palliative care is the active total care of the patient whose disease is incurable. The aim is to increase quality of life for the patient and her family. This involves addressing symptoms such as pain, nausea, bleeding and symptoms of intestinal obstruction, as well as meeting the patient's social, psychological and spiritual needs. Care therefore needs to be individualized. Important issues include the problems of prolongation of poor-quality life, euthanasia, symptom control versus drug side effects, making the transition from curative to palliative care, and resource allocation.

Organization of palliative care

Three levels of care are involved, usually working together: the general practitioner, specialist practitioners such as Macmillan nurses, and specialist hospices or gynaecology units.

Symptom control

Pain: The 'analgesic ladder' (Fig. 5.6) describes the differing analgesic strengths of drugs. Co-analgesics such as antidepressants, steroids and cytotoxics may be used too. Accurate appreciation of pain and drug side effects is important. Opioid analgesia can be 'patient controlled' and is normally accompanied by antiemetics. Alternative therapies such as acupuncture or behavioural techniques may allow greater patient control.

Nausea and vomiting affects 60% of patients with advanced carcinoma. It may be due to opiates, metabolic causes (e.g. uraemia), vagal stimulation (e.g. bowel distension) or psychological factors, all of which should be addressed. Antiemetics include anticholinergics, antihistamines, dopamine antagonists or 5HT-3 antagonists (e.g. ondansetron).

Heavy vaginal bleeding may occur with advanced cervical and endometrial carcinomas. High dose progestagens

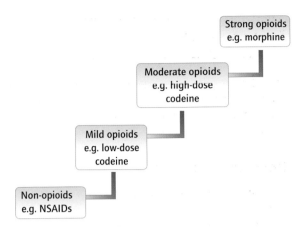

Fig. 5.6 The analgesic ladder. NSAIDs, non-steroidal anti-inflammatory drugs.

may be helpful; radiotherapy is often used if it has not been used before.

Ascites and bowel obstruction are particular features of advanced ovarian carcinoma. Ascites is best drained slowly by repeated paracentesis. Obstruction is ideally managed at home. Spontaneous resolution occurs in up to one-third of patients. If obstruction is partial, metoclopramide is used (pro-motility and antiemetic) and stool softeners, with enemas for constipation and a trial of dexamethasone to reduce tissue oedema. For com-plete obstruction cyclizine and ondansetron are used for nausea and vomiting, with hyoscine for spasm. The patient is encouraged to eat and drink small amounts as they feel able. Some may be managed for many months like this. Surgical palliation is indicated with acute, single site obstruction; stents may also be inserted low in the sigmoid colon or rectum.

Terminal distress: The last 24 h are often the memories the relatives will retain. The terminal stage should be managed sensitively with time for the patient and rela-tives in a quiet environment. Good symptom control with anxiolytics and analgesics without overly sedating can allow valuable time with the family.

Further reading

Cadron I, Leunen K, Van Gorp T, *et al.* Management of borderline ovarian neoplasms. *Journal of Clinical Oncology* 2007; **25**: 2928–37.

Gynaecological cancers information: http://www.oncolink.com

Levy-Lahad E, Friedman E. Cancer risks among *BRCA1* and *BRCA2* mutation carriers. *British Journal of Cancer* 2007, **96**. 11–5.

Kehoe S. Treatments for gynaecological cancers. *Best Practice & Research Clinical Obstetrics and Gynaecology* 2006; **20**: 985–1000.

Patient support website: http://www.ovacome.org.uk

Classification of Ovarian Tumours at a Glance		
Tumour-like conditions	Endometriotic cysts, follicular and lutein cysts	
Primary tumours	Benign, borderline and malignant types	
	Epithelial tumours:	Serous cystadenomas (benign or malignant)
		Mucinous cystadenomas (benign or malignant)
		Endometrioid carcinoma (malignant)
		Clear cell carcinoma (malignant)
		Brenner tumour (benign)
	Germ cell tumours:	Dermoid cyst (benign)
		Solid teratoma (malignant)
		Dysgerminoma (malignant)
	Sex cord tumours:	Granulosa cell tumours (benign or malignant)
		Thecomas (usually benign)
		Fibromas (benign)
Secondary malignancies	Usually from breast or bowel	

Carcinoma of the Ovary at a Glance

Epidemiology	Causes most gynaecological cancer deaths; postmenopausal, more common in the West
Pathology	Epithelial 90%, germ cell tumour if <30 years
Aetiology	Family history, nulliparity, early menarche, late menopause
Clinical features	Silent in early stage: 75% present in Stages 3–4, usually with abdominal distension or mass, pain or vaginal bleeding
Screening	Not routine and limited use. Studies awaited. Ultrasound scan (USS), CA 125 and family history/gene testing
Investigations	USS, chest X-ray, full blood count (FBC), urea and electrolytes (U&E), liver function tests, CA 125
Staging	1 Ovaries only; 1c with malignant cells in abdomen 2 Pelvis only 3 Abdomen and pelvis 4 Distant, including liver
Treatment	Surgery: total abdominal hysterectomy (TAH), bilateral salpingo-oöphorectomy (BSO), omentectomy, at staging laparotomy Debulk all advanced tumours Then chemotherapy unless 'borderline' or low risk Stage 1a Possible laparoscopy and oöphorectomy alone for young women wanting fertility (very close monitoring)
Prognosis	Poor (25% 5-year survival) because of late presentation

6 Disorders of the vulva and vagina

Anatomy

The vulva is the area of skin that stretches from the labia majora laterally, to the mons pubis anteriorly and the perineum posteriorly. It overlaps with the vestibule, the area between the labia minora and the hymen, which surrounds the urethral and vaginal orifices. The vagina is 7–10 cm long. It is lined by squamous epithelium. Anteriorly lie the bladder and urethra. Posteriorly to the upper third is the pouch of Douglas (peritoneal cavity). The lower posterior wall is close to the rectum. Most lymph drainage occurs via the inguinal lymph nodes, which drain to the femoral and thence to the external iliac nodes of the pelvis (Fig. 6.1). This is a route for metastatic spread of carcinoma of the vulva.

Vulval symptoms

The most common vulval symptoms are *pruritus* (itching), *soreness*, *burning* and *superficial dyspareunia* (pain on sexual penetration). Symptoms can be due to local problems including infection, dermatological disease, malignant and premalignant disease, and the vulval pain syndromes. Skin disease affects the vulva, but rarely in isolation. Systemic disease may predispose to certain vulval conditions (e.g. candidiasis with diabetes mellitus).

Obstetrics and Gynaecology, 3rd edition. By Lawrence Impey and Tim Child. Published 2008 by Blackwell Publishing, ISBN: 978-1-4051-6095-7.

Causes of pruritus vulvae
Infections: Candidiasis (± vaginal discharge)   Vulval warts (condylomata acuminata)   Pubic lice, scabies
Dermatological disease: Any condition, especially eczema, psoriasis, lichen simplex, lichen sclerosus, lichen planus, contact dermatitis
Neoplasia: Carcinoma   Premalignant disease (vulval intraepithelial neoplasia, VIN III) [→ p.51]

Miscellaneous benign disorders of the vulva and vagina

Lichen simplex (Fig. 6.2)

There is a long history of vulval itching and soreness. The area, typically the labia majora, is inflamed and thickened with hyper- and hypo-pigmentation. Vulval biopsy is indicated if the diagnosis is in doubt. Irritants such as soap should be avoided; emollients, moderately potent steroid creams and antihistamines are used.

Lichen planus

Of unknown aetiology, this causes irritation with flat, papular, purplish lesions in the anogenital area, but can affect hair, nails and mucous membranes. Treatment is with high potency steroid creams; surgery should be avoided.

Lichen sclerosus

The vulval epithelium is thin with loss of collagen.

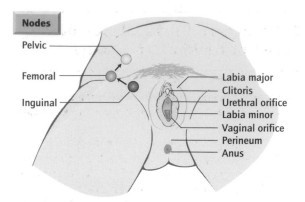

Fig. 6.1 Anatomy and lymph drainage of the vulva.

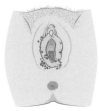

Fig. 6.3 Extensive vulval warts.

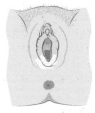

Fig. 6.2 Lichen simplex.

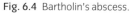

Fig. 6.4 Bartholin's abscess.

This may have an autoimmune basis and thyroid disease and vitiligo may coexist. The typical patient is post-menopausal, but much younger women are occasionally affected. Pruritus and soreness are usual. The appearance is of pink–white papules, which coalesce to form parchment-like skin with fissures. Vulval carcinoma can develop in 5% of cases. Biopsy is important to exclude carcinoma and to confirm the diagnosis. Treatment is with the ultra-potent topical steroids.

Vulvar dysaesthesia (vulvodynia) or the vulval pain syndromes

These are diagnoses of exclusion, with no evidence of organic vulval disease (*Curr Opin Obstet Gynecol* 2003; **15**: 497). They are now divided into provoked or sponta-neous vulvar dysaesthesia and subdivided according to site: local (e.g. vestibular) or generalized. They are asso-ciated with many factors including a history of genital tract infections, former use of oral contraceptives and psychosexual disorders. Spontaneous generalized vulvar

dysaesthesia (formerly essential vulvodynia) describes a burning pain that is more common in older patients. Vulvar dysaesthesia of the vestibule causes superficial dyspareunia or pain using tampons and is more common in younger women, in whom introital damage must be excluded. For both conditions, topical agents are seldom helpful and oral drugs such as amitriptyline or gabapen-tin are sometimes used.

Infections of the vulva and vestibule

Herpes simplex, vulval warts (condylomata acuminata) (Fig. 6.3), syphilis and donovanosis may all affect the vulva [→ p.73]. Candidiasis may affect the vulva if there has been prolonged exposure to moisture. Candi-diasis is common in diabetics, in pregnancy, when antibiotics have been used or when immunity is compromised.

Bartholin's gland cyst and abscess

The two glands behind the labia minora secrete lubricat-ing mucus for coitus. Blockage of the duct causes cyst formation. If infection occurs, commonly with *Staphy-lococcus* or *Escherichia coli*, an abscess forms (Fig. 6.4).

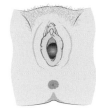

Fig. 6.5 Congenital vaginal cyst.

This is acutely painful and a large tender red swelling is evident. Treatment is with incision and drainage, and marsupialization, whereby the incision is sutured open to reduce the risk of re-formation.

Introital damage

This commonly follows childbirth. Overtightening, incorrect apposition at perineal repair or extensive scar tissue commonly present with superficial dyspareunia. Symptoms often resolve with time. If the introitus is too tight, vaginal dilators or surgery (Fenton's repair) are used.

Vaginal cysts

Congenital cysts commonly arise in the vagina (Fig. 6.5). They have a smooth white appearance, can be as large as a golf ball, and are often mistaken for a prolapse. They seldom cause symptoms, but if there is dyspareunia they should be excised.

Vaginal adenosis

When columnar epithelium is found in the normally squamous epithelium of the vagina it is called vaginal adenosis. It commonly occurs in women whose mothers received diethylstilboestrol (DES) in pregnancy, when it is associated with genital tract anomalies. Spontaneous resolution is usual, but it very occasionally turns malignant (clear cell carcinoma of the vagina). Women with DES exposure *in utero* are screened annually by colposcopy. It may also occur secondarily to trauma.

Vaginal wall prolapse and vaginal discharge are discussed in Chapters 7 and 10, respectively.

Premalignant disease of the vulva: vulval intraepithelial neoplasia

Vulval intraepithelial neoplasia (VIN) is the presence of atypical cells in the vulval epithelium. There are two main types:

1 VIN (usual type) is caused by human papilloma virus (HPV) and is responsible for most of the rare vulval cancers in women under the age of 45. The incidence is increasing. The lesion is warty and basaloid.

2 VIN (differentiated type) is due to lichen sclerosis and is the major cause of vulval cancer in women over the age of 45. The lesion is keratinizing.

The annual risk of vulval cancer in women with untreated carcinoma *in situ* (high-grade VIN) is at least 10%, while the risk of progression in treated lesions is 2–5%. VIN is also associated with smoking and immunosuppression. Pruritus or pain are common; lesions can be seen by the naked eye as papular, usually white, areas. Colposcopy is helpful, but biopsy is essential to confirm the diagnosis.

Management is to alleviate symptoms and to exclude, observe for, and prevent malignant change. Symptomatic high-grade VIN is treated with local excision, laser therapy or topical immunomodulators (e.g. imiquimod), although the recurrence rate is 30%. In the long term, serial examination and biopsy of suspicious areas is required.

Carcinoma of the vulva

Epidemiology

Carcinoma of the vulva accounts for 5% of genital tract cancers, with up to 1000 new cases each year in the UK and 400 deaths. It is most common after the age of 60 years.

Pathology

Ninety-five per cent of vulval malignancies are squamous cell carcinomas. Melanomas, basal cell carcinomas, adenocarcinomas and a variety of others, including sarcomas, account for the rest.

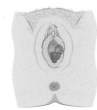

Fig. 6.6 Vulval carcinoma.

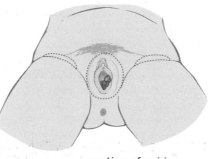

······· Lines of excision

Fig. 6.7 Skin sparing and separate incisions for a vulvectomy.

Spread and staging for carcinoma of the vulva	
Stage I	Tumour is <2 cm in diameter; no nodes are involved
	Ia Stromal invasion < 1 mm
	Ib Stromal invasion > 1 mm
Stage II	Tumour is >2 cm in diameter; no nodes are involved
Stage III	Tumour has spread beyond the vulva or perineum, to urethra, vagina or anus. Or nodes are involved on one side only
Stage IV	Tumour is in rectum, bladder, bone or distant metastases. And/or nodes are involved bilaterally

Aetiology

Although high-grade VIN is a premalignant stage of squamous carcinoma, carcinoma often arises *de novo*. It is also associated with lichen sclerosis, immunosuppression, smoking and Paget's disease of the vulva.

Clinical features

History: The patient experiences pruritus, bleeding or a discharge, or may find a mass, but malignancy often presents late as lesions go unnoticed or cause embarrassment.

Examination: This will reveal an ulcer or mass, most commonly on the labia majora or clitoris (Fig. 6.6). The inguinal lymph nodes may be enlarged, hard and immobile.

Spread and staging

Fifty per cent of patients present with Stage I disease. Vulval carcinoma spreads locally and via the lymph drainage of the vulva. Spread is to the superficial and then to the deep inguinal nodes, and thence to the femoral and subsequently external iliac nodes (Fig. 6.1). Contralateral spread may occur.

Staging is surgical and histological (i.e. after surgery).

Investigations

To establish the diagnosis and histological type, a biopsy is taken.

To assess fitness for surgery, a chest X-ray, electrocardiogram (ECG), full blood count (FBC) and urea and electrolytes (U&E) are required, as these patients are usually elderly. Blood is cross-matched.

Treatment

For Stage Ia disease, wide local excision is adequate, without inguinal lymphadenectomy.

For other stages, wide local excision and groin lymphadenectomy through separate 'skin sparing' incisions (Fig. 6.7) is performed—so-called triple incision radical vulvectomy. If the tumour does not extend to within 2 cm of the mid-line, unilateral excision and lymphadenectomy only are used. This approach has largely replaced the traditional radical vulvectomy through a 'butterfly incision' which dissected the entire vulva and groins en bloc. Complications include wound breakdown, infection, leg lymphoedema, lymphocyst formation and sexual and body image problems. *Radiotherapy* may be used to shrink large tumours prior to surgery, postoperatively if groin lymph nodes are positive, or palliatively to treat severe symptoms.

Prognosis

Many of these patients die from other diseases related to their age. Survival at 5 years in Stage I is >90%; in Stages III–IV the figure is 40%.

Malignancies of the vagina

Secondary vaginal carcinoma is common and arises from local infiltration from cervix, endometrium or vulva, or from metastatic spread from cervix, endometrium or gastrointestinal tumours.

Primary carcinoma of the vagina accounts for 2% of genital tract malignancies, affects older women and is usually squamous. Presentation is with bleeding or discharge and a mass or ulcer is evident. Treatment is with intravaginal radiotherapy or, occasionally, radical surgery. The average survival at 5 years is 50%.

Clear cell adenocarcinoma of the vagina is most common in the late teenage years. Most are a rare complication affecting the daughters of women prescribed DES during pregnancy to try to prevent miscarriage during the 1950s to early 1970s. With radical surgery and radiotherapy, survival rates are good.

Further reading

Cancer statistics: http://info.cancerresearchuk.org/cancerstats/types/vulva/

Dermatology guidelines: http://www.bad.org.uk/healthcare/guidelines/

Innamaa A, Nunns D. The management of vulval pain syndromes. *Hospital Medicine* 2005; **66**: 23–6.

Kehoe S. Treatments for gynaecological cancers. *Best Practice & Research in Clinical Obstetrics and Gynaecology* 2006; **20**: 985–1000.

Yesudian PD, Suqunendran H, Bates CM, *et al.* Lichen sclerosus. *International Journal of STD & AIDS* 2005; **16**: 465–73.

Carcinoma of the Vulva at a Glance

Epidemiology	1000 cases per year in UK. Age >60 years
Aetiology	Vulvar intraepithelial neoplasia (VIN) and oncogenic human papilloma viruses (HPVs), lichen sclerosis
Pathology	95% squamous cell carcinomas
Features	Pruritus, bleeding, discharge, mass
Spread	Local and lymph
Staging	I: <2 cm, no nodes: 1a stromal invasion <1 mm; 1b >1 mm II: >2 cm, no nodes III: Beyond vulva or unilateral nodes IV: In rectum/bone/bladder and/or bilateral nodes
Treatment	Biopsy, then wide local excision with separate groin node dissection, bilateral unless tumour >2 cm from mid-line Radiotherapy if lymph nodes involved
Prognosis	>90% 5-year survival in Stage I; 40% in Stages III–IV

Prolapse is descent of the uterus and/or vaginal walls within the vagina. Behind the vaginal walls, other pelvic organs descend and therefore produce a form of hernia.

Anatomy and physiology of the pelvic supports

The transverse cervical (cardinal) ligaments and the *uterosacral ligaments* are the most important (Fig. 7.1). These attach to the cervix and suspend the uterus from the pelvic side wall and sacrum, respectively; the upper vagina is also suspended. Laxity of these ligaments allows the uterus to prolapse and with it the upper vagina.

The levator ani muscle forms the floor of the pelvis from attachments on the bony pelvic walls and incorporates the perineal body in the perineum. The levator ani suspends the mid-vagina, urethra and rectum, which pass through it. Levator weakness allows prolapse of the vaginal walls and bladder or rectum. The round ligament has little role.

Types of prolapse

Uterine and vaginal prolapse often occur together as the causes are similar.

The uterus: Uterine prolapse (Fig. 7.2b) is graded 1–3. In first-degree prolapse, the cervix is still within the vagina. Second-degree prolapse is at the introitus, and in third-degree prolapse (procidentia) the entire uterus comes out of the vagina. If the uterus has been removed, the *vault*, or top of the vagina where the uterus used to be, can prolapse. This partially inverts the vagina.

The anterior vaginal wall: A *cystocoele* (Fig. 7.2c) is prolapse of the bladder forming a bulge in the anterior vaginal wall. A *urethrocoele* is when the 4-cm long urethra bulges in the lower anterior wall.

Obstetrics and Gynaecology, 3rd edition. By Lawrence Impey and Tim Child. Published 2008 by Blackwell Publishing, ISBN: 978-1-4051-6095-7.

The posterior vaginal wall: A *rectocoele* (Fig. 7.2d) is a prolapse of the rectum forming a bulge in the middle of the posterior wall. An *enterocoele* (Fig. 7.2e) is a prolapse of the pouch of Douglas, i.e. peritoneal cavity, bulging into the posterior vaginal wall just behind the uterus. It usually contains small bowel. The perineum may also be deficient, in that the posterior vaginal opening is lax.

Gynaecological prolapses
Uterine
Anterior wall: bladder (cystocoele) and/or urethra (urethrocoele)
Posterior wall: rectum (rectocoele) and/or pouch of Douglas (enterocoele)
Vaginal vault

Epidemiology

Half of all parous women have some degree of prolapse and 10–20% seek medical attention.

Aetiology of prolapse

Weakened support of pelvic organs

Vaginal delivery is the most important. It can cause both mechanical and neurological (pudendal nerve) injury. Further deliveries often worsen the problem. Prolonged labour, instrumental delivery, poor suturing of obstetric tears and bearing down before full dilatation are risk factors. *Oestrogen deficiency* after menopause causes partial atrophy of the pelvic supports and vaginal walls. *Iatrogenic* prolapse can follow hysterectomy as an inadequately supported vaginal vault will prolapse. *Genetic* predisposition to prolapse may be due to familial collagen weakness. Caesarean section before labour does not entirely protect against pelvic floor disorders (*Obstet Gynecol* 2006; **108**: 863).

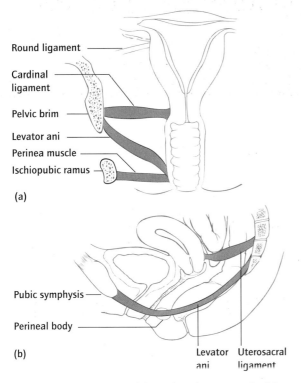

Round ligament

Cardinal ligament

Pelvic brim

Levator ani

Perinea muscle

Ischiopubic ramus

(a)

Pubic symphysis

Perineal body

(b)

Levator ani   Uterosacral ligament

Fig. 7.1 (a) Coronal view of the pelvis showing cardinal ligaments and the levator ani. (b) Lateral view of the pelvis showing the uterosacral ligaments and levator ani.

Increased strain on the supports

Obesity produces extra weight on the pelvic supports and they may weaken. *Pelvic masses* and a *chronic cough* have the same effect.

Causes of prolapse
Childbirth
Oestrogen deficiency
Obesity and chronic cough
Congenital weakness
Pelvic masses

Clinical features

History: Symptoms are often absent, but a dragging sensation or the sensation of a lump are common, usually worse at the end of the day or when standing up. Back pain is unusual. Severe prolapse interferes with inter-

course, may ulcerate and cause bleeding or discharge. A cystocoele can cause urinary frequency and incomplete bladder emptying. Stress incontinence [→ p.61] is common, but it may be incidental. A rectocoele often causes no symptoms, but occasionally causes difficulty in defaecating. Some women have to reduce the prolapse with their fingers to enable the passing of urine or stool.

Examination: includes the abdomen followed by bimanual examination to exclude pelvic masses. A large prolapse is visible from the outside (Fig. 7.3). A Sims' speculum [→ p.7] allows separate inspection of the anterior and posterior vaginal walls: the patient is asked to bear down to demonstrate prolapse. An enterocoele may be mistaken for a rectocoele, but a finger in the rectum will be seen to bulge into a rectocoele but not into an enterocoele, which does not contain rectum. Large polyps and vaginal cysts may be mistaken for a prolapse. Stress incontinence should be sought with the prolapse temporarily reduced by asking the patient to strain/cough.

Symptoms of prolapse
Often asymptomatic
General: Dragging sensation, lump
Cystocoele: Urinary frequency, incontinence
Rectocoele: Occasional difficulty in defaecating

Investigations

To look for a cause consider a pelvic ultrasound if a pelvic mass is suspected. Cystometry [→ p.60] is required if incontinence is the principal complaint.

To assess fitness for surgery (if appropriate) an electrocardiogram (ECG), chest X-ray, full blood count (FBC) and renal function may be required, as the women are often elderly.

Prevention

Prevention involves recognition of obstructed labour, adequate suturing of perineal lacerations and the avoidance of an excessively long second stage. Pelvic floor exercises after childbirth are encouraged.

Management

Treatment must be to alleviate symptoms and small prolapses often require no treatment. *Weight reduction* is

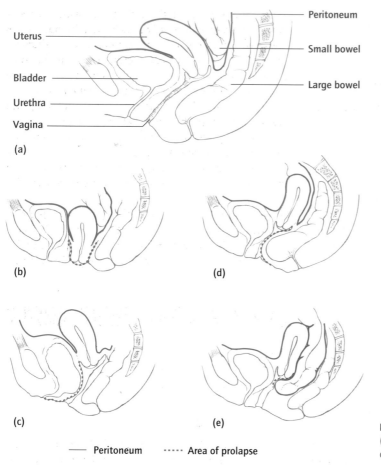

Uterus

Bladder

Urethra

Vagina

Peritoneum

Small bowel

Large bowel

(a)

(b)

(d)

(c)

(e)

—— Peritoneum   ····· Area of prolapse

Fig. 7.2 Types of prolapse. (a) Normal pelvis, (b) uterine prolapse, (c) cystocoele, (d) rectocoele, (e) enterocoele.

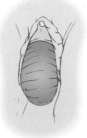

Fig. 7.3 Appearance of cystocoele.

often appropriate. Smoking is discouraged. *Physiotherapy* may help mild to moderate degrees of prolapse and reduce the stress incontinence that can be associated although evidence is limited (*Cochrane* 2006: CD003882).

Pessaries

These are used in the patient who is unwilling or unfit for surgery. They act like an artificial pelvic floor, placed in the vagina to stay behind the symphysis pubis and in front of the sacrum. The most commonly used is the ring pessary, but the shelf pessary is more effective for severe forms of prolapse (Fig. 7.4). They are changed every 9–12 months; postmenopausal women may require oes-

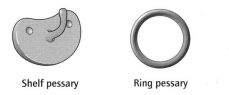

Shelf pessary   Ring pessary

Fig. 7.4 Pessaries for uterovaginal prolapse. (a) Shelf pessary; (b) ring pessary.

trogen replacement: either oestrogen alone as a vaginal topical preparation or as standard hormone repalcement therapy (HRT), to prevent vaginal ulceration. Occasionally, pessaries cause pain, urinary retention or infection, or fall out.

Surgical treatment

Prolapse may kink the urethra, masking stress incontinence. As repair could precipitate incontinence, concomitant surgery for stress incontinence may be required.

Uterine prolapse: For major degrees of uterine descent, *vaginal hysterectomy* will give the best results [→ p.126]. A *sacrohysteropexy*, attaching the prolapsed uterus to the sacrum, can be performed if the uterus is to be conserved (*BJOG* 2001; **108**: 629). This is uncommonly performed as most women with severe uterine prolapse have completed their family (older age and/or a number of deliveries) or are advised to complete their family before considering definitive surgery in the form of hysterectomy.

Vaginal vault prolapse can be repaired vaginally with *sacrospinous colpopexy* by suspension of the vault to the sacrospinous ligament. Complications include nerve or vessel injury, infection and buttock pain. The abdominal (open or laparoscopic) route involves a *sacrocolpopexy*, by fixation of the vault to the sacrum using a mesh. Complications include mesh erosion and haemorrhage. The abdominal route is more successful than vaginal (less recurrence and dyspareunia) but takes longer with slower recovery (*Cochrane* 2004: CD004014).

Vaginal wall prolapse: Anterior and *posterior 'repairs'* are used for the relevant prolapse but, as several prolapses may occur in one patient, these operations are often combined. Synthetic meshes are sometimes used for support.

Surgery for genuine stress incontinence: If this is present, the tension-free vaginal tape (TVT), trans-obturator tape (TOT) procedures, or *Burch colposuspension* may be performed at the same time as prolapse repair [→ p.128].

Prolapse: treatment options
Do nothing
Physiotherapy
Pessaries
Surgery

Further reading

Maher C, Baessler K, Glazener CMA, *et al*. Surgical management of pelvic organ prolapse in women. *Cochrane Database of Systematic Reviews* 2004: CD004014.

Onwude JL. Genital prolapse in women. *BMJ Clinical Evidence* [online web publication March 2007].

Thakar R, Stanton S. Management of genital prolapse. *BMJ (Clinical Research Ed.)* 2002; **324**: 1258–62.

Genital Prolapse at a Glance

Definition	Descent of vaginal walls and pelvic organs within the vagina
Types	Anterior wall (bladder) is a cystocoele Posterior wall is a rectocoele (rectum) or enterocoele (pouch of Douglas) Uterine prolapse graded 1–3, depending on descent Vault prolapse after hysterectomy
Epidemiology	Very common; older multiparous women
Aetiology	Pregnancy and vaginal delivery, oestrogen deficiency, obesity, chronic cough, pelvic masses, surgery, iatrogenic (vault)
Features	Often asymptomatic. Dragging sensation or lump coming down Bulge of vaginal wall visible from outside or with Sims' speculum
Prevention	Improved management of labour
Treatment	General: Lose weight, treat chest problems inc. smoking Pessaries: Ring or shelf, if frail. Change 9–12 monthly Surgery: Vaginal hysterectomy for uterine prolapse, anterior repair for cystocoele, posterior repair for rectocoele. Sacrocolpopexy for vault prolapse. Consider surgery for genuine stress incontinence

8 Disorders of the urinary tract

Anatomy and function of the female urinary system

Voluntary control of urine release is achieved by the bladder and urethra. The ureters bring urine to the bladder from the kidneys and enter the bladder obliquely. The bladder has a smooth muscle wall (detrusor muscle) and can normally 'store' about 400 mL urine, although the normal first urge to void is at about 200 mL. It is drained by the urethra. This is about 4 cm long and has a muscular wall and an external orifice in the vestibule just above the vaginal introitus.

Neural control of the bladder and urethra

Parasympathetic nerves aid voiding; sympathetic nerves prevent it. The voiding reflex consists of afferent fibres, which respond to distension of the bladder wall and pass to the spinal cord. Efferent parasympathetic fibres pass back to the detrusor muscle and cause contraction. They also enable opening of the bladder neck. Meanwhile, efferent sympathetic fibres to the detrusor muscle are inhibited. This 'micturition reflex' is controlled at the level of the pons. The cerebral cortex modifies the reflex and can relax or contract the pelvic floor and the striated muscle of the urethra.

Continence

Continence is dependent on the pressure in the urethra being greater than that in the bladder (Fig. 8.1). Bladder

Obstetrics and Gynaecology, 3rd edition. By Lawrence Impey and Tim Child. Published 2008 by Blackwell Publishing, ISBN: 978-1-4051-6095-7.

pressure is influenced by detrusor pressure and external (intra-abdominal) pressure. Urethral pressure is influenced by the inherent urethral muscle tone and also by external pressure, namely the pelvic floor and, normally, intra-abdominal pressure. The detrusor muscle is expandable: as the bladder fills, there is no increase in pressure. Increases in abdominal pressure such as coughing will be transmitted equally to the bladder and upper urethra because both lie within the abdomen. Normally, therefore, coughing does not alter the pressure difference and does not lead to incontinence.

Micturition

Micturition results when bladder pressure exceeds urethral pressure. This is achieved voluntarily by a simultaneous drop in urethral pressure (partly due to pelvic floor relaxation) and an increase in bladder pressure due to a detrusor muscle contraction.

Incontinence

Essentially there are two main causes of female incontinence:

1 Uncontrolled increases in detrusor pressure increasing bladder pressure beyond that of the normal urethra. 'Overactive bladder', previously called 'detrusor instability' is the most common cause of this mechanism.

2 Increased intra-abdominal pressure transmitted to bladder but not urethra, because the upper urethra neck has slipped from the abdomen. Bladder pressure therefore exceeds urethral pressure when intra-abdominal pressure is raised, for example when coughing. 'Genuine stress incontinence' (GSI) is the most common cause of this mechanism.

Much rarer causes include urine bypassing the sphincter through a fistula or the pressure of urine overwhelming the sphincter due to overfilling

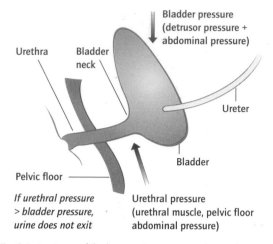

Urethra   Bladder neck

Bladder pressure (detrusor pressure + abdominal pressure)

Ureter

Pelvic floor

Bladder

If urethral pressure > bladder pressure, urine does not exit

Urethral pressure (urethral muscle, pelvic floor abdominal pressure)

Fig. 8.1 Anatomy of the lower urinary tract and contributors to bladder and urethral pressure.

Urinary symptoms	
Urgency:	A severe desire to void
Dysuria:	Pain on micturition
Frequency:	Micturition more than six times a day
Nocturia:	Micturition more than once a night
Nocturnal enuresis:	Incontinence during sleep
Stress incontinence:	Incontinence with raised intra-abdominal pressure
Urge incontinence:	Incontinence with urgency

of the bladder due to neurogenic causes or outlet obstruction.

Investigation of the urinary tract

Urine dipstick tests: Urine dipstick testing for blood, glucose, protein leucocytes and nitrites is essential whenever a patient presents with urinary symptoms. Leucocytes, and particularly nitrites, suggest the presence of infection. If positive then send a urine sample for microscopy and culture (confirm infection and type/sensitivity of organism). Glycosuria and haematuria can be detected: diabetes and bladder carcinoma or calculi can cause urinary symptoms.

Urinary diary: The patient keeps a record for a week of the time and volume of fluid intake and micturition. This gives invaluable information about drinking habits, frequency and bladder capacity.

Post-micturition ultrasound or catheterization: These exclude chronic retention of urine.

Urodynamic studies: These are necessary prior to surgery for GSI or for women whose *overactive bladder* symptoms do not respond to medical therapy. Urodynamics may be performed with or without video imaging.

Cystometry. This is the most important urodynamic study and directly measures, via a catheter, the pressure in the bladder (vesical pressure) whilst the bladder is filled and provoked with coughing. A pressure transducer is also placed in the rectum (or vagina) to measure abdominal pressure (Fig. 8.2). The true detrusor pressure (i.e. the pressure generated by true contraction of the detrusor muscle) can be automatically calculated by subtracting the abdominal pressure from the vesical pressure. The detrusor pressure does not normally alter with filling or provocation (raised intra-abdominal pressure). If leaking occurs with coughing, in the absence of a detrusor contraction, then the problem is likely to be GSI. If an involuntary detrusor contraction occurs, '*detrusor overactivity*' is diagnosed. Initially the patient experiences urgency and then incontinence if bladder pressure is increased beyond that of the urethra. Cystometry is widely used in the management of incontinence as both GSI and *detrusor overactivity* cause the symptom of stress incontinence, but their treatments are very different.

Intravenous pyelogram (IVP): This is useful for assessment and localization of fistulae and filling defects, and in women with recurrent infections or haematuria.

Computer tomography (CT) urogram: With the use of contrast the integrity and route of the ureter is examined.

Methylene dye test: Blue dye is instilled into the bladder. Dye leakage from places other than the urethra, i.e. fistulae, can be seen.

Cystoscopy: Inspection of the bladder cavity is useful to exclude tumours, stones, fistulae and interstitial cystitis but gives little indication of bladder performance.

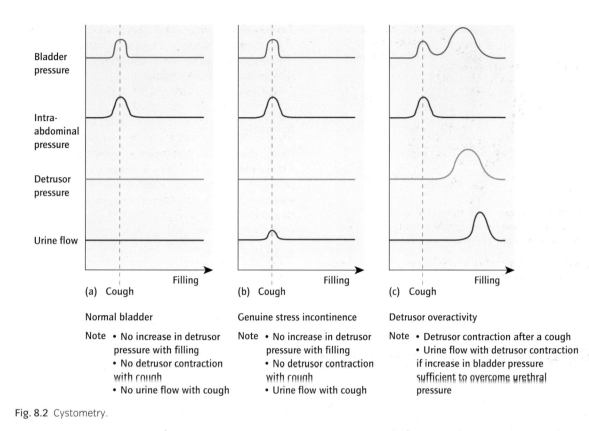

Fig. 8.2 Cystometry.

Genuine stress incontinence

Definition

This is defined as involuntary loss of urine when bladder pressure exceeds maximum urethral pressure in the absence of a detrusor (bladder muscle) contraction. The diagnosis can only be made with certainty after excluding an overactive bladder using cystometry (Fig. 8.2).

Epidemiology

Genuine stress incontinence accounts for almost 50% of causes of incontinence in the female and occurs to varying degrees in more than 10% of all women.

Aetiology

Important causes of GSI include pregnancy and vaginal delivery, particularly prolonged labour and forceps delivery, obesity and age (particularly postmenopausal). Prolapse commonly coexists but is not always related. Previous hysterectomy (not for prolapse or urine symptoms) may predispose to GSI (*Lancet* 2007; **370**: 1494).

Mechanism of incontinence

When there is an increase in intra-abdominal pressure ('stress'), the bladder is compressed and its pressure rises. In the normal woman, the bladder neck is equally compressed so that the pressure difference is unchanged. However, if the bladder neck has slipped below the pelvic floor because its supports are weak, it will not be

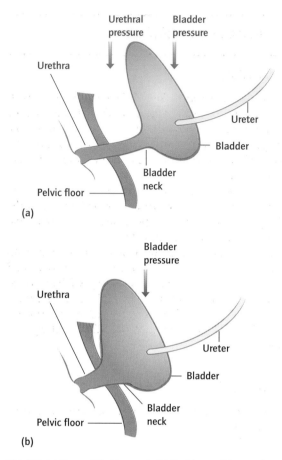

Fig. 8.3 (a) Normal bladder neck. (b) Bladder neck in genuine stress incontinence (GSI).

compressed and its pressure remains unchanged (Fig. 8.3). If the rest of the urethra and the pelvic floor are unable to compensate, the bladder pressure exceeds urethral pressure and incontinence results.

Clinical features

History: This must assess the degree to which the patient's life is disrupted. Stress incontinence predominates, but many patients also complain of frequency, urgency or urge incontinence. It is important to have the patient prioritize her symptoms as the treatment for GSI differs from that for the overactive bladder. Faecal incontinence [→ p.27], also due to childbirth injury, may coexist.

Examination with a Sims' speculum often, but not invariably, reveals a cystocoele or urethrocoele. Leakage of urine with coughing may be seen. The abdomen is palpated to exclude a distended bladder.

Investigations

Urine dipstick is important to exclude infection. Cystometry (Fig. 8.2b) is required to exclude overactive bladder if considering surgery or if *overactive bladder* symptoms fail to respond to medical treatment.

Management

If obese, the patient is encouraged to lose weight. Causes of a chronic cough (e.g. smoking) are addressed. She should reduce excessive fluid intake.

Conservative

Conservative treatment is aimed at strengthening the pelvic floor. Pelvic floor muscle training (PFMT) is an appropriate first line treatment for at least 3 months and is taught by a physiotherapist. The strength of pelvic floor muscle contraction should be digitally assessed before treatment. PFMT should consist of at least 8 contractions, 3 times per day. If PFMT is beneficial then continue an exercise programme. Vaginal 'cones' or sponges are used to alleviate incontinence adequately in more than half of patients. The 'cones' are inserted into the vagina and held in position by voluntary muscle contraction. Increasing sizes are used as muscle strength increases (*Cochrane* 2006: CD005654).

Drug treatment

Duloxetine (serotonin reuptake inhibitor) improves stress incontinence compared to placebo or PFMT but increases the risk of adverse effects such as headache and gastric problems. It appears to enhance pudendal nerve stimulation of the pelvic floor. Duloxetine is best offered as an alternative to surgical treatment, after a failed trial of PFMT. The US Food and Drug Administration denied approval of duloxetine for treatment of stress urinary incontinence because of an increase in suicide risk.

Oestrogen supplementation as hormone replacement therapy (HRT) improves stress incontinence compared to placebo but is less successful than PFMT.

Surgery

This is only performed after cystometry has excluded an overactive bladder. The primary aim is to allow transmission of raised intra-abdominal pressure to the bladder neck as well as the bladder. The traditional 'gold-standard' procedure is the open *Burch colposuspension* [→ p.128]. In this operation the bladder neck is 'lifted' using sutures placed via an abdominal incision. The operation can be performed laparoscopically and success rates appear similar.

Currently, 'mid-urethral sling' procedures such as the *tension-free vaginal tape (TVT)* and the *trans-obturator tape (TOT)* [→ p.128] are the most commonly performed first line surgical option, and have up to 90% cure rates. TVT and TOT are newer techniques and therefore long-term data over 5–10 years are lacking. However, these procedures have revolutionized surgical treatment of stress incontinence, are less invasive than colposuspension, can be performed under spinal or local anaesthesia and require a shorter hospital stay. All the operations can cause bleeding, infection, voiding difficulty and *de novo* overactive bladder. TVT and TOT have similar efficacy (*J Urol* 2007; **177**: 214). TVT is associated with an increased risk of bladder perforation compared to TOT but both procedures have lower morbidity than a colposuspension.

In the elderly or medically unfit, periurethral bulking injections of collagen may have a limited role. It is a minor procedure but around 50% of women will be leaking urine again within 2 years of surgery. Operations such as the anterior vaginal repair and the Stamey needle-suspension procedure are no longer recommended for GSI.

Distinction between genuine stress incontinence and stress incontinence

Genuine stress incontinence (GSI) is a *disorder* diagnosed only after cystometry, of which stress incontinence is the major symptom

Stress incontinence is a *symptom*: 'I leak when I cough'. It can be due to GSI, but it may also be the result of overactive bladder or overflow incontinence

---

Overactive bladder

Definition

The *overactive bladder* (OAB) is defined as urgency, with or without urge incontinence, usually with frequency or nocturia in the absence of proven infection. The symptom combinations are suggestive of *detrusor overactivity* but can be due to other forms of urinary tract dysfunction.

Detrusor overactivity is a urodynamic diagnosis characterized by involuntary detrusor contractions during the filling phase which may be spontaneous or provoked by, for instance, coughing (Fig. 8.2c).

These definitions recognize that not all women with symptoms of OAB will have *detrusor overactivity*, and not all women with *detrusor overactivity* will have symptoms of *overactive bladder*. The limitations of urodynamic studies should be remembered as the process, involving rapid retrograde bladder filling, is non-physiological.

Epidemiology

Overactive bladder causes 35% of cases of female incontinence.

Aetiology

It is most commonly idiopathic. The condition can follow operations for GSI and is then probably the result of bladder neck obstruction. Occasionally OAB is due to involuntary detrusor contractions (*detrusor overactivity*) occurring in the presence of underlying neuropathy such as multiple sclerosis or spinal cord injury.

Mechanism of incontinence

The detrusor contraction is normally felt as urgency. If strong enough, it causes the bladder pressure to overcome the urethral pressure and the patient leaks: urge incontinence. This can occur spontaneously or with provocation, for example, with a rise in intra-abdominal pressure or a running tap. Coughing may therefore lead to urine loss and be confused with stress incontinence.

Clinical features

History: Urgency and urge incontinence, frequency and nocturia are usual. Stress incontinence is common. Some patients leak at night or at orgasm. A history of childhood enuresis is common, as is faecal urgency.

Examination is often normal, but an incidental cysto-coele may be present.

Investigations

The urinary diary will show frequent passage of small volumes of urine, particularly at night, and may show high intake of caffeine-containing drinks such as tea/coffee or colas. With *detrusor overactivity* cystometry demonstrates contractions on filling or provocation (Fig. 8.2c). Occasionally, the bladder pressure merely rises steadily with filling. However, cystometry is generally not indicated until either there has been failure of lifestyle changes and drug management of OAB symptoms or if surgery for GSI is considered.

Treatment

Recommend caffeine and/or fluid intake reduction if excessive and commence *bladder training* for at least 6 weeks. Instead of voiding at first desire, the patient voids by the clock at increasing intervals. Evidence regarding its effectiveness is limited (*Cochrane* 2004: CD001308). If it is ineffective an antimuscarinic drug such as *tolterodine* and *oxybutynin* is used. These are anticholinergic and relax smooth muscle in the bladder. Equally effective, the side effect profile, principally a dry mouth, is better with *tolterodine* (*Cochrane* 2006: CD003193).

In postmenopausal women with vaginal atrophy, intravaginal *oestrogens* are beneficial. *Synthetic antidiuretic hormone* reduces severe nocturnal symptoms, although caution is required in the presence of comorbidities such as cardiac disease.

If conservative treatments have failed, botulinium toxin A ('botox') or sacral nerve stimulation may be used. Botox is administered into the detrusor muscle with a needle cystoscopically. Long-term data are lacking and there is a risk of total bladder paralysis needing self-catheterization. Botox treatment lasts for about 6 months. Very severe and resistant symptoms may be helped by surgery: *clam augmentation ileocystoplasty*.

Causes of incontinence	
Genuine stress incontinence (GSI)	50%
Overactive bladder	35.0%
Mixed	10.0%
Overflow incontinence	1.0%
Fistulae	0.3%
Unknown	4.0%

Causes of urgency and frequency
Urinary infection
Bladder pathology
Pelvic mass compressing the bladder
Overactive bladder
Genuine stress incontinence (GSI)

Other urinary disorders

'Mixed' GSI and overactive bladder

This accounts for about 10% of all cases of incontinence. The diagnosis is made at cystometry. The overactive bladder is treated first.

Acute urinary retention

The patient is unable to pass urine for 12 h or more, catheterization producing as much or more urine than the normal bladder capacity. It is painful, except when due to epidural anaesthesia or failure of the afferent pathways. Causes include childbirth, particularly with an epidural, vulval or perineal pain (e.g. herpes simplex), surgery, drugs such as anticholinergics, the retroverted gravid uterus, pelvic masses and neurological disease (e.g. multiple sclerosis or cerebrovascular accident). Catheterization is maintained for 48 h whilst the cause is treated.

Chronic retention and urinary overflow

This accounts for only 1% of cases of incontinence. Leaking occurs because bladder overdistension eventually causes overflow. It can be due to either urethral obstruction or detrusor inactivity. Pelvic masses and incontinence surgery are common causes of urethral obstruction. Autonomic neuropathies (e.g. diabetes) and previous overdistension of the bladder (e.g. unrecognized acute retention after epidural anaesthesia)

[→ p.242] cause detrusor inactivity. Presentation may mimic stress incontinence or urinary loss may be continuous. Examination reveals a distended non-tender bladder. The diagnosis is confirmed by ultrasound or catheterization after micturition. Intermittent self-catheterization is commonly required.

Painful bladder syndrome and interstitial cystitis

Painful bladder syndrome (PBS) is a condition in which a patient experiences suprapubic pain related to bladder filling, accompanied by other symptoms such as frequency in the absence of proven urinary tract infection (UTI) or other obvious pathology. The diagnosis of interstitial cystitis is confined to patients with painful bladder symptoms who have characteristic cystoscopic and histological features. The aetiology is unknown. Treatments include dietary changes, bladder training, tricyclic antidepressants, analgesics and intravesical infusion of various drugs.

Fistulae

These are abnormal connections between the urinary tract and other organs (Fig. 8.4). The most common are the vesico-vaginal and urethro-vaginal fistulae. In the developing world they are common as a result of obstructed labour: in the West they are rare and usually due to surgery, radiotherapy or malignancy. Whilst small fistulae may resolve spontaneously, surgery is usually required, the timing depending on the site and the cause. Investigate with a CT urogram or an IVP.

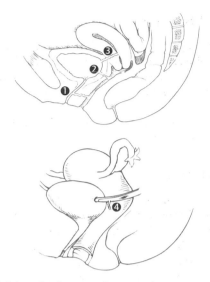

Fig. 8.4 Urinary fistulae: 1, urethro-vaginal; 2, vesico-vaginal; 3, vesico-uterine; 4, uretero-vaginal.

Further reading

http://www.continence-foundation.org.uk

National Institute for Clinical Excellence (NICE). *Urinary Incontinence*. Clinical Guideline No 40. 2006.

Onwude J. Stress incontinence. *BMJ Clinical Evidence* [online web publication Nov 2006].

Smith PP, McCrery RJ, Appell RA. Current trends in the evaluation and management of female urinary incontinence. *Canadian Medical Association Journal* 2006; **175**: 1233–40.

Genuine Stress Incontinence (GSI) at a Glance	
Definition	Leakage of urine with raised bladder pressure in the absence of a detrusor contraction
Epidemiology	10% of women, varying severity. More common with age
Aetiology	Childbirth and the menopause
Clinical features	Stress incontinence, also frequency and urgency. Prolapse common
Investigations	Urine dipstick; diary; cystometry before surgery to confirm diagnosis
Treatment	Conservative: Physiotherapy Medical: Duloxetine Surgical: Tension-free vaginal tape (TVT) or trans-obturator tape (TOT). Colposuspension if fails

Endometriosis and chronic pelvic pain

Endometriosis

Definition and epidemiology

Endometriosis is the presence and growth of tissue similar to endometrium outside the uterus. Some 1–2% of women are diagnosed as having endometriosis, particularly between the ages of 30 and 45 years although endometriotic lesions may occur in 1–20% of all women, albeit asymptomatically in most. It is more common in nulliparous women.

Pathology

Endometriosis, like normal endometrium, is oestrogen dependent: it regresses after the menopause and during pregnancy. It can occur throughout the pelvis, particularly in the uterosacral ligaments, and on or behind the ovaries (Fig. 9.1). Occasionally it affects the umbilicus or abdominal wound scars, the vagina, bladder, rectum and even the lungs. Accumulated altered blood is dark brown and can form a 'chocolate cyst' or endometrioma in the ovaries. Endometriosis causes inflammation, with progressive fibrosis and adhesions. In its most severe form, the entire pelvis is 'frozen', the pelvic organs rendered immobile by adhesions. Symptoms, particularly pain, correlate poorly with the extent of the disease.

Aetiology

Endometriosis in the pelvis is probably a result of retrograde menstruation. More distant foci may result from mechanical, lymphatic or blood-borne spread. As retro-

grade menstruation is common, but is not always associated with endometriosis, unknown individual factors appear to determine whether the retrograde menstrual endometrium implants and grows. Genetic linkage studies suggest a degree of inherited predisposition (*Hum Reprod* 2007; **22**: 717). A currently less popular theory is that endometriosis is the result of metaplasia of coelomic cells. It is also not understood why symptoms correlate poorly with the extent of the disease.

Clinical features

History: Symptoms are often absent, but endometriosis is an important cause of chronic pelvic pain. This is usually cyclical. Presenting complaints include dysmenorrhoea before the onset of menstruation, deep dyspareunia, subfertility, pain on passing stool (dyschezia) during menses, and, occasionally, menstrual problems. Rupture of a chocolate cyst causes acute pain, and this may be the first symptom. Cyclical haematuria, rectal bleeding or bleeding from the umbilicus are uncommon and suggest severe disease.

Examination: Common findings on vaginal examination are tenderness and/or thickening behind the uterus or in the adnexa. In advanced cases, the uterus is retroverted and immobile (due to adhesions) and a rectovaginal nodule of endometriosis may be apparent. With mild endometriosis the pelvis often feels normal.

Investigations

Laparoscopy: The diagnosis is only made with certainty after visualization ± biopsy, usually at laparoscopy. Active lesions are red vesicles or punctate marks on the peritoneum. White scars or brown spots ('powder burn') represent less active endometriosis, while exten-

Obstetrics and Gynaecology, 3rd edition. By Lawrence Impey and Tim Child. Published 2008 by Blackwell Publishing, ISBN: 978-1-4051-6095-7.

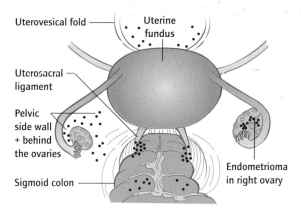

Fig. 9.1 Common sites of endometriosis in the pelvis.

Symptoms of endometriosis
None
Dysmenorrhoea
Chronic pelvic pain
Deep dyspareunia
Subfertility
Cyclical bowel or bladder symptoms
Dyschezia (pain on defaecation)

Differential diagnosis of endometriosis
Adenomyosis
Chronic pelvic inflammatory disease [→ p.76]
Chronic pelvic pain [→ p.69]
Other causes of pelvic masses
Irritable bowel syndrome

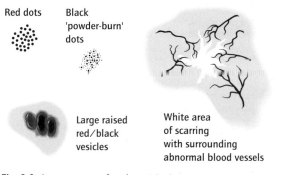

Fig. 9.2 Appearances of endometriosis.

Treatment

Endometriosis is a common incidental finding at laparoscopy. In more than 50% of women the disease regresses or does not progress (*BMJ* 1987; **294**: 272). Asymptomatic endometriosis does not require treatment although consideration should be given to removing endometriomata in view of the (very low) risk of misdiagnosing ovarian cancer. Symptoms should be ascribed to endometriosis with caution and the diagnosis reviewed if treatment does not relieve the patient's symptoms. Pain that is suggestive of endometriosis can be treated with a therapeutic 'trial' of a hormonal drug to suppress ovarian activity and is appropriate without a definitive diagnosis.

Medical treatment

Some women prefer to avoid hormonal therapy and can manage pain symptoms effectively with *analgesia* (e.g. non-steroidal anti-inflammatory drugs [NSAIDs]) and/or a complementary medicine approach.

Hormonal treatment is used based upon the observations that symptoms regress during pregnancy, in the postmenopausal period and under the influence of androgens. Treatment therefore mimics pregnancy (e.g. the 'pill' or progestogens) or the menopause (e.g. gonadotrophin-releasing hormone [GnRH] analogues) or is androgenic (e.g. danazol). Suppression of ovarian function with these hormonal drugs reduces endometriosis-associated pain. The hormonal drugs are equally effective but differ in their adverse effect and cost profiles.

sive adhesions and endometriomata indicate severe disease (Fig. 9.2). *Transvaginal ultrasound* is useful to make and to exclude the diagnosis of an ovarian endometrioma and may also suggest the presence of adenomyosis (although magnetic resonance imaging [MRI] may be a better investigation if adenomyosis is suspected). Peritoneal endometriosis will not be visualized on ultrasound scan but may be on MRI. If there is clinical evidence of deeply infiltrating endometriosis, ureteric, bladder and bowel involvement should be assessed with a MRI ± intravenous pyelogram (IVP) and barium studies (RCOG Guideline No. 24, 2006). Serum carcinoma/cancer antigen 125 (CA 125) levels [→ p.43] are sometimes raised but have little diagnostic value.

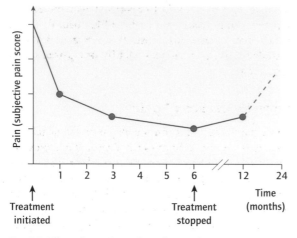

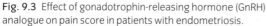

Fig. 9.3 Effect of gonadotrophin-releasing hormone (GnRH) analogue on pain score in patients with endometriosis.

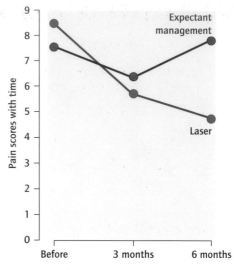

Fig. 9.4 Pain scores over time following laparoscopic removal or observation of minimal to moderate endometriosis. (From Sutton CJ *et al. Fertil Steril* 1994; **62**: 696–700.)

Symptom recurrence is common following medical treatment. The treatments are contraceptive so are not suitable for women who, in addition to experiencing pain, are trying to conceive.

The combined oral contraceptive is widely used and has high acceptability. It is not suitable for older women and/or smokers [→ p.95]. It is often used in a back-to-back or in a 'tricycling' regime when two or three pill packets are taken without a break to reduce the frequency of painful withdrawal bleeds.

Progestogen preparations are used on a cyclical or continuous basis. Although generally well tolerated, the side effects of fluid retention, weight gain, erratic bleeding and premenstrual syndrome-like symptoms are severe in a few patients.

GnRH analogues act by inducing a temporary menopausal state: overstimulation of the pituitary leads to down-regulation of its GnRH receptors (Fig. 9.3). Pituitary gonadotrophin and therefore ovarian hormone production are inhibited. Side effects mimic the menopause [→ p.105]: reversible bone demineralization limits therapy to 6 months, although it can be extended for up to 2 years or more using 'add-back' hormone replacement therapy (HRT) [→ p.109], which prevents bone loss and reduces menopausal side effects.

Danazol and *gestrinone*, synthetic compounds with androgenic effects, are seldom used now because of their severe side effects.

An alternative to systemic hormone treatment is the progestogen *intrauterine system* (IUS) that reduces pain with symptom control maintained over 5 years (*Hum Reprod* 2005; **20**: 789).

Surgical treatment

The *laser* or *bipolar diathermy* can be used laparoscopically at the time of diagnosis to destroy endometriotic lesions ('see and treat') (Fig. 9.4). Surgery may also improve conception rates so is preferable to medical treatment for women with endometriosis-related pain and infertility. More *radical surgery* involves dissection of adhesions and removal of ovarian endometriomata, or even a hysterectomy with bilateral salpingo-oöphorectomy (BSO). Surgery can be very difficult due to the severity of adhesions and anatomic distortion; there are risks of damaging bowel, bladder, blood vessels and the ureters. In expert hands, symptomatic improvement is seen in 70% of patients: this may be longer term than with medical therapy. Hysterectomy should be considered a 'last resort'; it is only appropriate in the woman whose family is complete. HRT will be required if the ovaries are removed, and only exceptionally causes a reactivation.

Treatment of endometriosis	
Medical:	Analgesia
	Combined oral contraceptives
	Progestogens
	Gonadotrophin-releasing hormone (GnRH) analogues ± hormone replacement therapy (HRT)
	Intrauterine system (IUS)
Surgical:	Laparoscopic laser ablation/diathermy ± adhesiolysis
	Hysterectomy and bilateral salpingo-oöphorectomy (BSO)

Endometriosis and fertility [→ p.88]

The more severe the endometriosis, the greater the chance of subfertility. Endometriosis is found in 25% of laparoscopies for investigation of subfertility. If the fallopian tubes are unaffected, medical treatment will not increase fertility, but laparoscopic ablation may, particularly when adhesions are present (*Cochrane* 2002: CD001398). Excision of ovarian endometrioma cysts improves fertility compared to cyst drainage alone. With severe disease affecting the fallopian tubes surgery may have a limited benefit and *in vitro* fertilization (IVF) will be the best option [→ p.90].

Chronic pelvic pain

Definition

Chronic pelvic pain (CPP) is defined as intermittent or constant pain in the lower abdomen or pelvis of at least 6 months' duration, not occurring exclusively with menstruation or intercourse. CPP presents in primary care as often as migraine or low back pain and affects about 15% of adult women. It carries a heavy social and economic price.

Assessment and investigation

This needs time. The woman's own ideas on the cause of the pain need to be elicited and discussed. There is frequently more than one component to the pain. A full history will prevent non-gynaecological diagnoses being missed. Psychological evaluation is helpful with some patients. It is obvious, but essential to remember, that just because no cause can be found for pain does not mean that it does not exist. Possible investigations include transvaginal ultrasound, MRI or laparoscopy as appropriate.

Possible causes of pain

Pelvic pain that varies considerably over the menstrual cycle may be due to hormonally driven gynaecological conditions including *endometriosis* or *adenomyosis*. Oestrogen activity appears to be important as postmenopausal pain is rare (and more likely to be due to malignancy) and suppression of ovarian activity appears to cure two-thirds of cases. There may be gynaecological or pelvic adhesions, although these may be incidental findings and evidence for pain benefit of dividing adhesions is lacking (*Lancet* 2003; **361**: 1247). However, ovarian tissue can become trapped within adhesions (e.g. following previous surgery such as hysterectomy or ovarian cystectomy) and cause cyclical pain treated by oöphorectomy or adhesiolysis.

Symptoms suggestive of *irritable bowel syndrome* or *interstitial cystitis* are often present in women with CPP. These conditions may be a primary cause or a component of the pain. *Psychological factors* are important. Depression and sleep disorders are common. A substantial number give a history of childhood and/or ongoing sexual or physical abuse. *Other possible theories* include the 'pelvic congestion syndrome', in which venous congestion in the pelvis is said to cause chronic pain and the 'myofascial syndrome', in which, it is said, the pain originates in muscle trigger points or trapped nerves.

Management

If symptoms are suggestive of irritable bowel syndrome then dietary change and a trial of antispasmodics should be tried first (*Ann Intern Med* 2000; **133**: 136). Appropriate analgesia should be arranged for the pain. Women with cyclical pain should be offered a therapeutic trial using the combined oral contraceptive pill or a GnRH agonist for a period of 3–6 months before having a diagnostic laparoscopy if the pain is unresolved. Progestogen IUS could also be considered.

Laparoscopy may have a role in developing a woman's beliefs about her pain, even if the findings are normal, but further invasive investigation is usually counterproductive. Counselling and psychotherapy are useful and pain management programmes involve relaxation techniques, sex therapy, diet and exercise. Even if no explanation for the pain can be found, attempts should be made to treat the pain empirically and to develop a management plan 'in partnership' with the woman. Drugs such as amitriptyline or gabapentin may be used to manage the pain.

Further reading

http://www.endometriosis.org/support
Johnson N, Farquhar C. Endometriosis. *BMJ Clinical Evidence* [online web publication March 2007].

Royal College of Obstetricians and Gynaecologists. The initial management of chronic pelvic pain. 2005. RCOG Guideline No. 41. http://www.rcog.org.uk
Royal College of Obstetricians and Gynaecologists. The investigation and management of endometriosis. RCOG Green-top Guideline. 2006. http://www.rcog.org.uk

Endometriosis at a Glance	
Definition	Endometrium outside the uterus
Epidemiology	Common (1–20%). More prevalent in nulliparous women, diagnosed at 35–40 years
Aetiology	Poorly understood. Probably retrograde menstruation that implants. Genetic susceptibility
Pathology	Peritoneal inflammation causes fibrosis, adhesions, 'chocolate cysts'
Clinical features	Pelvic pain, dysmenorrhoea, dyspareunia, dyschezia, subfertility
Investigations	Laparoscopy, biopsy. Transvaginal ultrasound
Medical treatment	Ovarian suppression (combined pill, progestogens, gonadotrophin-releasing hormone [GnRH] analogues ± hormone replacement therapy [HRT]). Progestogen-releasing intrauterine system (IUS) Medical treatment does not improve fertility
Surgical treatment	Laparoscopic ablation ± adhesiolysis. May improve symptoms and fertility. Ovarian cystectomy. Hysterectomy and bilateral salpingo-oöphorectomy (BSO) if severe in older woman
Prognosis	Disease usually recurs after cessation of medical treatment

10 Genital tract infections

The normal vagina is lined by squamous epithelium. It is richly colonized by a bacterial flora, predominantly *Lactobacillus*, and has an acidic pH (<4.5). This normal flora has a significant role in defence against infection by pathogens. In prepubertal girls and postmenopausal women, lack of oestrogen results in a thin, atrophic epithelium, a higher pH (6.5–7.5) and reduced resistance to infection.

Genital infections, several of which are sexually transmitted, are a common cause of gynaecological symptoms, but may also be asymptomatic. In recent years the incidence of major sexually transmitted infections (STIs) has risen in the UK as a result of changes in sexual behaviour, particularly frequent partner change, among young people.

Infections of the vulva and vagina

Non-sexually transmitted infections

Candidiasis (thrush)

Infection with *Candida albicans*, a yeast-like fungus (Fig. 10.1), is the most common cause of vaginal infection and is found in up to 20% of women, often without symptoms. Pregnancy, diabetes and the use of antibiotics are risk factors. There is little evidence that it is sexually transmitted. If symptomatic, there is a 'cottage cheese' discharge with vulval irritation and itching. Superficial dyspareunia and dysuria may occur. The vagina and/or vulva are inflamed and red. The diagnosis is established by culture and treatment is with topical imidazoles (e.g. Canesten) or oral fluconazole. Recurrent candidiasis is more common and more severe in the immunocompromised.

Obstetrics and Gynaecology, 3rd edition. By Lawrence Impey and Tim Child. Published 2008 by Blackwell Publishing, ISBN: 978-1-4051-6095-7.

Bacterial vaginosis (formerly *Gardnerella* or anaerobic vaginosis)

This is when the normal lactobacilli are overgrown by a mixed flora including anaerobes, *Gardnerella* and *Mycoplasma hominis*. It is found in 12% of women, but why it occurs is poorly understood. A grey–white discharge is present, but the vagina is not red or itchy. There is a characteristic fishy odour from amines released by bacterial proteolysis. The diagnosis is established by a raised vaginal pH, the typical discharge, a positive 'whiff' test (fishy odour when 10% potassium hydroxide [KOH] is added to the secretions) and the presence of 'clue cells' (epithelial cells studded with Gram-variable coccobacilli) on microscopy. Treatment of symptomatic women is with metronidazole or clindamycin cream. These bacteria can cause secondary infection in pelvic inflammatory disease (PID; [→ p.75]). There is also an association with preterm labour [→ p.191].

Infection associated with foreign bodies

Infection and discharge in children is often due to a foreign body. Sexual abuse must also be considered, but discharge is more often due to atrophic vaginitis due to low oestrogen levels. *Toxic shock syndrome* usually occurs as a rare complication of the retained, particularly hyperabsorbable tampon. A toxin-producing *Staphylococcus aureus* is responsible: a high fever, hypotension and multisystem failure can occur. Treatment is with antibiotics and intensive care.

Sexually acquired infections

Principles in the management of STIs

Screening for concurrent disease is important because more than one STI may be present.
The regular sexual partner should be treated and screened for other infections.

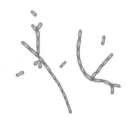

Fig. 10.1 *Candida albicans* showing budding hyphae and oval spores.

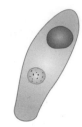

Fig. 10.2 *Chlamydia trachomatis.*

Partner notification (contact tracing) involves identification and contacting recent sexual contacts, for screening and treatment. This is usually performed by the patient. *Confidentiality* should be maintained. The doctor is breaching confidentiality if he/she informs sexual contacts of his/her patient of her diagnosis without her permission. Sexually transmitted infections can occur within monogamous relationships (e.g. genital herpes following orogenital sex). The diagnosis of an STI is emotive and patients need to be handled sensitively and with adequate explanation.

Education: Frequently changing partners increases the risk of acquiring STIs, including human immunodeficiency virus (HIV).

Barrier methods of contraception greatly reduce the risk of acquiring STIs, including HIV.

Chlamydia

Chlamydia trachomatis is a small bacterium (Fig. 10.2) and is now the most common sexually transmitted bacterial organism in the developed world. Some 5–10% of women aged 20–30 years have been infected. This is usually asymptomatic, but urethritis and a vaginal discharge can occur. The principal complication is pelvic infection, which may also be silent. This can cause tubal damage leading to subfertility and/or chronic pelvic pain. *Chlamydia* infection also causes Reiter's syndrome, characterized by a triad of urethritis, conjunctivitis and arthritis. Nucleic acid amplification tests (NAATs), e.g. polymerase chain reaction (PCR), are best and can be used on urine for screening purposes. Treatment is with doxycycline or azithromycin.

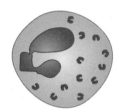

Fig. 10.3 Gram-negative *Neisseria gonorrhoeae* in pairs in a human neutrophil.

Gonorrhoea

This is caused by *Neisseria gonorrhoeae*, a Gram-negative diplococcus (Fig. 10.3). It is common, particularly so in the developing world. It is commonly asymptomatic in women, although vaginal discharge, urethritis, bartholinitis and cervicitis can occur and the pelvis is commonly infected. Men usually develop urethritis. Systemic complications include bacteraemia and acute, usually monoarticular, septic arthritis. Diagnosis is from culture of endocervical swabs. In the UK, penicillin and even ciprofloxacin resistance is increasing: ceftriaxone is often required, particularly for 'imported' infections. Partner notification and treatment is essential.

Genital warts (condylomata acuminata)

These are caused by the human papilloma virus (HPV). They are extremely common. Appearances vary from tiny flat patches on the vulval skin to small papilliform

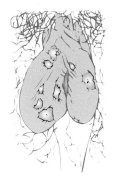

Fig. 10.5 *Treponema pallidum.*

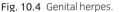

Fig. 10.4 Genital herpes.

(cauliflower-like) swellings. Warts are usually multiple and may affect the cervix, where certain oncogenic types (16 and 18) are associated with the development of cervical intraepithelial neoplasia (CIN; [→ p.33]) (*Lancet* 2007; **370**: 890). Treatment is with topical podophyllin or imiquimod cream (external warts only). Cryotherapy or electrocautery is used for resistant warts. There is a high recurrence rate (up to 25%). A vaccine against HPV is now available [→ p.33] for the purpose of preventing cervical neoplasia.

Genital herpes

Genital infection is mostly with the herpes simplex virus (HSV) type 2, although type 1, the cause of cold sores, is increasingly implicated (Fig. 10.4). The primary infection is the worst, with multiple small painful vesicles and ulcers around the introitus. Local lymphadenopathy, dysuria and systemic symptoms are common; secondary bacterial infection, aseptic meningitis or acute urinary retention are rarer. The virus then lies dormant in the dorsal root ganglia: in about 75% of patients reactivations occur. These attacks are less painful, less severe, and often preceded by localized tingling. The diagnosis is established from examination and with viral swabs. Aciclovir (also valaciclovir or famciclovir) is used in severe infections and will also reduce the duration of symptoms if started early in a reactivation. Neonatal herpes has a high mortality and can be prevented [→ p.158].

Syphilis

Infection by the spirochaete *Treponema pallidum* (Fig. 10.5) is common in the developing world, and although relatively rare in developed countries the incidence is rising in the UK. *Primary syphilis* is characterized by a solitary painless vulval ulcer (chancre). Untreated, *secondary syphilis* may develop weeks later, often with a rash, influenza-like symptoms and warty genital or perioral growths (condylomata lata). At this stage the spirochaete infiltrates other organs and can cause a variety of symptoms. *Latent syphilis* follows as this phase resolves spontaneously. Primary or secondary syphilis during pregnancy carries a high risk of *congenital infection*. *Tertiary syphilis* is now very rare. It develops many years later and virtually any organ can be affected. Aortic regurgitation, dementia, tabes dorsalis and gummata in skin and bone are the best-known complications. A variety of diagnostic tests are used (including enzyme immunoassay (syphilis EIA) and Venereal Disease Research Laboratories (VDRL) test). Treatment of all stages is with parenteral (usually intramuscular) penicillin.

Trichomoniasis

Trichomonas vaginalis is a flagellate protozoan (Fig. 10.6) that is common worldwide but relatively rare in the UK. Typical symptoms are an offensive grey–green discharge, vulval irritation and superficial dyspareunia, but it can be asymptomatic. Cervicitis has a punctate erythematous ('strawberry') appearance. Diagnosis is from wet film microscopy, special staining or culture of vaginal swabs. Treatment is with metronidazole.

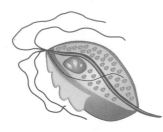

Fig. 10.6 *Trichomonas vaginalis.*

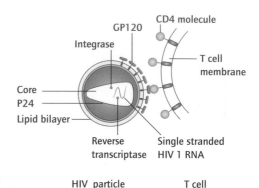

Fig. 10.7 Human immunodeficiency virus (HIV) particle attaching to a T lymphocyte.

Other STIs causing genital ulcers

Other than herpes and syphilis, chancroid (*Haemophilus ducreyi*), lymphogranuloma venereum (subtypes of *Chlamydia trachomatis*) and donovanosis (*Calymmatobacterium granulomatis*)—formerly called granuloma inguinale—all cause genital ulceration. They are rare in the UK but not in the tropics and are occasionally seen as 'imported' diseases.

Human immunodeficiency virus

Infection with this retrovirus (Fig. 10.7) is the cause of the clinical syndrome acquired immune deficiency syndrome (AIDS). The numbers of heterosexually acquired HIV infections is increasing markedly and now outnumbers infection from sex between men (Fig. 10.8). Consequently, the numbers of women infected are also increasing. The male:female ratio for all new infections diagnosed in 1985/6 was 14:1 whereas in 2004/5 it was 1.4:1. Over 80% of those diagnosed in the UK who acquired HIV heterosexually were infected abroad, the majority in Africa (www.hpa.org.uk/infections).

Risk factors are multiple sexual partners, migration from high prevalence countries (particularly sub-Saharan Africa), failure to use barrier contraception and the presence of other STIs, as well as intravenous drug abuse and sexual contact with high-risk males. Seroconversion is often accompanied by an influenza-like illness with a rash, but most HIV-positive women are asymptomatic. The development of opportunistic infections or malignancy (including cervical carcinoma) or a CD4 count <200 cells/mm^3 are diagnostic of AIDS. CIN [→ p.33] is more common in HIV-infected women, affecting one-third. Yearly smears are recommended as progression to malignancy is more rapid. Genital infections, particularly candidiasis and menstrual disturbances, are more common. Vertical transmission to the fetus [→ p.161] is virtually prevented by antiretroviral therapy, elective Caesarean and avoidance of breastfeeding. With current combination antiretroviral regimes (termed highly active antiretroviral therapy [HAART]) HIV is increasingly considered as a chronic controllable condition in a similar manner to diabetes.

Infections of the uterus and pelvis

Endometritis

This is infection confined to the cavity of the uterus alone. Untreated, spread of infection to the pelvis is common. Endometritis is often the result either of *instrumentation of the uterus* or as a *complication of pregnancy*, or *both*. Infecting organisms include *Chlamydia* and gonococcus if these are present in the genital tract. However, the organisms of bacterial vaginosis and organisms such as *Escherichia coli*, staphylococci and even clostridia may be implicated. It is common after Caesarean section; it also occurs after miscarriage or termination of pregnancy, particularly if some 'products of conception' are retained. Illegal terminations are rare in the West but are particularly prone to sepsis.

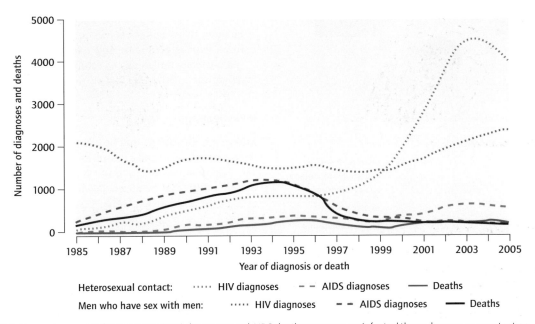

Fig. 10.8 Human immunodeficiency virus (HIV) diagnoses and AIDS deaths among men infected through same-sex contact or individuals infected through heterosexual contact, UK.

Endometritis presents with persistent and often heavy vaginal bleeding, usually accompanied by pain. The uterus is tender and the cervical os is commonly open. A fever may initially be absent but septicaemia can ensue. Investigations include vaginal and cervical swabs and a full blood count (FBC); pelvic ultrasound is not very reliable. Broad-spectrum antibiotics are given. An evacuation of retained products of conception (ERPC; [→ pp.117,127]) is then performed if symptoms do not subside or if there are 'products' in the uterus at ultrasound examination.

Acute pelvic infection and pelvic inflammatory disease

Definition and epidemiology

Pelvic inflammatory disease (PID) or salpingitis traditionally describes sexually transmitted pelvic infection, but pelvic infection is best considered as a single entity. Endometritis usually coexists. The incidence is increas-

ing: 2% of women will be affected. Younger, poorer, sexually active nulliparous women are at most risk. Pelvic infection almost never occurs in the presence of a viable pregnancy.

Aetiology

Ascending infection of bacteria in the vagina and cervix: *Sexual factors* account for 80%. These are more common in women with multiple partners, not using barrier contraception. The combined oral contraceptive is partly protective. Spread of previously asymptomatic STIs to the pelvis is usually spontaneous but can be the result of *uterine instrumentation* (e.g. termination of pregnancy, ERPC, laparoscopy and dye test, and intrauterine devices) and/or *complications of childbirth and miscarriage*. In these latter instances, infection is often due to introduction of non-sexually transmitted bacteria. *Descending infection* from local organs such as the appendix can also occur.

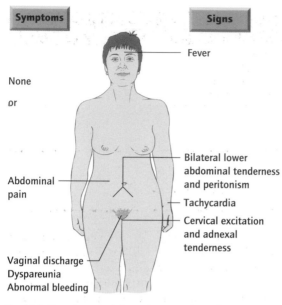

Symptoms	Signs
None	Fever
or	
Abdominal pain	Bilateral lower abdominal tenderness and peritonism
	Tachycardia
	Cervical excitation and adnexal tenderness
Vaginal discharge	
Dyspareunia	
Abnormal bleeding	

Fig. 10.9 Symptoms and signs of acute pelvic inflammatory disease (PID).

Pathology and bacteriology

Infection is frequently polymicrobial. *Chlamydia* (up to 60%) and gonococcus are the principal sexually transmitted culprits. The latter causes an acute presentation; the former is often asymptomatic and symptoms, if present, may be due to secondary infection. Endometritis and a bilateral salpingitis and parametritis occur; the ovaries are rarely affected. Perihepatitis (Fitz-Hugh–Curtis syndrome) affects 10% and causes right upper quadrant pain due to adhesions, easily visible at laparoscopy, between the liver and the anterior abdominal wall.

Clinical features

History: Many have no symptoms and present later with subfertility or menstrual problems. Bilateral lower abdominal pain with deep dyspareunia is the hallmark, usually with abnormal vaginal bleeding or discharge (Fig. 10.9).

Examination: In severe cases examination reveals a tachycardia and high fever, signs of lower abdominal peritonism with bilateral adnexal tenderness and cervical excitation (pain on moving the cervix). A mass (pelvic abscess) may be palpable vaginally. More frequently, the diagnosis is less clear and may be confused with appendicitis and ovarian cyst accidents (pain usually unilateral) or ectopic pregnancy (pregnancy test positive plus usually unilateral pain).

Investigations

Endocervical swabs should be taken for *Chlamydia* and gonococcus, and blood cultures sent if there is a fever. The white blood cell count (WBC) and C-reactive protein (CRP) may be raised. Pelvic ultrasound helps to exclude an abscess or ovarian cyst. Laparoscopy with fimbrial biopsy and culture is the 'gold standard' although not commonly performed.

Treatment

Analgesics and either a parenteral cephalosporin, e.g. intramuscular ceftriaxone, followed by doxycycline and metronidazole, or ofloxacin with metronidazole are most effective (*BMJ* 2001; **322**: 251). Febrile patients should be admitted for intravenous therapy. The diagnosis should be reviewed after 24 h if there is no significant improvement and a laparoscopy performed. Pelvic abscess may not respond to antibiotic therapy and may require drainage either under ultrasound guidance or laparoscopically. Rupture of a large pelvic abscess can be life-threatening.

Complications

The main early complication is the formation of an abscess or pyosalpinx. Later, many women develop tubal obstruction and subfertility, chronic pelvic infection or chronic pelvic pain [→ p.88]. Ectopic pregnancy is six times more common after pelvic infection. The chance of tubal damage following one episode of acute PID is around 12%.

Chronic pelvic inflammatory disease

This is a persisting infection and is the result of non-treatment or inadequate treatment of acute PID. Typically, there are dense pelvic adhesions and the fallopian tubes may be obstructed and dilated with fluid (hydrosalpinx) or pus (pyosalpinx) (Fig. 10.10). Common symptoms are chronic pelvic pain or dysmenorrhoea, deep dyspareunia [→ p.69], heavy and irregular men-

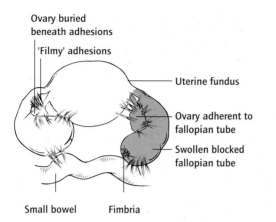

Fig. 10.10 View of pelvis affected by chronic pelvic inflammatory disease (PID).

struation, chronic vaginal discharge and subfertility. Examination may reveal features similar to endometriosis: abdominal and adnexal tenderness and a fixed retroverted uterus. Transvaginal ultrasound may reveal fluid collections within the fallopian tubes or surrounding adhesions. Laparoscopy is the best diagnostic tool; culture is often negative. Treatment is with analgesics and antibiotics if there is evidence of active infection. Severe cases occasionally respond to cutting of the adhesions (adhesiolysis), but sometimes removal of affected tubes (salpingectomy) is required.

Features of pelvic inflammatory disease (PID)
Silent (particularly chlamydial)
Bilateral pain
Vaginal discharge
Cervical excitation
Adnexal tenderness
Fever
White blood cell count (WBC) and C-reactive protein (CRP) raised

Late complications of pelvic inflammatory disease (PID)
Subfertility
Chronic PID
Chronic pelvic pain
Ectopic pregnancy

Vaginal discharge: causes and treatment

Discharge from the vagina is a common complaint which, despite often being labelled as 'intractable', can usually be treated if properly evaluated:

Physiological discharge is the most common cause and is usually non-offensive. It increases around ovulation, during pregnancy and in women taking the combined oral contraceptive. Exposure of columnar epithelium in cervical eversion and ectropion [→ p.31] may cause discharge and can be treated by cryotherapy or diathermy once infection (cervicitis) has been excluded with swabs.

Infection: Bacterial vaginosis and candidiasis are the most common; chlamydial infection, gonorrhoea and *Trichomonas vaginalis* all can cause a discharge, particularly with cervicitis [→ p.31] and PID. Many other organisms can be present in the presence of a foreign body.

Atrophic vaginitis: This is due to oestrogen deficiency and is common before the menarche, during lactation and after the menopause. Treatment of symptomatic discharge is with oestrogen cream; systemic hormone replacement therapy (HRT) may be preferred in the postmenopausal woman.

Differential diagnosis of vaginal discharge						
Cause	*Itching*	*Discharge*	*pH*	*Redness*	*Odour*	*Treatment*
Ectropion/eversion	No	Clear	Normal	No	Normal	Cryotherapy
Bacterial vaginosis	No	Grey–white	Raised	No	Fishy	Antibiotics
Candidiasis	Yes	White	Normal	Yes	Normal	Imidazoles
Trichomoniasis	Yes	Grey–green	Raised	Yes	Yes	Antibiotics
Malignancy	No	Red–brown	Variable	No	Yes	Biopsy
Atrophic	No	Clear	Raised	Yes	No	Oestrogen

Foreign body: Retained tampons or swabs after childbirth are all too common. Foreign bodies are not uncommon in the young child. Discharge is usually very offensive.

Malignancy: A bloody and offensive discharge is suggestive of cervical carcinoma, but any genital tract malignancy can be responsible. The very rare fallopian tube carcinoma typically presents with a watery discharge in the postmenopausal women.

Common causes of vaginal discharge
Physiological
Candidiasis
Bacterial vaginosis
Atrophic vaginitis
Cervical eversion and ectropion
Occasionally foreign body

Further reading

Barrett S, Taylor C. A review on pelvic inflammatory disease. *International Journal of STD & AIDS* 2005; **16**: 715–20.

British Association for Sexual Health and HIV (clinical effectiveness guidelines). http://www.bashh.org/guidelines.asp

Faculty of Family Planning and Reproductive Healthcare. The management of women of reproductive age attending non-genitourinary medicine settings complaining of vaginal discharge. 2006. http://www ffprhc.org.uk/admin/uploads/326_VaginalDischargeGuidance.pdf

Mitchell H. Vaginal discharge—causes, diagnosis, and treatment. *British Medical Journal* 2004; **328**: 1306–8.

Pisani E, Garnett GP, Grassly NC, *et al.* Back to basics in HIV prevention: focus on exposure. *British Medical Journal* 2003; **326**: 1384–7.

Whitely RJ, Roizman B. Herpes simplex virus infections. *Lancet* 2001; **357**: 1513–8.

Acute Pelvic Inflammatory Disease (PID) at a Glance	
Definition	Infection of the pelvis, usually sexually transmitted
Epidemiology	2% lifetime risk, younger, multiple partners
Aetiology	Ascending: Sexually transmitted infections (STIs): *Chlamydia* and gonorrhoea spontaneous or after childbirth/uterine instrumentation. Non-STIs: seldom spontaneous Descending: Rarer; from other organs or blood
Clinical features	Chlamydial PID often silent. Bilateral abdominal pain, vaginal discharge, fever, erratic menstrual bleeding
Investigations	Swabs, full blood count (FBC), C-reactive protein (CRP). Laparoscopy if doubt or poor response to treatment. Pregnancy test
Treatment	Analgesia and antibiotics, e.g. metronidazole and ofloxacin
Complications	Pelvic abscess, chronic PID, chronic pelvic pain, subfertility, ectopic pregnancy

11 Fertility and subfertility

Definitions

A couple are 'subfertile' if conception has not occurred after a year of regular unprotected intercourse. Fifteen per cent of couples are affected. Most couples do not have 'infertility' since they continue to have a monthly chance of conception, even though this may be lower than normal. Failure to conceive may be *primary*, meaning that the female partner has never conceived, or *secondary*, indicating that she has previously conceived, even if the pregnancy ended in miscarriage or termination.

Conditions for pregnancy

Four basic conditions are required for pregnancy:
1 An egg must be produced. Failure is 'anovulation' (30% of cases). Management of subfertility involves finding out if ovulation is occurring and, if not, why.
2 Adequate sperm must be released. 'Male factor' problems contribute to 25% of cases. The history, examination and investigations should involve the male, or at least examination of his semen.
3 The sperm must reach the egg. Most commonly the fallopian tubes are damaged (25% of cases). Sexual (5%) and cervical (<5%) problems may also prevent fertilization.
4 The fertilized egg (embryo) must implant. The incidence of defective implantation is unknown. This may account for much of the 30% of couples with 'unexplained subfertility'.

Counselling and support for the subfertile couple

A trained counsellor should be available in every fertility clinic. Reproduction is a fundamental body function

Obstetrics and Gynaecology, 3rd edition. By Lawrence Impey and Tim Child. Published 2008 by Blackwell Publishing, ISBN: 978-1-4051-6095-7.

that these couples have not achieved and over which they have little control. One partner may feel responsible, or guilty about past pregnancy terminations or sexually transmitted disease. Many men feel disempowered and less 'male'. The relationship may suffer and intercourse becomes clinical. Counsellors allow couples to talk about these problems. They can also educate the couple and may even uncover a hidden (e.g. sexual) problem.

Contributors to subfertility	
Ovulatory problems	30%
Male problems	25%
Tubal problems	25%
Coital problems	5%
Cervical problems	<5%
Unexplained	30%

N.B. Because more than one cause may be present, the percentage total is more than 100%.

Disorders of ovulation

Ovulatory dysfunction is a contributory cause in 30% of subfertile couples. Fertility declines with increasing female age due mainly to the reduced genetic 'quality' of remaining oocytes rather than ovulatory problems.

Physiology of ovulation

At the beginning of each cycle, *low* oestrogen levels exert a positive feedback to cause hypothalamic gonadotrophin-releasing hormone (GnRH) pulses to stimulate the anterior pituitary gland to produce gonadotrophins: follicle-stimulating hormone (FSH) and luteinizing hormone (LH) (Fig. 11.1). These cause growth and initiate maturation of several of the follicles of the ovary, each of which contains an immature oocyte. These follicles also start producing oestradiol. The resulting

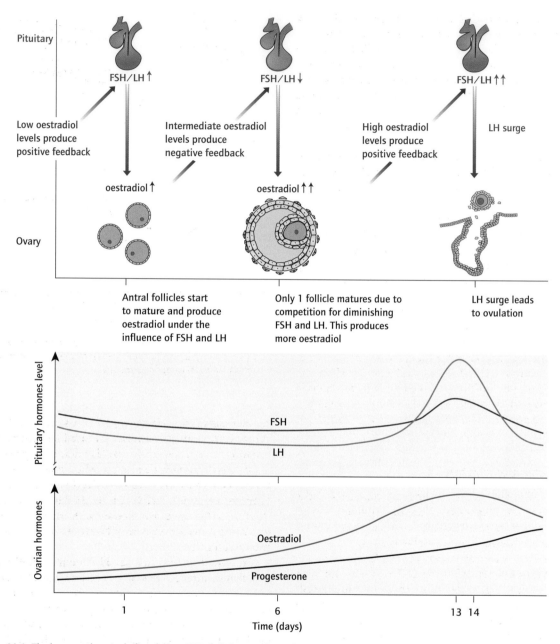

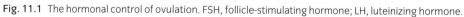

Fig. 11.1 The hormonal control of ovulation. FSH, follicle-stimulating hormone; LH, luteinizing hormone.

intermediate oestradiol level has a negative feedback effect on the hypothalamus, such that less FSH and LH are produced. Therefore, the maturing follicles compete for less stimulating hormones. Usually only one (the *dominant follicle*) is large enough with sufficient gonadotrophin receptors to be able to survive and continue growth. The development of this dominant follicle is also co-regulated by inhibin B, which also suppresses FSH.

As this follicle matures, its oestradiol output increases considerably. When a *high* 'threshold' level of oestradiol is attained, the negative feedback is reversed and positive feedback now causes LH and FSH levels to again increase and dramatically so: it is the peak of the former that ultimately leads to rupture of the now ripe follicle when it is around 2 cm diameter. This is ovulation and the egg spills onto the ovarian surface where it can be picked up by the fallopian tube. Following ovulation the follicle becomes a corpus luteum and releases oestrogen and progesterone to maintain a secretory endometrium suitable for embryo implantation. If this does not occur the corpus luteum involutes and hormone levels fall, leading to menstruation around 14 days after ovulation. If embryo implantation does occur, the human chorionic gonadotrophin (hCG) produced by the trophoblast tissue acts on the corpus luteum to maintain oestrogen and progesterone production until the fetoplacental unit takes over at 8–10 weeks' gestation.

Detection of ovulation

History: The vast majority of women with regular cycles are ovulatory. Some experience vaginal spotting or an increase in vaginal discharge or pelvic pain ('mittelschmertz') around the time of ovulation.

Examination: Cervical mucus pre-ovulation is normally acellular, will 'fern' (form fern-like patterns) when on a dry slide (Fig. 11.2a) and will form 'spinnbarkeit' (elastic-like strings) of up to 15 cm (Fig. 11.2b). The body temperature normally drops some 0.2°C pre-ovulation and then rises 0.5°C in the luteal phase. If the woman is asked to record her temperature every day, the pattern can be seen on a temperature chart (Fig. 11.2c). These examinations are generally not requested or performed.

Investigations are more reliable and are used more frequently. The only proof of ovulation is conception but positive investigations are strongly suggestive.

1 Elevated serum progesterone levels in the mid-luteal

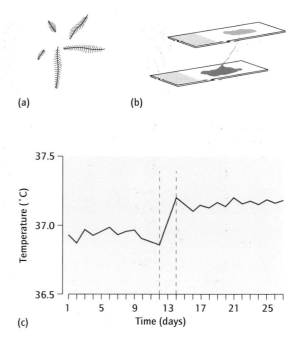

(a) (b)

(c)

Fig. 11.2 Evidence of ovulation: (a) cervical mucus showing fern-like pattern; (b) spinnbarkeit formation of mucus between two glass slides; (c) temperature chart.

phase usually indicate that ovulation has occurred. The luteal phase (time from ovulation to subsequent menstruation) is constant at 14 days. Therefore a low progesterone result can only be interpreted as showing lack of ovulation if it was taken around 7 days before the subsequent menstruation, i.e. day 21 of a 28-day cycle or day 28 of a 35-day cycle. For women with irregular cycles repeat progesterone tests may be required until menstruation starts.

2 Ultrasound scans can serially monitor follicular growth and, after ovulation, demonstrate the fall in size and haemorrhagic nature of the corpus luteum. This is time-consuming and generally not performed.

3 Over-the-counter urine predictor kits will indicate if the LH surge has taken place. Ovulation should then follow.

Detection of ovulation
Mid-luteal phase serum progesterone (the standard test)
Ultrasound follicular tracking (time-consuming)
Temperature charts (not recommended)
Luteinizing hormone (LH) -based urine predictor kits

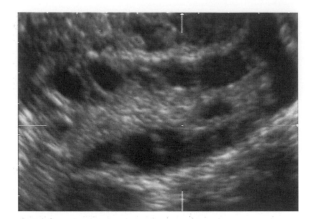

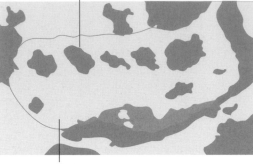

Multiple small follicles

Ovary

Fig. 11.3 Ultrasound of a polycystic ovary (PCO).

Causes of anovulation: polycystic ovary syndrome

Polycystic ovary syndrome (PCOS) is a diagnosis of exclusion. Other causes of irregular or absent periods need to be considered and investigated as appropriate [→ p.15].

Definitions and epidemiology

Polycystic ovary (PCO) describes a characteristic trans-vaginal ultrasound appearance of multiple (12 or more) small (2–8 mm) follicles in an enlarged (>10 mL volume) ovary. PCO is found in about 20% of women (Fig. 11.3), the majority of whom have regular ovulatory cycles. Women with PCO may develop other features of the full syndrome if they put on weight (see below).

Polycystic ovary syndrome: PCOS affects around 5% of women and causes over 80% of cases of anovulatory infertility. It is diagnosed when at least two out of the following three criteria are met (*JCEM* 2006: **91**; 786):
1 PCO on ultrasound;
2 Irregular periods (>35 days apart);
3 Hirsutism: clinical (acne or excess body hair) and/or biochemical (raised serum testosterone).

Pathology/aetiology

Susceptibility to PCO is mainly genetic. Affected women demonstrate disordered LH production and peripheral insulin resistance with compensatory raised insulin levels. The combination of raised levels of LH and insulin acting on the PCO lead to increased ovarian androgen production. Raised insulin levels also increase adrenal androgen production and reduce hepatic production of steroid hormone binding globulin (SHBG) which leads to increased free androgen levels. Increased intraovarian androgens disrupt folliculogenesis leading to excess small ovarian follicles (and the PCO picture) and irregular or absent ovulation. Raised peripheral androgens cause hirsutism (acne and/or excess body hair). Increasing body weight leads to increased insulin and consequently androgen levels. Hence environmental factors (weight) can modify the phenotype of PCOS. Many women have a family history of type II diabetes.

Clinical features

PCO: Polycystic ovaries without the syndrome are generally asymptomatic.

PCOS: The stereotypical patient with the syndrome is obese, has acne, hirsutism and oligomenorrhoea or amenorrhoea: these may therefore be the presenting symptoms (Fig. 11.4). However, since only two out of the three criteria are necessary presentation can vary. Although many women with severe PCOS have normal body weight, changes in weight over time will alter insulin levels and severity of the syndrome. Miscarriage is more common in PCOS and may be related to the increased levels of LH and/or insulin and also increased body weight.

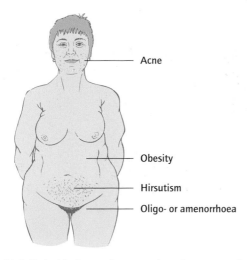

Acne

Obesity

Hirsutism

Oligo- or amenorrhoea

Fig. 11.4 Typical features of severe polycystic ovary syndrome (PCOS).

Clinical features of polycystic ovary syndrome (PCOS)
None
Subfertility
Oligomenorrhoea or amenorrhoea
Hirsutism and/or acne
Obesity
Miscarriage

Investigations for polycystic ovary syndrome (PCOS)
Transvaginal ultrasound scan
Follicle-stimulating hormone (FSH), luteinizing hormone (LH), testosterone, prolactin, thyroid-stimulating hormone (TSH)
Fasting lipids and glucose to screen for complications

Diagnosis of polycystic ovary syndrome
Two or more out of:
● Ovaries polycystic morphology on ultrasound
● Irregular periods 5 weeks or more apart
● Hirsutism (clinical and/or biochemical)

Investigations

Alternative causes for the symptoms need to be excluded.

Blood tests: Anovulation is investigated with FSH (raised in ovarian failure, low in hypothalamic disease, normal in PCOS), prolactin (to exclude a prolactinoma) and thyroid-stimulating hormone (TSH). Hirsutism is investigated with serum testosterone levels (possibility of androgen-secreting tumour or congenital adrenal hyperplasia if very raised). LH is measured (often raised in PCOS but not diagnostic).

Ultrasound: (transvaginal scan) is used to look for polycystic ovaries (Fig. 11.3).

Other: Screening for diabetes and abnormal lipids is also advised.

Complications of PCOS

Up to 50% of women with PCOS develop *type II diabetes* in later life; 30% develop gestational diabetes [→ p.174] during pregnancy. This risk is reduced by weight reduction. *Endometrial cancer* is more common in women with many years of amenorrhoea due to unopposed oestrogen action. In spite of a number of risk factors (weight, insulin resistance, diabetes, abnormal lipids) increased mortality rates have not been demonstrated in women with PCOS. As women with PCOS have normal oestrogen levels, even when amenorrhoeic, they are not at increased risk of osteoporosis.

Treatment of symptoms other than infertility

Advice regarding diet and exercise are given. Normalization of weight should result in reduction in insulin levels and improvement in all PCOS symptoms. If fertility is not required, treatment with the combined oral contraceptive will regulate menstruation and treat hirsutism. At least three to four bleeds per year, whether spontaneous or induced, are necessary to protect the endometrium. The antiandrogens cyproterone acetate (also available combined as a contraceptive pill) or spironolactone are effective treatments for hirsutism but conception must be avoided. The insulin sensitizer metformin reduces insulin levels and therefore androgens and hirsutism (and also promotes ovulation). Eflornithine is a topical antiandrogen used for facial hirsutism.

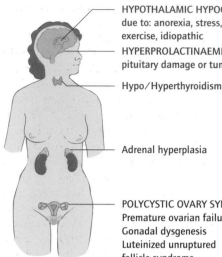

HYPOTHALAMIC HYPOGONADISM
due to: anorexia, stress,
exercise, idiopathic
HYPERPROLACTINAEMIA
pituitary damage or tumour

Hypo/Hyperthyroidism

Adrenal hyperplasia

POLYCYSTIC OVARY SYNDROME
Premature ovarian failure
Gonadal dysgenesis
Luteinized unruptured
follicle syndrome

Fig. 11.5 Causes of anovulation (common causes shown in capital letters).

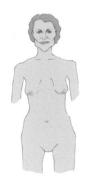

Fig. 11.6 Anorexia nervosa causes amenorrhoea and subfertility.

Other causes of anovulation

These may originate in the ovary, the pituitary or hypothalamus, or in other parts of the endocrine system (Fig. 11.5). Remember to consider pregnancy as a cause of amenorrhoea.

Hypothalamic causes

Hypothalamic hypogonadism: A reduction in hypothalamic GnRH release causes amenorrhoea, because reduced stimulation of the pituitary reduces FSH and LH levels, which in turn reduces oestradiol levels. This is usual with anorexia nervosa (Fig. 11.6) and common in women on diets, athletes and those under stress. Restoration of body weight, if appropriate, restores hypothalamic function. *Kallmann's syndrome* occurs when GnRH secreting neurones fail to develop; in other patients, the cause is obscure. Exogenous gonadotrophins or a GnRH pump will induce ovulation. Bone protection with the contraceptive pill or hormone replacement therapy (HRT) is required.

Pituitary causes

Hyperprolactinaemia is excess prolactin secretion, which reduces GnRH release. It is usually caused by benign

tumours (adenomas) or hyperplasia of pituitary cells, but is also associated with PCOS and the use of psychotropic drugs. It accounts for 10% of anovulatory women, who commonly have oligomenorrhoea or amenorrhoea, galactorrhoea and, if a pituitary tumour is enlarging, headaches and a bitemporal hemianopia. Prolactin levels are elevated. Computed tomography (CT) imaging is indicated if neurological symptoms occur. Treatment with a dopamine agonist (bromocriptine or cabergoline) usually restores ovulation, because dopamine inhibits prolactin release. Surgery is needed if this fails or neurological symptoms warrant it. Primary hypothyroidism can cause raised prolactin levels so thyroid function test are indicated.

Pituitary damage can reduce FSH and LH release. Production of GnRH is normal. This results from pressure from tumours, or infarction following severe postpartum haemorrhage (Sheehan's syndrome).

Ovarian causes of anovulation (in addition to PCOS)

The luteinized unruptured follicle syndrome is present when a follicle develops but the egg is never released. It is unlikely to occur every month so does not cause persistent problems.

Premature ovarian failure [→ p.105]: As the ovary fails, oestradiol and inhibin levels are low, so reduced negative feedback on the pituitary causes FSH and LH levels to rise. Exogenous gonadotrophins are of no use, since there are no ovarian follicles to respond, and donor eggs are required for pregnancy. Bone protection with HRT or the oral contraceptive pill is required.

Gonadal dysgenesis: These rare conditions usually present with primary amenorrhoea [→ p.17].

Other causes

Hypo- or *hyperthyroidism* reduces fertility. Menstrual disturbances are usual.
Androgen-secreting tumours [→ p.17] cause amenorrhoea and virilization.

Common causes of anovulation
Polycystic ovary syndrome (PCOS)
Hypothalamic hypogonadism
Hyperprolactinaemia
Thyroid disease

Induction of ovulation

Lifestyle changes and treatment of associated disease

Treatment of fertility involves health advice regarding pregnancy, the risks of multiple pregnancy with ovulation induction and the use of folic acid [→ p.142]. Restoration of normal weight is advised: this alone may restore ovulation. Treatment of specific causes, such as a thyroid abnormality or hyperprolactinaemia, usually leads to restoration of ovulation. Smoking should cease.

Treatment of PCOS

Clomifene is the traditional first line ovulation induction drug in PCOS. It is limited to 6 months' use and results in ovulation and live birth rates of around 70% and 40%, respectively. Clomifene is an anti-oestrogen, blocking oestrogen receptors in the hypothalamus and pituitary. As gonadotrophin release is normally inhibited by oestrogen, its effect is to increase the release of FSH and LH. Effectively, therefore, it 'fools' the pituitary into 'believing' there is no oestrogen. As it is only given at the start of the cycle, from days 2 to 6, it can initiate the process of follicular maturation which is thereafter self-perpetuating for that cycle. Clomifene cycles should be monitored by ultrasound, at least in the first month, to reduce the risk of multiple follicle maturation and multiple pregnancy (10%, mostly twins).

If ovulation does not occur ('clomifene resistance') then second line treatments include:
Metformin is an oral insulin sensitizing drug which aims to restore ovulation. It is not licensed for use in non-diabetics but is increasingly used 'off-licence' in PCOS. It does not promote multiple ovulation so there is no increase in multiple pregnancies (and no need for scan monitoring). When used alone it has a significantly lower live birth rate compared to clomifene, so clomifene continues to be the first line treatment of choice (*NEJM* 2007; **356**: 551). Metformin increases the effectiveness of clomifene in clomifene-resistant women. It treats hirsutism so may be a suitable first line fertility treatment for anovulatory women who want hirsutism treated and to avoid multiple pregnancy. Additional unproven benefits, when metformin is continued during pregnancy, may include a reduction in early miscarriage and the development of gestational diabetes, both of which are more common with PCOS.
Gonadotrophins (see below).
Laparoscopic ovarian diathermy is as effective as gonadotrophins (*Cochrane* 2007: CD001122) and with a lower multiple pregnancy rate. Each ovary is monopolar diathermied at a few points for a few seconds. During the same operation tubal patency can be tested using methylene blue insufflation and any comorbidities such as endometriosis treated. If successful then regular ovulations can continue for years.

Gonadotrophin induction of ovulation

These are used when clomiphene has failed, but also in hypothalamic hypogonadism if the weight is normal. Recombinant or purified urinary FSH $\pm$ LH acts as a substitute for the normal pituitary production and is given by daily subcutaneous injection to stimulate follicular growth. The result is often maturation of more than one follicle. Follicular development is monitored with ultrasound. Once a follicle is of a size adequate for ovulation (about 17 mm), the process can be artificially stimulated by injection of hCG (which is structurally similar to LH) or recombinant LH.

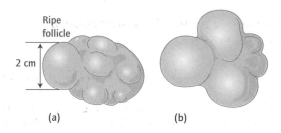

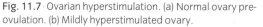

Fig. 11.7 Ovarian hyperstimulation. (a) Normal ovary pre-ovulation. (b) Mildly hyperstimulated ovary.

Inducing ovulation	
If polycystic ovary syndrome (PCOS):	Weight loss and lifestyle changes. If inappropriate/fails . . . Clomiphene. If fails . . . Add metformin Gonadotrophins Ovarian diathermy. If no success . . . *In vitro* fertilization (IVF)
If hypothalamic hypogonadism:	Restore weight Gonadotrophins if weight normal
If hyperprolactinaemia:	Bromocriptine or cabergoline
If ovulation or pregnancy does not occur following second line treatments then *in vitro* fertilization (IVF) [→ p.90] is the next step.	

Side effects of ovulation induction

Multiple pregnancy is more likely with clomifene or gonadotrophins (but not metformin) as more than one follicle may mature. Multiple pregnancy increases perinatal complication rates [→ p.217]. High order multiple pregnancies now more commonly follow ovulation induction alone than IVF, since with the latter a maximum of two embryos are replaced in the majority of women, and in the former follicular growth and ovulation are less controlled.

Ovarian hyperstimulation syndrome (OHSS): Gonadotrophin (and rarely clomifene) stimulation 'overstimulates' the follicles, which can get very large and painful (Fig. 11.7). It is more common during IVF (approximately 4% of cycles) than standard ovulation induction.

In severe cases, hypovolaemia, electrolyte disturbances, ascites, thromboembolism and pulmonary oedema may develop. OHSS can be fatal. Prevention involves use of the lowest effective gonadotrophin doses, ultrasound monitoring of follicular growth, and if this is excessive, 'coasting' (withdrawing gonadotrophins but continuing pituitary down-regulation) or cancellation of IVF cycle (withholding hCG injection). If severe OHSS develops hospitalization is required for restoration of intravascular volume, electrolyte monitoring and correction, analgesia and thromboprophylaxis [→ p.128]. Drainage of ascitic fluid is occasionally necessary to increase comfort and breathing.

Ovarian and breast carcinoma: The evidence is conflicting but generally reassuring (*Reprod Biomed Online* 2007; **15**: 38).

Male subfertility

Male factors contribute in 25% of subfertile couples.

Physiology of sperm production

Spermatogenesis in the testis is dependent on pituitary LH and FSH, the former largely acting via testosterone production in the Leydig cells of the testis. FSH and testosterone control Sertoli cells, which are involved in synthesis and transport of sperm. Testosterone and other steroids inhibit the release of LH, completing a negative feedback control mechanism with the hypothalamic–pituitary axis. It takes about 70 days for sperm to develop fully.

Detection of adequate sperm production: semen analysis

A normal semen analysis result virtually excludes a male cause for infertility. The sample should be produced by masturbation with the last ejaculation having occurred 2–7 days previously. The sample must be analysed within 1–2 h of production. An abnormal analysis result must be repeated after 70 days. If persistently abnormal, examination and investigation of the male must follow (Fig. 11.8).

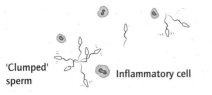

'Clumped' sperm   Inflammatory cell

Fig. 11.8 Semen analysis. Antisperm antibodies causing clumping.

Normal semen analysis	
Volume	>2 mL
Sperm count	>20 million/mL
Progressive motility	>50%

Definitions of terms describing abnormal semen	
Azoospermia:	No sperm present
Oligospermia:	<20 million/mL
Severe oligospermia:	<5 million/mL
Asthenospermia:	Absent or low motility

Common causes of abnormal semen analysis
Unknown
Smoking/alcohol/drugs/chemicals/inadequate local cooling
Genetic factors
Antisperm antibodies

Male factor investigations and treatment

Semen analysis
If abnormal repeat and:
   Examine the scrotum
   Optimize lifestyle factors

If oligospermic then:
   Intrauterine insemination

If moderate to severe oligospermia then:
   In vitro fertilization (IVF) ± intracytoplasmic sperm injection (ICSI)

If azoospermic then;
   Examine for presence of vas deferens
   Check karyotype, cystic fibrosis, hormone profile
   Surgical sperm retrieval then IVF + ICSI or donor insemination

Common causes of abnormal/absent sperm release

Idiopathic oligospermia and *asthenozoospermia* are common. Sperm numbers and/or motility are low but not absent.

Drug exposure: Alcohol, smoking, drugs (e.g. sulfasalazine or anabolic steroids), and exposure to industrial chemicals, particularly solvents, can impair male fertility.

Varicocoele: This refers to varicosities of the pampiniform venous plexus and usually occurs on the left side. It is present in about 25% of infertile men (but 15% of all men). It is not fully understood how it impairs fertility.

Antisperm antibodies are present in about 5% of infertile men and are common after vasectomy reversal. Poor motility and 'clumping' together of the sperm are evident on the semen analysis.

Other causes include infections (e.g. epididymitis), mumps orchitis, testicular abnormalities (e.g. in Klinefelter's syndrome XXY), obstruction to delivery (e.g. congenital absence of the vas), hypothalamic problems, Kallmann's syndrome and hyperprolactinaemia and retrograde ejaculation.

Management of male factor subfertility

General advice: Lifestyle changes and drug exposures are addressed. The testicles should be below body temperature: advice on wearing loose clothing and testicular cooling is given.

Specific measures: Ligation of a varicocoele does not significantly improve fertility so is not recommended (*Lancet* 2003; **361**: 1849). Gonadotrophin treatment of hypopituitary disease may be required.

Assisted conception techniques: *Intrauterine insemination* (IUI) may help if there is mild to moderate sperm dysfunction. If more severe oligospermia is present then *IVF* is used; if this very severe then *intracytoplasmic sperm injection* (ICSI) is used as part of an IVF cycle. If there is azoospermia, sperm can be extracted direct from the testis (surgical sperm retrieval [SSR]) in 50–80% of men and then used for ICSI-IVF (*Fertil Steril* 2007; **88**: 374). Or, donor sperm may be used, after appropriate counselling; this is called donor insemination (DI). Frozen-thawed sperm is injected into the uterus during a natural menstrual or mildly stimulated cycle at the time of ovulation. Children born from current sperm or oocyte donations in the UK can contact the donor from the age of 18, and there is a critical national shortage of sperm (and oocyte) donors.

Disorders of fertilization

The egg and sperm are unable to meet in 30% of subfertile couples.

Physiology of fertilization

At ovulation, the fallopian tube moves so that the fimbrial end collects the oocyte from the ovary. The tube must have adequate mobility to move onto the ovary to achieve this. Peristaltic contractions and cilia in the tube help sweep the oocyte along toward the sperm. Blockage or ciliary damage will impair this. At ejaculation, millions of sperm enter the vagina. The cervical mucus helps them get through the cervix.

Why the sperm might not meet the egg	
Tubal damage:	Infection
	Endometriosis
	Surgery/adhesions
Cervical problems	
Sexual problems	

Causes of failure to fertilize: tubal damage

This contributes in 25% of subfertile couples.

Infection

Pelvic inflammatory disease (PID) [→ p.75], particularly due to sexually transmitted infections (e.g. *Chlamydia*), causes adhesion formation within and around the fallopian tubes (Fig. 11.9). It is the main cause of tubal damage and 12% of women will be infertile after one episode of infection. Infection at the time of insertion of intrauterine contraceptive devices or a ruptured appendix may also be responsible. Most women will have had no symptoms, but some give a previous history of pelvic pain, vaginal discharge or abnormal menstruation.

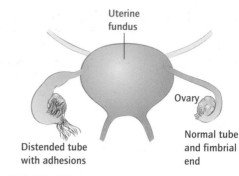

Fig. 11.9 Tubal blockage.

If there are peritubal adhesions or 'clubbed' and closed fimbrial ends of otherwise normal looking tubes then laparoscopic adhesiolysis and salpingostomy can be performed. Ectopic pregnancy rates are increased. Success rates are very poor if the tube is damaged proximal to the fimbrial ends. Under these circumstances or if conception does not occur after surgery, IVF is indicated.

Endometriosis [→ p.66]

This is found in 25% of subfertile women, but is probably contributory in many fewer. Its role in subfertility is more than simply mechanical (*Fertil Steril* 2006; **86**(5S): S156), but this is poorly understood. Laparoscopic surgery to remove endometriotic deposits improves fertility even in mild cases; medical treatment is not used since it suppresses ovulation. IVF is the next step if this fails.

Previous surgery/sterilization

Any pelvic surgery may cause adhesion formation. The now obsolete 'wedge resection' of the ovaries in PCOS patients was notorious for this. Treatment is as for infectious causes but IVF is often needed. If women have undergone tubal clip sterilization but now want pregnancy the options are IVF or open microsurgical tubal reanastomosis (increased ectopic risk).

Other causes of failure to fertilize

Cervical problems

'Cervical factors' rarely contribute to subfertility and the postcoital test is no longer recommended. Cervical problems can be due to *antibody production* by the woman, whereby antibodies agglutinate or kill the sperm, *infection* in the vagina or cervix that prevents adequate mucus production or *cone biopsy* for microinvasive cervical carcinoma [→ p.36]. IUI to bypass the cervix is often used.

Sexual problems

These occur in about 5% of subfertile couples. Impotence can be psychological or organic. Ignorance or discomfort can also prevent coitus. Counselling with a trained psychosexual counsellor is required, after exclusion of organic disease.

Detection of problems with fertilization

Detection of tubal damage

As pelvic infection and endometriosis are often symptomless, only limited information can be gained from the history and examination. One or other of the following tests is necessary for full assessment of subfertility. However, if severe male factor infertility is present, IVF ± ICSI will be required in any event and patency of the tubes is irrelevant and investigation is not required.

Laparoscopy and dye test [→ p.125] allows visualization and assessment of the fallopian tubes. Methylene blue dye is injected through the cervix from the outside. Whether it enters or spills from the tubes can then be seen, demonstrating whether the tubes are patent. *Hysteroscopy* is performed first to assess the uterine cavity for abnormalities.

Hysterosalpingogram (HSG): Without anaesthetic, radio-opaque contrast is injected through the cervix. Spillage from the fimbrial end (and filling defects) can be seen on X-ray. A variant of this test can be performed using transvaginal ultrasound and an ultrasound opaque liquid (HyCoSy). These tests are preferred in women with no risk factors for tubal disease and no symptoms or signs suggestive of endometriosis, as they are less invasive and safer than laparoscopy.

Assisted conception

Recent advances have greatly increased the success of fertility treatment. Over 1% of babies now born in the

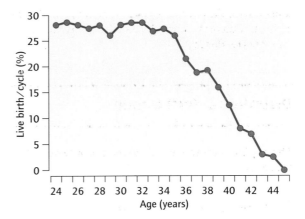

Fig. 11.10 Live birth rate per *in vitro* fertilization (IVF) cycle by female age.

UK are conceived through assisted conception. The current methods are IVF, ICSI, frozen embryo replacement (FER), IUI, oocyte donation and preimplantation genetic diagnosis (PGD). They are often unavailable on the National Health Service. Success is best measured by the live birth rate: this declines after 35 years, and considerably after 40 years of age (Fig. 11.10). Sperm quality is important but ICSI has rendered this less significant. Oocyte or embryo donation is now possible for premature ovarian failure, inherited genetic disorders or advanced maternal age.

Indications for assisted conception
When any/all other methods have failed
Unexplained subfertility
Male factor subfertility (intracytoplasmic sperm injection [ICSI])
Tubal blockage (standard *in vitro* fertilization [IVF])
Genetic disorders

Intrauterine insemination: superovulation

Method: At the time of gonadotrophin superovulation, washed sperm are injected directly into the cavity of the uterus.

Criteria: The tubes should be patent, as the oocyte(s) still need to travel from the ovary to the sperm. This is suitable for couples with unexplained subfertility, cervical

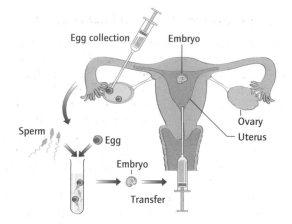

Fig. 11.11 Process of an *in vitro* fertilization (IVF) cycle.

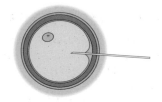

Fig. 11.12 Intracytoplasmic sperm injection (ICSI).

and sexual, and some male factors, and is cheaper but less successful than IVF.

Results: The live birth rate is about 10% per stimulated cycle with a 15% risk of multiple pregnancy.

In vitro fertilization

Method: During 'long-protocol' IVF the pituitary gonadotrophins are suppressed using 2–3 weeks of *GnRH agonist*. This prevents an endogenous LH surge and premature ovulation before oocyte collection. Multiple follicular development is then achieved with 2 weeks of daily subcutaneous gonadotrophin injections (FSH ± LH). The eggs are collected under intravenous sedation by aspirating follicles transvaginally under ultrasound control (Fig. 11.11). They are then incubated with washed sperm and transferred to a growth medium. Trans-cervical replacement of embryos into the uterus takes place 2–5 days later. Transferring no more than two embryos is mandatory in women <40 years of age to reduce the obstetric and paediatric complications associated with high order multiples. There is a move towards single embryo transfer to reduce the number of twin pregnancies (25% of live births are twins when two embryos are replaced). Spare, good quality embryos can be frozen for future thawing and FER. Luteal phase support, using progesterone or hCG, is given until 4–8 weeks' gestation.

Criteria: The fallopian tubes need not be patent. Normal 'ovarian reserve' (i.e. a FSH level <12 mIU/L) is needed

so that sufficient oocytes will be collected for fertilization and transfer. Therefore IVF is not possible for women with ovarian failure.

Results: The live birth rate per cycle in women <36 years in good centres is about 35% per stimulated cycle.

Intracytoplasmic sperm injection

This is the injection, with a very fine needle, of one sperm right into the oocyte cytoplasm (Fig. 11.12). It is a laboratory adjunct to IVF. It is useful for severe male factor infertility when there are not enough motile sperm available to incubate a sufficiently high concentration with each oocyte for standard IVF. Prior to the development of ICSI in the 1990s such couples could only be treated with DI. Now they can achieve the same pregnancy rates as couples with no male factor infertility undergoing IVF. Sperm can be retrieved from the testes with SSR and used for ICSI.

Oocyte donation

Some women cannot conceive with their own eggs either naturally or with IVF because of ovarian failure, older age (>43 years) or genetic disease. With oocyte donation another woman, the donor, goes through a full stimulated IVF cycle. Her retrieved oocytes are fertilized with the sperm of the recipient woman's partner. The recipient woman receives oestrogen and progesterone to prepare her endometrium for transfer of the fresh embryos. As there is a shortage of anonymous oocyte donors 'egg sharing' is commonly performed in which women who themselves need IVF agree to share or donate half of their oocytes anonymously to a recipient couple. The costs of treatment for the sharing couple are generally reduced.

Preimplantation genetic diagnosis

Day 3 preimplantation embryos generally contain about eight cells. With PGD one or two cells are removed from the embryo and the DNA examined using the techniques of polymerase chain reaction (PCR) or fluorescence *in situ* hybridization (FISH) to look for genetic abnormalities. Unaffected embryos are then replaced in the uterus 2 days later. PGD may be indicated for couples who are carriers of single gene defects such as cystic fibrosis or who have chromosome translocations placing them at a high risk of conceiving a child with aneuploidy. Embryos can also be sexed to avoid the replacement of male embryos that may be affected by, for example, haemophilia. Embryo sexing for 'social reasons' such as desire for a child of a particular sex is not permitted in the UK.

As women age they produce a higher proportion of embryos with abnormal numbers of chromosomes (this explains the increased rate of both miscarriage and Down's syndrome with female age). Women over the age of 37 can have all of their IVF embryos 'screened' using PGD to identify and replace only 'normal' embryos in an attempt to overcome the age-related decline in IVF success rates. Unfortunately, studies have not shown this technique of preimplantation genetic screening (PGS) to be beneficial when the indication is advanced maternal age (*BMJ* 2007; **335**: 752).

Surrogacy

Some women are unable to carry a pregnancy because of problems with their uterus (absent due to congenital anomaly or hysterectomy) or health (e.g. renal failure or immunological disease requiring teratogenic drugs). Surrogacy can be used in which another woman, the surrogate, carries the pregnancy and delivers the child who is then adopted by the commissioning couple. Either the surrogate's own eggs can be fertilized by insemination of the patient's partner's sperm (straight surrogacy) or, if the patient's ovaries are functioning she can go through IVF, have her oocytes collected and fertilized, and the embryos are then transferred to the womb of the surrogate (host surrogacy). There are a number of difficult ethical issues surrounding surrogacy.

Complications of assisted conception

Superovulation: Multiple pregnancy (25% of live births from IVF) and ovarian hyperstimulation are discussed above. The former are producing a significant impact on obstetric and neonatal services. A legislated move towards elective single embryo transfer (eSET) for certain groups of patients undergoing IVF is likely.

Egg collection: Intraperitoneal haemorrhage and pelvic infection may complicate the ultrasound-guided aspiration of mature follicles necessary for IVF although the risk is low (<1%).

Pregnancy: In addition to increased multiple pregnancies the rates of ectopic pregnancy are also higher. Recent data suggest a slight but significant increase in perinatal mortality and morbidity following IVF, even allowing for multiple pregnancies, although the cause is unclear. It may be that couples who require IVF have an inherently higher risk of adverse outcome than those who conceive naturally. A small increase in chromosomal and gene abnormalities is reported with ICSI although this appears to be related to a higher rate of genetic abnormality in men with severe male factor infertility (*NEJM* 2007; **356**: 579).

Ethics and regulation of assisted conception

The many ethical and practical problems in subfertility treatment are regulated by the Human Fertilization and Embryology Authority (HFEA) (www.hfea.gov.uk). All centres offering IVF must be licensed and their outcome data collected and reported for public use.

Rapid advances have occurred in reproductive medicine in the last 30 years and ethical dilemmas have followed. These include those of surrogacy, oocyte donation, embryo selection, storage of and research on embryos and their use after divorce or death. In the future, the practical possibilities of genetic testing, manipulation and even human cloning are likely to pose even greater problems.

Further reading

Braude P, Flinter F. Use and misuse of preimplantation genetic testing. *British Medical Journal* 2007; **335**: 752–4.

National Institute for Clinical Excellence. Fertility

assessment and treatment for people with fertility problems. Clinical Guidelines. 2004. http://www.NICE.org.uk

Norman RJ, Dewailly D, Legro RS, Hickey TE. Polycystic ovary syndrome. *Lancet* 2007; **370**: 685–97.

Tournaye H. Evidence-based management of male subfertility. *Current Opinions in Obstetrics and Gynaecology* 2006; **18**: 253–9.

Van Voorhis BJ. *In vitro* fertilization. *New England Journal of Medicine* 2007; **356**: 379–86.

Subfertility at a Glance

Definition	Failure to conceive after a year	
	Primary: female never conceived. Secondary: previously conceived	
Epidemiology	15% of couples	
Aetiology	Anovulation (30%):	Polycystic ovary syndrome (PCOS), hypothalamic hypogonadism, hyperprolactinaemia, thyroid dysfunction, ovarian failure
	Male factor (25%):	Idiopathic, varicocoele, antibodies, genetic, drug/chemical exposure, many others
	No fertilization:	Tubal factor (25%): infection, endometriosis, surgery
		Cervical factor (<5%)
		Sexual factor (5%)
	Unexplained (30%)	
Investigations	Detect ovulation:	Mid-luteal phase progesterone, ultrasound scan, urine luteinizing hormone (LH) testing
	Cause of anovulation:	Follicle-stimulating hormone (FSH), LH, testosterone, prolactin, thyroid-stimulating hormone (TSH)
	Detect male factor:	Semen analysis
	Detect tubal factor:	Laparoscopy and dye or hysterosalpingogram/HyCoSy
Treatment	General:	Ensure correct weight. Give folic acid
	If anovulation:	Treat specific disorder
		PCOS: clomifene, metformin, gonadotrophins, ovarian diathermy
	If male factor:	Treat specific disorder (generally not possible). Intrauterine insemination (IUI), *in vitro* fertilization (IVF) with or without intracytoplasmic sperm injection (ICSI), donor insemination (DI)
	If tubal factor:	Laparoscopic surgery if mild/endometriosis
		IVF if fails or with severe disease
	If unexplained:	IUI/IVF

Polycystic ovary syndrome (PCOS) at a Glance

Definition	Polycystic ovary (PCO) is multiple (>12) small follicles within enlarged ovaries PCOS is 2 out of 3 of: PCO on scan; irregular periods; hirsutism (raised serum androgens and/or acne/excess body hair)
Epidemiology	20% of women have PCO; 5% have PCOS; 80% of anovulatory infertility due to PCOS
Aetiology	PCO is genetic. Development of the syndrome is incompletely understood. Many have peripheral insulin resistance so raised fasting insulin (worsened by obesity). Increased luteinizing hormone (LH) secretion and increased androgen production
Features	Asymptomatic, anovulatory infertility, oligo-/amenorrhoea, obesity, hirsutism, acne
Investigations	Ultrasound scan of ovaries Blood: Often raised testosterone Normal follicle stimulating hormone (FSH) (high with ovarian failure and low with anorexia) Low luteal phase progesterone if anovulatory
Treatment	None if chance finding. Weight loss if appropriate If infertility: Clomifene; ovarian diathermy, metformin, gonadotrophins if failed; *in vitro* fertilization (IVF) If menstrual problems: Combined oral contraceptive If acne/hirsutism: Cosmetic treatments, contraceptive pill ± cyproterone acetate, spironolactone, eflornithine facial cream
Complications	Infertility, obesity, miscarriage Long-term risks: diabetes, endometrial carcinoma if persistent anovulation

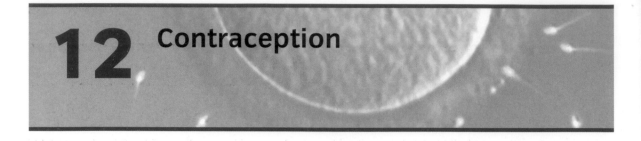

12 Contraception

Contraception is the prevention of pregnancy. On an individual basis it is important to ensure that all pregnancies are wanted or intended (www.fpa.org.uk). It is also important on a global scale because the world population is rapidly increasing. Contraceptive methods may help reduce the spread of disease, e.g. human immunodeficiency virus (HIV) [→ p.74] and *Chlamydia* [→ p.72].

The ideal contraceptive

The ideal contraceptive does not exist. If it did it would have the characteristics listed below. Long-acting reversible contraceptives (LARC) may come closest:
- 100% effective
- 100% safe
- 100% reversible
- Free from side effects
- Independent of intercourse
- Cheap/free
- Free from medical intervention
- Acceptable to all cultures and religions
- Prevents sexually transmitted infections
- Non-contraceptive benefits

Efficacy of contraception

This is measured as the risk of pregnancy per 100 woman years of using the given method, and is called the Pearl index (PI). If the PI of a contraceptive is 2 then, of 100 women using it for a year, two will be pregnant by the end. The effectiveness of a contraceptive is also determined by the user's compliance. With user-dependent contraceptives such as the pill, and particularly condoms, efficacy with 'perfect use' will be greater than with 'typical use'.

Obstetrics and Gynaecology, 3rd edition. By Lawrence Impey and Tim Child. Published 2008 by Blackwell Publishing, ISBN: 978-1-4051-6095-7.

Safety of contraception

Most methods of contraception have been the subject of adverse publicity. Some are less safe than others, or are contraindicated in particular women. By taking a full medical history, the doctor can consider and discuss with the woman whether the benefits of a particular method outweigh the risks. It is important that measurements of safety are compared with the safety of pregnancy; for instance, the diabetic woman is at increased risk of complications with the 'pill', but pregnancy risks more complications. Similarly, smoking is considerably more hazardous than using the 'pill'.

Compliance with contraception

This is a major problem. Contraception must be appropriate to the woman's lifestyle; if it is disliked or misunderstood it will not be used. The woman must be fully counselled about any proposed contraceptive: its major problems and minor side effects. This will enable the woman to know what to expect, and may prevent discontinuation of the chosen method. Media 'scares' over the 'pill' have led to inappropriate discontinuation and unwanted pregnancies.

Contraception for the adolescent

One in 100 of 13- to 15-year-olds become pregnant every year in the UK, and this figure has only fallen by 10% since 1998. The current Department of Health target aims to reduce the under-18 years conception rate by 50% by the year 2010; by 2005 the reduction was 11%. Infant mortality rates for babies born to mothers under the age of 18 are twice the national average. Sex education and public awareness of family planning services will need to increase. It may be too late to prevent intercourse, but the implications, including sexually transmitted disease and unwanted pregnancy, should be discussed. The combined oral contraceptive or depot preparations are usually indicated, but should be used in conjunction with a condom to prevent sexually transmitted disease.

It is acceptable to prescribe contraception to sexually mature girls <16 years, and there is no obligation to tell her parents if she cannot be persuaded to do so. The General Medical Council guidelines permit a doctor to breach the young woman's confidentiality where it is essential to her medical interests, but she must be told before information is disclosed.

Contraception in later life

Although fertility is reduced after 40 years of age (mainly due to increased oocyte and embryo aneuploidy), most women with regular cycles still ovulate. All methods of contraception can be used; including a low-dose combined oral contraceptive in non-smoking women with no other risk factors. Intrauterine devices (IUDs) are particularly appropriate and, if fitted after the age of 40 years, may not need to be replaced. The hormone-releasing intrauterine system (IUS) [→ p.13] will, in addition, greatly reduce menstrual loss. Despite this, many women seek sterilization.

Contraception in the developing world

Where education and access to health care is poor, the practical requirements of a contraceptive are different. Minimal medical supervision, prevention of sexually transmitted disease, cost and duration of treatment are important. This means reversible depot methods, such as Implanon and vaccines have more potential. Breast-feeding has important contraceptive benefits where contraception is scarce, although around 2% of women will fall pregnant in the first 6 months if no additional contraception is used.

Organization and planning of family planning services

In the UK, contraception is available from general practitioners and family planning clinics. In addition, emergency contraception [→ p.98] can be purchased over-the-counter from pharmacies.

The concept of the 'sexual health clinic' has developed, with contraception, genitourinary medicine, and even colposcopy and menopause services alongside each other.

Hormonal contraception

Oestrogens and progestogens can be used for contraception in the following ways:

1 Progestogen as a tablet: the progestogen-only pill ('mini pill').
2 Progestogen as a depot: Implanon, Depo-Provera or in the levonorgestrel-containing intrauterine system (IUS).
3 Oestrogen and progestogen: the combined oral contraceptive (the 'pill'): mono/bi/triphasic.
4 Novel methods include patch or vaginal ring combinations of oestrogen and progestogen.

Combined oral contraceptives (the 'pill')

Combined oral contraceptives (COCs) act mainly by exerting a negative feedback effect [→ p.9] on gonadotrophin release and thereby inhibiting ovulation. A single tablet, containing both an oestrogen and a progestogen, is taken every day for 3 weeks and then stopped for 1 week (Fig. 12.1). Vaginal bleeding then occurs as a result of withdrawal of the hormonal stimulus on the endometrium. The cycle is then restarted. Pill packets can be taken consecutively without break ('back-to-back') to reduce the frequency of the withdrawal bleed although increased irregular spotting may occur.

Types

Monophasic pills deliver the same dose of oestrogen and progestogen every day. The synthetic oestrogen (ethinyloestradiol) content may range from 20 to 50 µg. The usual preparations of choice are the 30 or 35 µg pills (e.g. Microgynon 30). In *biphasic* or *triphasic pills*, the doses of both hormones alter two and three times, respectively.

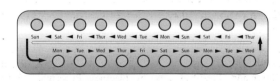

Fig. 12.1 The combined oral contraceptive.

They are more expensive and have no clear advantages over standard *monophasic* preparations (*Cochrane* 2006: CD 003283; CD 002032).

Contraceptive efficacy

Taken properly, the combined pill is highly effective, with a failure rate of 0.2 per 100 woman years. If less care is taken, failure rates are much higher.

Common side effects of sex hormones	
Progestogenic	*Oestrogenic*
Depression	Nausea
Postmenstrual tension-like symptoms	Headaches
	Increased mucus
Bleeding; amenorrhoea	Fluid retention and weight gain
Acne	Occasionally hypertension
Breast discomfort	Breast tenderness and fullness
Weight gain	Bleeding
Reduced libido	

Indications

All women without major contraindications may use it ('from menarche to menopause'). It is suitable for the teenager (in conjunction with condoms) and the older woman with no cardiovascular risk factors until the age of 50. It is also useful for menstrual cycle control, menorrhagia, premenstrual symptoms, dysmenorrhoea, acne/hirsutism and prevention of recurrent simple ovarian cysts.

The 'pill' in practice

Reduced absorption of the 'pill' can occur if suffering from diarrhoea, vomiting or if taking some oral antibiotics. If the woman has diarrhoea she should continue taking the pills but follow the missed-pill instructions (below) for each day of the illness. If she vomits within 2 h of taking the pill she should take another or follow the rules for missed pills. If she is taking broad-spectrum antibiotics (penicillin, ampicillin, tetracycline, cefalosporins) then she should continue the pills but use condoms during and for 7 days after the antibiotic course. If using liver enzyme inducing drugs (e.g. anticonvulsants or St John's Wort), the pill oestrogen dose may need to be increased.

The missed 'pill': For standard strength preparations (30–35 μg ethinyloestradiol) one or two missed pills anywhere in the pack are not a problem. For very low dose preparations (20 μg) only one pill can be missed. The forgotten pill should be taken as soon as possible and then the packet continued as normal. If more pills have been missed then continue the packet as normal but condoms should be used for 7 days. If there are less than seven pills remaining in the packet avoid a pill-free break by running straight into the next packet.

The 'pill' and surgery: The pill is normally stopped 4 weeks before major surgery because of its prothrombotic risks, but the risks of pregnancy should also be considered. The pill is not discontinued prior to minor surgery.

Counselling the woman starting on the 'pill'
Advise of major complications and benefits
Advise to stop smoking
Advise to see doctor if symptoms suggestive of major complications
Advise about poor absorption with antibiotics and sickness and what to do about missed pill(s) (give leaflet)
Stress the importance of follow-up and blood pressure measurement

Disadvantages

Major: complications

These are very rare. In general, the risks of pregnancy (including termination of an unwanted pregnancy) outweigh the risks of oral contraception. The estimated excess annual risk of death for women taking the pill is 2–5 per million users for women <35 years of age. This can be minimized by careful selection and follow-up of women (paying particular attention to establishing if there are any pre-existing risks for cardiovascular or hepatic disease, or migraine with focal neurological symptoms). *Venous thrombosis* and *myocardial infarction* are the most important complications (http://www.ffprhc.org.uk/). The risk is further multiplied by smoking, increased age and obesity (absolute contraindication if body mass index [BMI] >40, or age >35 years and smokes >15 cigarettes per day; relative contraindication if BMI 35–39).

Venous thromboembolism is more common with 'third generation' pills containing the progestogens *gestodene* or *desogestrel* than with the more widely prescribed second generation preparations containing *norithisterone* or *levonorgestrel* although the absolute risk remains low. Other problems include a slightly increased risk

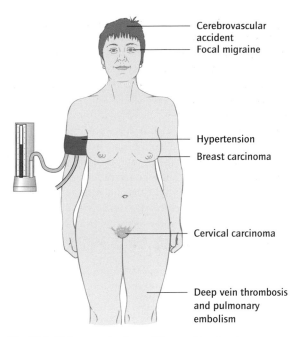

Fig. 12.2 Major complications of the combined oral contraceptive.

Non-contraceptive benefits: Useful effects include more regular, less painful and lighter menstruation. There is protection against simple ovarian cysts, benign breast cysts, fibroids and endometriosis. Hirsutism and acne may improve: the 'pill' need not be prescribed merely for contraception. The risk of pelvic inflammatory disease (PID), but not HIV, is reduced possibly because of thicker cervical mucus. Longer term, there is reduction in the incidence of ovarian, endometrial and bowel cancer.

Contraindications to the combined oral contraceptives (COCs)	
Absolute:	History of venous thrombosis
	History of cerebrovascular accident, ischaemic heart disease, severe hypertension
	Migraine with aura
	Active breast/endometrial cancer
	Inherited thrombophilia
	Pregnancy
	Smokers >35 years and smoking >15 cigarettes/day
	Body mass index (BMI) >40
	Diabetes with vascular complications
	Active/chronic liver disease
Relative:	Smokers
	Chronic inflammatory disease
	Renal impairment, diabetes
	Age >40 years
	BMI 35–40
	Breastfeeding up to 6 months postpartum

of *cerebrovascular accidents, focal migraine, hypertension, jaundice,* and *liver, cervical and breast carcinoma* (Fig. 12.2).

Minor: side effects

Both oestrogenic and progestogenic side effects may occur. The most common are nausea, headaches and breast tenderness. Breakthrough bleeding is common in the first few months, but has usually settled after 3 months. If not then consider changing the pill to one containing a more potent progestogen or if using a 20 µg ethinyloestradiol pill increase it to a 30 µg preparation. Lactation is partly suppressed so the pill is contraindicated during the first 6 weeks of breastfeeding (relative contraindication from 6 weeks to 6 months postpartum and no restriction beyond 6 months).

Advantages

Contraceptive: Despite the rare complications, the 'pill' is a very effective and acceptable method of contraception: it has been the subject of considerable research and in appropriate women it is very safe.

Risk of non-fatal venous thromboembolism for users of combined oral contraceptives (COCs)	
User category	Incidence per 100 000 women per year
All women not using 'pill'	5
Pregnant women	60
Women using older 30 µg 'pill'	15
Women using new 30 µg 'pill'	25
Women smoking and using 'pill'	60

Counselling before using the 'mini pill'
Advise woman about bleeding patterns
Emphasize the importance of meticulous timekeeping

Progestogen-only pill (the 'mini pill')

Used by 5% of women aged 16–50 years. The standard progestogen-only pill (POP) contains a low dose (e.g. 350 mg norethisterone: Micronor) and must be taken every day without a break and at the same time (±3 h). It makes cervical mucus hostile to sperm and in 50% of women inhibits ovulation too. Failure rates are 1 per 100 woman years: higher than the combined pill. Side effects are progestogenic: vaginal spotting (breakthrough bleeding), weight gain, mastalgia and premenstrual-like symptoms are most common. Functional ovarian cysts can occur. It is less effective than the combined pill, and the need for meticulous timing can spell failure, particularly in younger women. It is particularly suitable for older women and those in whom the combined pill is contraindicated. It is also used for lactating mothers. There is no increased risk of thrombosis and it can be used in almost all the situations where the combined pill is contraindicated.

A newer preparation (Cerazette) contains a higher dose of the progestogen *desogestrel* and inhibits ovulation in over 95% of cycles. It is more effective than the standard POP and can be taken within a 12-h window.

If a pill is missed by more than 3 h (12 h for Cerazette) then another should be taken as soon as possible and condoms used for 2 days. The POPs are not affected by broad-spectrum antibiotics.

Long-acting reversible contraceptives

With depot administration methods, progestogens are slowly released, bypassing the portal circulation. The mode of action is similar to that of the 'mini pill', but ovulation is normally also prevented. The LARCs demonstrate many of the features of an ideal contraceptive. In particular they are not user-dependent and have high efficacy rates (*Curr Opin Obstet Gynecol* 2007; **19**: 453). The LARC methods are more cost-effective than the combined oral contraceptive after 12 months of use. However, current usage rates are low.

Depo-Provera and Noristerat

Depo-Provera, containing medroxyprogesterone acetate (150 mg), is administered by intramuscular injection every 3 months. The failure rate is <1.0 per 100 woman years. It often causes irregular bleeding in the first weeks, but this is usually followed by amenorrhoea. Other pro-

← 3.9 cm →

Fig. 12.3 Implanon.

gestogenic side effects may occur. Prolonged amenorrhoea may follow its cessation and women should be warned of this, particularly if they are considering pregnancy in the near future. Bone density decreases although is regained after stopping. Consequently other contraceptives may be preferable in teenagers (before peak bone mass is achieved) and women over 45 when nearing the menopause. It is useful during lactation and when compliance is a problem. An alternative depot preparation with similar efficacy is Noristerat (*Cochrane* 2006: CD005214), containing norethisterone, which is given every 8 weeks.

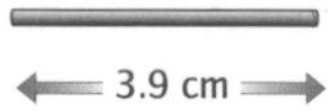

Implanon

This consists of a single 60-mm rod containing progestogen (etonogestrel), which is inserted in the upper arm subdermally with local anaesthetic (Fig. 12.3). The failure rate is <1.0 per 100 woman years. It will last 3 years and female satisfaction is high (*Cochrane* 2007: CD001326). Side effects include progestogenic symptoms, particularly irregular bleeding in the first year. There is no drop in bone density. Removal is usually easy and there is a rapid resumption of fertility. Because it is simple and long-acting, it may have a particular role in the developing world.

Progestogen-impregnated intrauterine system

This is discussed below.

Emergency contraception

In emergency contraception a drug or IUD is used shortly after unprotected intercourse in an attempt to prevent pregnancy. A number of different regimes are available (*Cochrane* 2004: CD001324).

The 'morning-after pill'

The chances of conception after unprotected intercourse can be reduced by taking the 'morning-after pill'. A

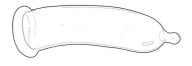

Fig. 12.4 The male condom.

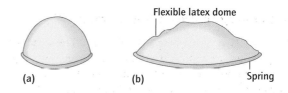

Fig. 12.5 (a) The cervical cap. (b) The diaphragm.

single dose of 1.5 mg of the progestogen levonorgestrel (Levonelle) is taken, preferably within 24 h and no later than 72 h, after unprotected intercourse (*Lancet* 2002; **360**: 1803). It is available over-the-counter from pharmacists. Levonelle affects sperm function and endometrial receptivity and, if given just prior to ovulation, may prevent follicular rupture. The method has a 95% success rate if used within 24 h, reduced to 58% if delayed until 72 h. The levonorgestrel does not provide contraception for the rest of the cycle. Vomiting can occur plus menstrual disturbances in the following cycle.

Intrauterine device

If beyond 72 h since unprotected intercourse insertion of an IUD usually prevents implantation. The IUD can be inserted up to 5 days after the expected day of ovulation. Mifepristone [→ p.118] may be taken orally but is more likely to cause cycle disturbance and is unlicensed for emergency contraception.

When discussing emergency contraception it is vital to arrange future contraception and to consider screening for sexually transmitted infections (STIs) depending on circumstances such as whether the episode occurred outside of a relationship. If the next period is late the woman should be advised to perform a pregnancy test.

Barrier contraception

Barrier methods physically prevent the sperm from getting through the cervix. A principal advantage, especially with condoms, is the protection against STIs.

Male condom

This consists of a sheath (latex or not) that fits onto the erect penis (Fig. 12.4). The failure rate is 2–15 per 100 woman years; this is dependent on using it properly. It

affords the best protection against disease, including HIV, and should always be used for casual intercourse, even if in conjunction with other methods.

Female condom

This fits inside the vagina. Failure rates are similar to the condom but it is less well accepted. It too protects against STIs.

Diaphragms and caps

These are fitted before intercourse and must remain *in situ* for at least 6 h afterwards. Cervical caps fit over the cervix (Fig. 12.5a), whilst the spring of the latex dome of the diaphragm holds it between the pubic bone and the sacral curve, covering the cervix (Fig. 12.5b). Types and sizes vary, and selection should be determined by trained personnel. Failure rates are about 5 per 100 woman years and dependent on the type used (*Cochrane* 2002: CD003551). Although some protection against PID is gained, there is less protection against HIV. Some women find them inconvenient, and they are best suited to a woman with good motivation.

Spermicides

Barrier methods are used in conjunction with a spermicide containing nonoxynol-9, in the form of a jelly, cream or pessary. Spermicides are not recommended for use on their own (*Cochrane* 2005: CD005218).

Intrauterine contraceptive devices ('the coil')

These devices are inserted into the uterine cavity and are

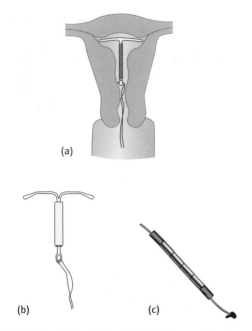

Fig. 12.6 Intrauterine devices (IUDs). (a) Copper T in uterus, (b) intrauterine system (IUS), (c) Gynefix.

of two types: copper or progestogen-bearing. Thin plastic strings protrude through the cervix and are pulled to remove the device. They are normally changed every 5–10 years.

Types of IUDs

Copper-containing devices operate primarily by preventing fertilization, the copper ion being toxic to sperm. They also act to block implantation. The copper is either wound around an inert frame which sits within the uterine cavity (Fig. 12.6a) or threads which are attached to the fundus (Fig. 12.6c) (*Contraception* 2007; **75**(6S): S82).

Hormone-containing devices contain the progestogen levonorgestrel (Mirena), which is slowly released locally over 5 years (Fig. 12.6b). This is now called the intrauterine system (IUS). Its main contraceptive effects are local, through changes to the cervical mucus and utero-tubal fluid which impair sperm migration, backed by endometrial changes impeding implantation. It has the additional benefit of reducing menstrual loss and pain [→ p.12]. The blood levels of levonorgestrel are less than

half that of the progestogen mini-pill so systemic side effects are low. Irregular light bleeding is the main problem. Return of fertility after removal is rapid and complete.

Contraceptive efficacy

With high copper content and progestogen-releasing devices, the failure rate is <0.5 per 100 woman years. A major advantage is the lack of user dependence.

Indications

The IUD is used by 20% of sexually active French women but only 5% in the UK. They are safe, effective and reversible and can be used in a number of situations when hormonal contraception is contraindicated, particularly in older women. Coils are normally inserted during the first half of the cycle, but can be used straight after delivery of the placenta or 6 weeks post-delivery, or at termination of pregnancy. The progestogen-releasing IUS is also used for non-contraceptive indications such as menorrhagia or dysmenorrhoea.

Complications

Pain or cervical shock (due to increased vagal tone) can complicate insertion. The device can be *expelled*, usually within the first month. *Perforation* of the uterine wall (<0.5%) can occur at insertion, or the device may migrate through the wall afterwards. Expulsion or perforation will cause the threads to disappear, but they may also have been cut too short. If the threads are not visible at the cervix an ultrasound scan is performed to look for the IUD within the uterus. If it is not present then an abdominal X-ray will reveal the IUD if it is within the abdomen—if so then a laparoscopy is indicated to remove it. *Heavier or more painful menstruation* can occur (except with progestogen devices). Women with asymptomatic STIs in the cervix are at increased risk of PID during the first 20 days after insertion. The risk of *infection* (10%) is mainly limited to younger women with multiple partners and is reduced by screening for infection first. If pregnancy occurs despite the presence of an IUD, it is more likely to be *ectopic*, but the overall ectopic rate is still lower than in a woman using no contraception. If ectopic pregnancy has been excluded, the IUD should be removed early so as to reduce the risk of miscarriage.

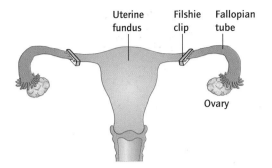

Fig. 12.7 Female sterilization. View of uterine fundus with Filshie clips on tubes.

Contraindications to the intrauterine device (IUD)	
Absolute:	Endometrial or cervical cancer Undiagnosed vaginal bleeding Active/recent pelvic infection Current breast cancer (for progestogen intrauterine system [IUS]) Pregnancy

Relative:	Previous ectopic pregnancy
	Excessive menstrual loss (unless progestogen
	   IUS)
	Multiple sexual partners
	Young/nulliparous
	Immunocompromised, including human
	   immunodeficiency virus (HIV)-positive

Advantages

The IUD is extremely safe. The woman does not need to remember to use other contraception. Menstrual loss is reduced if progestogen-containing devices are used (IUS). The IUD can be used as emergency contraception if inserted within 5 days of ovulation.

Counselling before inserting an intrauterine device (IUD)	
Advise of the major risks	

Advise to inform her
   doctor if:
	She bleeds intermenstrually
	She experiences pelvic pain or a
	   vaginal discharge, or if she
	   feels she might be pregnant

Advise about checking for strings after each period	

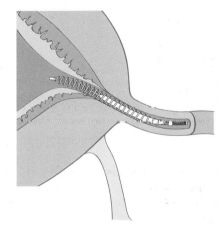

Fig. 12.8 Female sterilization: Microinserts placed hysteroscopically into fallopian tubes.

Female sterilization

Twenty-five per cent of couples rely on male or female sterilization. The minimum that needs to be done for female sterilization is interruption of the fallopian tubes so that sperm and egg cannot meet. More radical procedures such as hysterectomy should only be performed if specific indications are present. The most common technique uses clips (e.g. Filshie clip; Fig. 12.7). These are applied to the tubes laparoscopically [→ p.125], completely occluding the lumen. This normally involves a general anaesthetic.

A recent alternative is trans-cervical sterilization involving the hysteroscopic placement of microinserts into the proximal part of each tubal lumen (e.g. Essure; Fig. 12.8) (*Curr Opin Obstet Gynecol* 2007; **19**: 325). The inserts expand and cause fibrosis and occlusion of the lumen confirmed, 3 months later, with a hysterosalpingogram.

Contraceptive efficacy

The Filshie clip and Essure both have failure rates of around 0.5%, i.e. about 1 in 200 women will become pregnant at some time. Long-term data on Essure are lacking.

Indications

Both doctor and woman must be satisfied that there will be no regret: therefore it is usually used in an older woman whose family is complete, or when disease contraindicates pregnancy.

Counselling a woman before sterilization
The woman, and preferably her partner, must be certain Alternative contraception is discussed Warn of 1 in 200 lifetime risk of failure Risk of ectopic if pregnancy Reversal not possible with hysteroscopic sterilization and not guaranteed with Filshie clips. Reversal unavailable on the National Health Service (NHS) Risks of surgery [→ p.125] and of possible laparotomy

Complications

Laparoscopic sterilization is a safe procedure (*Cochrane* 2002: CD003034), but perioperative complications include the risks of laparoscopy (primarily visceral damage) and inadequate access to the tubes. Postoperative pain is reduced by using local anaesthetic on the tubes and in the skin incisions. If pregnancy does occur, it is more likely to be ectopic. Requests for reversal should be rare with adequate woman selection and counselling. Reversal is performed using microsurgical techniques via a laparotomy or, occasionally, laparoscopy. *In vitro* fertilization (IVF) is an alternative to reversal (*Cochrane* 2006: CD004144).

Trans-cervical hysteroscopic sterilization is associated with a fallopian tube perforation rate and device expulsion rate of 2% and a 14% chance of failure to correctly insert the devices at the first procedure. Other methods of contraception are used until the hysterosalpingogram has confirmed bilateral tubal occlusion at 3 months. The technique is not reversible and IVF would be required for conception.

Male sterilization

Vasectomy is more effective than female sterilization (1 in 2000 lifetime risk after two negative semen analyses) and involves ligation and removal of a small segment of the vas deferens, thereby preventing release of sperm. It can be performed under local anaesthetic. Sterility is not assured until azoospermia is confirmed by two semen analyses and may take up to 6 months to achieve. Complications (5%) include failure, postoperative haematomas and infection, and chronic pain. Natural conception following successful reversal is often prevented by antisperm antibody formation which restricts motility. Such sperm can be washed and used during an insemination or IVF cycle [→ p.90]. Surgical sperm retrieval followed by IVF of retrieved oocytes is an alternative to vasectomy reversal.

Male hormonal contraception

Spermatogenesis can be halted by depot administration of progestogens through central effects at the hypothalamus and pituitary. The gonadotrophin drive to the testes is reduced (in a similar way to the effects of depot progestogen in women causing anovulation). However, this also switches off androgen production so additional exogenous testosterone replacement therapy is required. Trial results are promising and the development of a reliable male hormonal contraception is likely (*Cochrane* 2007: CD004316).

Natural contraception

This is less reliable than most methods and offers no protection against STIs. It is only suitable for monogamous women who would not be concerned by pregnancy. *Lactation* has a major contraceptive role in the developing world. The *'rhythm' method* avoids the fertile period around ovulation and over-the-counter kits can help this. Some kits (e.g. Persona) measure urine levels of luteinizing hormone and oestrogen and from this calculate 'safe' days for intercourse. *'Withdrawal'* involves removal of the penis just before ejaculation, but is not recommended because sperm can be released before orgasm.

Further reading

Faculty of Sexual and Reproductive Healthcare, Royal College of Obstetricians and Gynaecologists. http://www.ffprhc.org.uk (source of excellent contraception guidelines and reviews)

Family Planning Association: http://www.fpa.org.uk

Ornstein RM, Fisher MM. Hormonal contraception in adolescents: special considerations. *Paediatric Drugs* 2006; **8**: 25–45.

Royal College of Obstetricians and Gynaecologists. Male and female sterilisation. Clinical Guideline No. 4. 2004. http://www.rcog.org.uk

Contraception at a Glance

Combined oral contraceptive	Women:	Any, except smoker >35 years, BMI >40, history of venous thromboembolism, cerebrovascular disease and cerebrovascular accident, hypertension or inherited thrombophilia, current breast cancer.
	Failure:	Pearl index (PI) 0.1 (perfect use); 5.0 (typical use)
	Mode of action:	Inhibits ovulation
	How to use:	Start on day 1 of cycle, 3 weeks, then 1 week break
	Rare major problems:	Deep vein thromboses, ischaemic heart disease, cerebrovascular accident, hypertension, breast and cervical carcinoma
	Common side effects:	Breast tenderness, bleeding, headaches, nausea
	Benefits:	Good contraception, cycle control, well accepted. Reduces risk of developing fibroids, and ovarian, endometrial, bowel cancer.
	Drawbacks:	Major side effects and contraindications. User dependent so failure rate increased
Progestogen-only pill	Women:	Any. Need to be well motivated
	Failure:	PI 0.5 (perfect use); 5.0 (typical use) [Cerazette similar to combined pill]
	Mode of action:	Cervical mucus and sometimes inhibition of ovulation
	How to use:	Continuous, every day at same time [Cerazette 12 h window]
	Side effects:	Vaginal spotting, other progestogenic effects
	Benefits:	Few contraindications, lactation
	Drawbacks:	Compliance and failure rate. User dependent
Depot progestogens	Women:	Any. When compliance a problem
	Failure:	PI <0.5
	Mode of action:	As above, and ovulation usually inhibited
	How to use:	Depo-Provera intramuscularly every 3 months, Noristerat every 8 weeks, Implanon every 3 years
	Side effects:	Progestogenic; prolonged amenorrhoea and reversible bone loss with Depo-Provera
	Benefits:	Woman can 'forget about it' (i.e. no user-dependent failures)
	Drawbacks:	Progestogenic side effects
Intrauterine devices (IUDs)	Women:	Older, multiparous, monogamous
	Failure:	PI <1.0 depending on type (PI 0.1 for Mirena IUS)
	Mode of action:	Prevents implantation/fertilization
	How to use:	Insert into uterus, change every 5–10 years
	Side effects:	Pelvic infection, menstrual disturbance, perforation
	Benefits:	Woman can 'forget about it', intrauterine system (IUS) reduces blood loss
	Drawbacks:	Pelvic infection

(Continued)

Contraception at a Glance (Continued)

Condoms	Person:	Any, essential for casual intercourse
	Failure:	PI 2.0 (perfect use); 15 (typical use)
	Benefits:	Non-hormonal, safe, protection against sexually transmitted infection (STIs)
	Drawbacks:	Inconvenience, poor technique
Caps/diaphragms	Woman:	Any, well motivated, usually monogamous
	Failure:	PI 5.0 (perfect use); 15 (typical use)
	How to use:	Insert before intercourse, with spermicide, remove 6 h later
	Benefits:	Non-hormonal, woman has control
	Drawbacks:	Failure rates, inconvenience, limited protection against STIs
Sterilization	Person:	Older, multiparous, family finished
	Failure:	1 in 200 (female); 1 in 2000 (male) lifetime risk
	How to do:	Female: laparoscopic clip or hysteroscopic insert occlusion of fallopian tubes
		Male: ligation and removal of segment of vas deferens (vasectomy)
	Side effects:	Perioperative complications
	Benefits:	'Permanent'
	Drawbacks:	Reversal expensive and limited success. Common source of litigation

13 The menopause and post-reproductive health

Definitions

Menopause is the permanent cessation of menstruation resulting from loss of ovarian follicular activity. It occurs at a median age of 52 years. Natural menopause is recognized to have occurred after 12 consecutive months of amenorrhoea (Fig. 13.1).

Perimenopause includes the time beginning with the first features of the approaching menopause, such as vasomotor symptoms and menstrual irregularity, and ends 12 months after the last menstrual period.

Postmenopause should be defined as dating from the final menstrual period. However, it cannot be determined until after 12 months of spontaneous amenorrhoea.

Premature menopause is arbitrarily defined as menopause occurring before the age of 40 and affects 1% of women. In most women no cause is found. Some will have a *surgical menopause* following bilateral oöphorectomy perhaps performed during hysterectomy. Other causes include infections, autoimmune disorders, chemotherapy, ovarian dysgenesis and metabolic diseases. Hormone replacement therapy (HRT) is indicated at least until the age of 50. Oocyte donation is required for fertility treatment.

Postmenopausal bleeding

Definition

Vaginal bleeding occurring at least 12 months after the last menstrual period.

Obstetrics and Gynaecology, 3rd edition. By Lawrence Impey and Tim Child. Published 2008 by Blackwell Publishing, ISBN: 978-1-4051-6095-7.

Causes

Postmenopausal bleeding is an important clinical problem. The main onus is to exclude carcinoma of the endometrium or cervix and premaligant endometrial hyperplasia with cytological atypia. Carcinoma of the endometrium and atypical hyperplasia account for about 20% of cases. Withdrawal bleeds occur with sequential HRT and, so long as they are regular, do not warrant investigation. Bleeding may also occur from a poorly oestrogenized vaginal wall: 'atrophic vaginitis', but this should be a diagnosis of exclusion. A purulent blood-stained vaginal discharge in a postmenopausal woman should be investigated to rule out endometrial cancer or, uncommonly, a diverticular abscess draining via the uterus or vagina.

Causes of postmenopausal bleeding (PMB)
Endometrial carcinoma
Endometrial hyperplasia ± atypia and polyps
Cervical carcinoma
Atrophic vaginitis
Cervicitis
Ovarian carcinoma
Cervical polyps

Management

All women should undergo a bimanual and speculum examination and a cervical smear taken if one has not been taken according to the national screening programme. Transvaginal sonography (TVS) has become a routine procedure for initial assessment. It measures endometrial thickness and also gives information on other pelvic pathology, such as fibroids and ovarian cysts. TVS is less invasive than endometrial biopsy or hysteroscopy but does not give a histological diagnosis. A thickened endometrium or a cavity filled with fluid indicates an increased risk of malignancy or other pathology (hyperplasia or polyps).

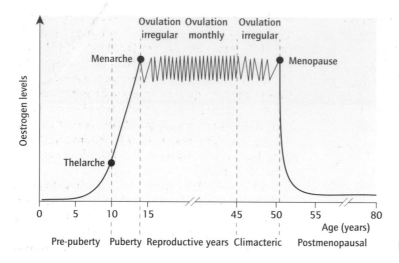

Fig. 13.1 Oestrogen levels in a lifetime.

If the endometrial thickness is 4 mm or less on TVS and there was only a single episode of PMB then endometrial biopsy is not required. If the endometrium is thicker or there have been multiple bleeds an endometrial biopsy is performed. This can be as an outpatient procedure using a Pipelle suction device, or as a hysteroscopy and biopsy/curettage under local or general anaesthetic. If a Pipelle biopsy is normal but bleeding persists then a formal hysteroscopy and curettage is performed. Once malignancy is excluded, atrophic vaginitis can be treated with HRT or topical oestrogen.

Symptoms and consequences of the menopause (Fig. 13.2)

Cardiovascular disease

The major cause of death in developed countries in women over the age of 60 years is cardiovascular disease (coronary heart disease and stroke) (Fig. 13.3). While it is difficult to differentiate the effects of age and oestrogen deficiency, oöphorectomized women are at two to three times higher risk of coronary heart disease than age-matched premenopausal women.

Vasomotor symptoms

Hot flushes and night sweats are the most common

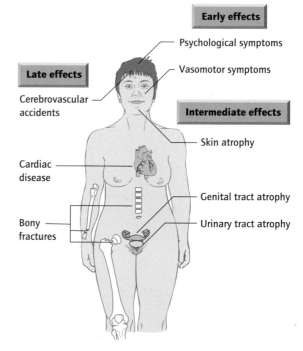

Fig. 13.2 Changes and clinical features of oestrogen deficiency.

symptoms of the menopause and affect about 70% of Western women. Night sweats can cause sleep disturbance leading to tiredness and irritability. They may begin before periods stop and usually are present for less

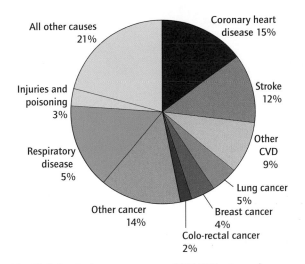

Fig. 13.3 Deaths by cause, women, 2005, UK (redrawn from the British Heart Foundation). CVD, cardiovascular disease.

than 5 years. However, some women will continue to flush in their 60s and 70s.

Urogenital problems

Oestrogen deficiency can cause vaginal atrophy and urinary problems. Vaginal atrophy can also affect women taking systemic HRT. It can be extremely uncomfortable and can result in dyspareunia, cessation of sexual activity, itching, burning and dryness. Urinary symptoms include frequency, urgency, nocturia, incontinence and recurrent infection. Women may suffer in silence and not seek medical help.

Sexual problems

Sexual problems affect about half of all women and become more common with age. Interest in sex declines in both sexes with increasing age and this change is more pronounced in women. The term female sexual dysfunction (FSD) is now used and an international classification system employed. Sexual problems are classified into various types: loss of sexual desire, loss of sexual arousal, problems with orgasm and sexual pain such as painful sex (dyspareunia).

Osteoporosis

Osteoporosis is defined as 'a skeletal disorder character-

ized by compromised bone strength predisposing to an increased risk of fracture'. It is a major problem with 1 in 3 women over 50 years (and 1 in 12 men) having one or more osteoporotic fractures. Bone strength reflects the integration of two main features: bone density and bone quality. *Bone density* is expressed as grams of mineral per area or volume and, in any given individual, is determined by peak bone mass and amount of bone loss. *Bone quality* refers to architecture, turnover, damage accumulation (e.g. microfractures) and mineralization.

The World Health Organization (WHO) definitions of osteoporosis, classified according to bone mineral density (BMD) are shown below. The T score is that number of standard deviations (SD) by which a particular bone differs from the young normal mean.

Definitions of osteoporosis according to the World Health Organization (WHO)	
Description	*Definition*
Normal:	BMD value between −1 SD and +1 SD of the young adult mean (T score −1 to +1)
Osteopenia:	BMD reduced between −1 and −2.5 SD from the young adult mean (T score −1 to −2.5)
Osteoporosis:	BMD reduced by equal to or more than −2.5 SD from the young adult mean (T score −2.5 or lower)

Osteoporotic fractures

Fractures are the clinical consequences of osteoporosis. The most common sites are the wrist or Colles' fracture, the hip and the spine. Fractures have a major impact on quality of life, result in a significant economic burden and, particularly in the case of hip fractures, are associated with considerable excess mortality: mortality is about 30% in the year after a hip fracture.

Risk factors for the development of osteoporosis

The risk factors most important in clinical practice are parental history of fracture (particularly hip fracture), early menopause, chronic use of corticosteroids (oral and possibly inhaled), prolonged immobilization and prior fracture.

Risk factors for osteoporosis	
Genetic:	Family history of fracture (particularly a first degree relative with hip fracture)
Constitutional:	Low body mass index Early menopause (<45 years of age)
Environmental:	Cigarette smoking Alcohol abuse Low calcium intake Sedentary life style
Drugs:	Corticosteroids, >5 mg/day prednisolone or equivalent
Diseases:	Rheumatoid arthritis Neuromuscular disease Chronic liver disease Malabsorption syndromes Hyperparathyroidism Hyperthyroidism Hypogonadism

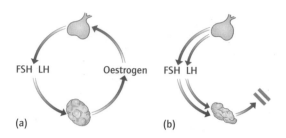

Fig. 13.4 Ovarian responsiveness to pituitary hormones. (a) Reproductive years: feedback control between ovary and hypothalamic–pituitary axis. (b) Postmenopausal years: unresponsive ovaries produce no oestrogen or inhibin. Lack of feedback on hypothalamus–pituitary axis causes high levels of follicle-stimulating hormone (FSH) and luteinizing hormone (LH).

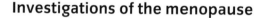

Investigations of the menopause

Follicle-stimulating hormone

Follicle-stimulating hormone (FSH) levels give an estimate of the degree of ovarian reserve remaining (Fig. 13.4). Increased FSH levels suggest fewer oocytes remaining in the ovaries. Levels are helpful with suspected *premature ovarian failure*, but in women over the age of 45 who are having hot flushes is pointless as the diagnosis is usually clear. FSH levels vary markedly on a daily basis during the perimenopause and levels are not a guide to fertility status or when the last period is likely to occur.

FSH levels can be measured in women whether or not they have had a hysterectomy. If not, they are best measured between days 2 and 5 of the cycle (day 1 is the first day of menstruation) in order to avoid the mid-cycle preovulatory increase and the luteal phase suppression of FSH. In women with oligomenorrhoea or amenorrhoea or who have undergone hysterectomy two samples separated by an interval of 2 weeks should be obtained. FSH levels are of little value in monitoring HRT.

Luteinizing hormone, oestradiol and progesterone

Measuring these hormones is of no value in diagnosing ovarian failure. Oestradiol is naturally low early in the menstrual cycle in women with normal ovarian function. A low progesterone level indicates anovulation which can be secondary to many causes, most commonly polycystic ovary syndrome (PCOS).

Thyroid function tests (free T4 and thyroid-stimulating hormone)

Thyroid disease can cause hot flushes. Therefore thyroid function tests should be checked in women with an inadequate symptomatic response to HRT.

Catecholamines and 5-hydroxyindolacetic acid

Twenty-four hour urine levels of catecholamines and 5-hydroxyindolacetic acid are used to diagnose phaeochromocytoma and carcinoid syndrome, respectively. Both are rare cause of hot flushes.

Bone density estimation

Population screening is of little value and it is best to target women at risk of osteoporosis (see box above).

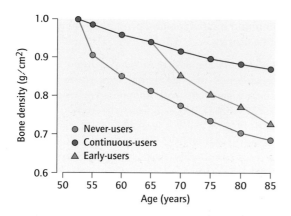

Fig. 13.5 Bone density in oestrogen users and non-users.

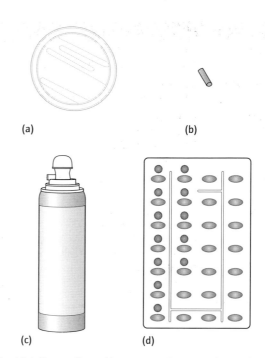

Fig. 13.6 Preparations of hormone replacement therapy (HRT): (a) patch, (b) implant, (c) gel and (d) pills.

The main sites for measurement are the lumbar spine and the hip. Since the spine may have falsely increased values due to osteophytes from osteoarthritis, kyphosis, scoliosis and aortic calcification, the best site to measure is the hip. Bone density changes slowly and the frequency of follow-up scans is controversial. Initially, follow-up scans may be undertaken at 2 years to assess response to treatment and, in general, should not be done more frequently than every 3 years thereafter.

Dual energy X-ray absorptometry (DEXA) is an X-ray based system that uses two different energies to differentiate between soft tissue and bone. Values for BMD may be quoted as g/cm^2 (Fig. 13.5) or converted into values that relate to either the average female (or male) peak bone mass (T score) or that of the patient's age group (Z score).

Biochemical markers of bone metabolism

Biochemical markers of bone turnover are classified as markers of resorption or formation. Biochemical markers of bone turnover can be used to monitor response to therapy such as bisphosphonates (see below) because significant suppression of bone turnover occurs far more rapidly than detectable changes in bone mineral density. Significant changes can occur within 3–6 months of initiation of therapy. Bone markers are not used to diagnose osteoporosis.

Treatment: Hormone replacement therapy

HRT consists of oestrogen alone in women who have had a hysterectomy but is combined with a progestogen in those who have not. Progestogens are given cyclically or continuously with the oestrogen. Systemic oestrogens can be delivered orally, transdermally (patch or gel) or subcutaneously (implant) (Fig. 13.6). Topical oestrogens are given vaginally. Progestogens can be delivered orally, transdermally (patch) or directly into the uterus (intrauterine system [IUS]). Many preparations are available with different combinations, strengths and routes of administration. Regimens may vary between countries.

Oestrogens

Two types of oestrogen are available: synthetic and natural. Natural oestrogens include oestradiol, oestrone and oestriol. These are synthesized from soya beans or yams and are chemically identical to the natural human hormones. Conjugated equine oestrogens are derived from pregnant mares' urine. Synthetic oestrogens, such as ethinyl oestradiol used in the combined oral contraceptive pill, are not used for HRT because of their greater metabolic impact.

Progestogens

The progestogens used in HRT, such as levonorgestrel and norethisterone, are also derived from plant sources such as soya beans or yams. The levonorgesterone intrauterine system (Mirena IUS) delivers 20 μg/day. This method of delivery also provides a solution to the problem of contraception in the perimenopause and is also the only way in which a 'no bleed' HRT regimen can be achieved in perimenopausal women.

Tibolone

Tibolone is a synthetic steroid compound that itself is inert but is converted *in vivo* to metabolites with oestrogenic, progestogenic and androgenic actions. It is used in postmenopausal women who wish to have amenorrhoea and treats vasomotor, psychological and libido problems. The daily dose is 2.5 mg. It conserves bone mass, and reduces the risk of vertebral fracture.

Androgens

Testosterone can be administered either as a patch or a subcutaneous implant. It can be used to improve libido but is not successful in all women, as other factors, such as marital problems, may be involved.

Regimens of HRT

Oestrogen alone: women after hysterectomy

These women should be given oestrogen alone and have no need for a progestogen. There may be concerns about a remnant of endometrium in the cervical stump in women who have had a subtotal hysterectomy. If this is suspected, the presence or absence of bleeding induced by monthly sequential HRT may be a useful diagnostic test.

Combined oestrogen and progestogen: women with a uterus

Progestogens are added to oestrogens to reduce the increased risk of endometrial hyperplasia and carcinoma, which occurs with unopposed oestrogen (*NEJM* 1975; **293**: 1164). Progestogen can be given 'sequentially' for 10–14 days every 4 weeks or for 14 days every 13 weeks, or it can be used 'continuously': every day. The first leads to monthly bleeds, the second to 3-monthly bleeds and the last aims to achieve amenorrhoea and is called 'no-bleed' or 'continuous combined' HRT. Progestogen must still be given to women who have undergone endometrial ablative techniques for menorrhagia such as transcervical resection of endometrium (TCRE), as not all the endometrium may have been removed.

Menopausal status: perimenopausal women

Women receiving HRT who are still menstruating or are within 12 months of their last spontaneous menstrual period can be given sequential or cyclic therapy. Alternatively, intrauterine levonorgestrel can be given: this is useful in women with heavy menstrual bleeding or needing contraception.

Menopausal status: postmenopausal women

Women are considered to be postmenopausal 12 months after their last menstrual period, although this definition is difficult to apply in clinical practice (e.g. especially in women who started HRT in the perimenopause). Continuous combined regimens should be used in these women because of the lack of induced bleeding and because it may have a reduced risk of endometrial cancer compared with sequential regimens. Continuous combined therapy induces endometrial atrophy. Intrauterine delivery of levonorgestrel can be continued but it may be technically more difficult to insert the intrauterine device in older women.

Topical oestrogens

These are used to treat urogenital symptoms. The options available are vaginally administered low-dose natural oestrogens, such as oestriol by cream or pessary, or oestradiol by tablet or ring. Long-term treatment is required since symptoms return on cessation of therapy. These low-dose preparations have not been shown to elevate systemic oestrogen levels significantly, so additional progestogen to protect the endometrium is not required.

Benefits, risks and uncertainties of oestrogen-based HRT

Benefits

Menopausal symptoms: Oestrogen is effective in treating hot flushes: improvement is usually noted within 4 weeks. Relief of hot flushes is the most common indication for HRT and is often used for less than 5 years. Vaginal dryness, soreness, superficial dyspareunia, urinary frequency and urgency respond well to oestrogens, which may be given either topically or systemically. Sexuality may be improved with oestrogen alone but may need testosterone in addition, especially in young oöphorectomized women. This can be given either by patches or implants.

Osteoporosis: HRT reduces the risk of both spine and hip as well as other osteoporotic fractures.

Colorectal cancer: HRT reduces the risk of colorectal cancer by about one-third. However, little is known about colorectal cancer risk when treatment is stopped. There is no information about HRT in high-risk populations and current data do not allow prevention as a recommendation.

Risks

Breast cancer: HRT slightly increases the risk. This equates to 2 extra breast cancers per 1000 women who use HRT from the age of 50 for 5 years. Such an effect is not seen in women who start HRT early for a premature menopause indicating that it is the duration of lifetime sex hormone exposure that is relevant. The increased breast cancer risk is not seen with oestrogen-alone regimes: it is the addition of progestogen that is the problem. However, this has to be balanced against the reduction in risk of endometrial cancer provided by combined therapy. Breast cancer risk falls on stopping therapy, the risk being no greater than that in women who have never taken HRT after 5 years.

Endometrial cancer: Unopposed oestrogen replacement therapy increases endometrial cancer risk. This is why a progestogen is added to regimens for non-hysterectomized women to reduce this risk.

Venous thromboembolism: HRT increases risk of venous thromboembolism (VTE) twofold from a background (not taking HRT) risk of 1.7 per 1000 in women over 50, with the highest risk occurring in the first year of use. Advancing age, obesity and an underlying thrombophilia significantly increase the risk.

Gallbladder disease: HRT increases the risk of gallbladder disease. However, gallbladder disease increases with ageing and with obesity.

Uncertainties

Cardiovascular disease (coronary heart disease and stroke): The role of HRT either in primary or secondary prevention remains uncertain and currently should not be used primarily for this indication. However, the timing, dose and possibly type of HRT (tablets or patches) may be critical in determining cardiovascular effects.

Dementia and cognition: While oestrogen may delay or reduce the risk of Alzheimer's disease (AD), it does not seem to improve established disease. It is unclear whether there is a critical age or duration of treatment for exposure to oestrogen to have an effect in prevention, but there may be a window of opportunity in the early postmenopause when the pathological processes that lead to AD (and cardiovascular disease) are being initiated and when HRT may have a preventive effect.

Ovarian cancer: The evidence is conflicting, with some studies showing an increased risk and others not. If there is an increased risk it is very small and only after long durations of use such as greater than 10 years.

Quality of life: The evidence is conflicting. While some studies have shown improvement in both symptomatic and asymptomatic women, others have not.

Duration of therapy

Menopausal symptoms: Treatment can be continued for up to 5 years and then stopped to evaluate whether symptoms recur with sufficient severity to warrant continuation.

Osteoporosis: Treatment may need to be lifelong. Bone mineral density falls when treatments are stopped (Fig. 13.5). Younger women commencing treatment with HRT may wish to change to other agents, such as bisphosphonates or raloxifene, because of the increased risk of breast cancer with longer-term combined HRT.

Premature menopause: Women are usually advised to continue with HRT until the median age of the natural menopause (i.e. 52 years).

Other treatments for the menopause

Non-oestrogen-based therapy

These should be considered for women who do not wish to take HRT or have a contraindication to therapy.

Hot flushes and night sweats

Progestogens such as 5 mg/day norethisterone or 40 mg/day megestrol acetate can be effective.
Clonidine is a centrally acting alpha-adrenoceptor agonist originally developed as an antihypertensive but is of limited value.
Selective serotonin reuptake inhibitors (SSRIs) and serotonin and noradrenaline reuptake inhibitors, such as paroxetine, fluoxetine, citalopram and venlafaxine, are effective in treating hot flushes in short-term studies.
Gabapentin is used to treat epilepsy, neuropathic pain and migraine. Limited evidence shows that it may be effective.

Vaginal atrophy

A variety of lubricants and moisturizers are available without prescription but tend to be less effective than oestrogen.

Prevention and treatment of osteoporosis

All pharmacological interventions except for parathyroid hormone and strontium ranelate act mainly by inhibiting bone resorption. Most of the studies have been undertaken in postmenopausal women with osteoporosis or at increased risk of the disease, and information on their use by perimenopausal women or those with premature ovarian failure is scant.
Bisphosphonates, such as alendronate, risedronate and ibandronate, are used in the prevention and treatment of osteoporosis. All bisphosphonates are absorbed poorly from the gastrointestinal tract and must be given on an empty stomach. The principal side effect of all bisphos-phonates is irritation of the upper gastrointestinal tract. Symptoms resolve quickly after drug withdrawal and are reduced by using weekly or monthly rather than daily administration. Bisphosphonates remain in bone for many years, may affect the fetal skeleton and are not advised in women with fertility aspirations.
Strontium ranelate decreases the risk of vertebral and hip fractures. It is administered daily, dissolved in water; it should be taken at least 2 h after food. The most common side effects are mild and transient nausea and diarrhoea but these are rare in absolute terms.
Raloxifene, a selective oestrogen receptor modulator, is licensed for the prevention of osteoporosis-related vertebral fracture. It reduces the incidence of vertebral fracture by 30–50%, depending on the dose, in women with established osteoporosis.
Parathyroid hormone peptides reduce the risk of vertebral but not hip fractures and are given by subcutaneous injection. Because they cost more than other options, they are reserved for patients with severe osteoporosis who are unable to tolerate or seem to be unresponsive to other treatments.
Calcium and vitamin D supplements may be relevant when evidence of insufficiency exists, especially in the elderly. Most studies show that about 1.5 g/day of elemental calcium is necessary to preserve bone health in postmenopausal women and elderly women who are not taking HRT. In women who use HRT, 1 g/day is sufficient to maintain calcium balance. The effects on fracture of calcium and vitamin D supplements, alone or in combination, however, are contradictory.

Alternative and complementary therapies

The evidence that alternative and complementary therapies improve menopausal symptoms or have the same benefits as HRT or non-oestrogen-based treatments is poor, but they are nevertheless widely used. Concerns include quality of production, interactions with other treatments and the presence, in some, of oestrogenic compounds.
Phytoestrogens are plant substances with effects similar to oestrogens. The most important groups are called isoflavones and lignans. Isoflavones are found in soya beans and chickpeas, lignans particularly in oilseeds.

Herbal remedies include black cohosh, kava kava, evening primrose, dong quai, gingko, ginseng and wild yam cream.

Progesterone transdermal creams have not been proven to be effective for menopausal symptoms or skeletal protection, and are not protective on the endometrium.

Further reading

British Menopause Society: http://www.thebms.org.uk/
PRODIGY Guidance—Menopause: http://www.prodigy.nhs.uk/guidance.asp?gt=Menopause
Rees M, Purdie DW. Management of the menopause. *The Handbook.* Royal Society of Medicine Press. London, 2006.

The Menopause at a Glance

Definition	The last menstrual period
Median age	52 years. Premature if <40 years
Perimenopause	Time preceding menopause, menstruation often erratic
Features	Early changes: Hot flushes, insomnia, psychological Later changes: Skin and breast atrophy, hair loss, atrophic vaginitis, prolapse, urinary symptoms, osteoporosis, cardiovascular disease
Investigations	Follicle-stimulating hormone (FSH) raised, but may be normal initially
Treatment	Not mandatory or universal. Consider hormone replacement therapy (HRT) to alleviate symptoms and prevent osteoporosis (or bisphosphonates), but beware of risks

Hormone Replacement Therapy (HRT) at a Glance

Definition	Use of exogenous oestrogens when endogenous secretion is absent
Preparations	Progesterone used with oestrogen or as synthetic combination (oestrogen alone if patient has had hysterectomy) Oral, patch, gel, implant, spray or vaginal ring
Advantages	Short-term relief from menopausal symptoms May regulate erratic bleeding during perimenopause Protects against and partly reverses osteoporosis Reduces urinary symptoms; improved skin and hair appearance Reduces risk of bowel carcinoma
Disadvantages	Menstruation unless 'period-free' preparation Oestrogenic and progestogenic side effects Increased risk of breast cancer (with progestogen HRT) and venous thromboembolism

Physiology of early pregnancy

The oocyte is fertilized in the ampulla of the fallopian tube to form a zygote. Mitotic division occurs as the zygote is swept toward the uterus by ciliary action and peristalsis (Fig. 14.1a). Tubal damage will impair movement and render tubal implantation and ectopic pregnancy more likely. The zygote normally enters the uterus on day 4, at the eight-cell (morula) stage. The morula becomes a blastocyst by developing a fluid-filled cavity within. Its outer layer becomes trophoblast, which will form the placenta, and from the sixth to twelfth day, this invades the endometrium to achieve implantation (Fig. 14.1b). Fifteen per cent of embryos are lost at this stage though this is too early to be considered a miscarriage.

The trophoblast produces hormones almost immediately, notably human chorionic gonadotrophin (hCG) (detected in pregnancy tests), which will peak at 12 weeks. This ability to invade and produce hCG is reflected in gestational trophoblastic disease. Nutrients are gained from the secretory endometrium, which turns deciduous (rich in glycogen and lipids) under the influence of oestrogen and progesterone from the corpus luteum which is maintained by hCG from the trophoblast. Trophoblastic proliferation leads to formation of chorionic villi. On the endometrial surface of the embryo, this villous system proliferates (chorion frondosum) and will ultimately form the surface area for nutrient transfer, in the cotyledons of the placenta. Placental morphology is complete at 12 weeks. A heartbeat is established at 4–5 weeks and is visible on ultrasound a week later.

Obstetrics and Gynaecology, 3rd edition. By Lawrence Impey and Tim Child. Published 2008 by Blackwell Publishing, ISBN: 978-1-4051-6095-7.

Spontaneous miscarriage

Definition and epidemiology

The fetus dies or delivers dead before 24 completed weeks of pregnancy. The majority occur before 12 weeks. Fifteen per cent of clinically recognized pregnancies spontaneously miscarry; more will be so early as to go unrecognized. The rate of miscarriage increases with maternal age (Fig. 14.2).

Types of miscarriage

Threatened miscarriage: There is bleeding but the fetus is still alive, the uterus is the size expected from the dates and the os is closed (Fig. 14.3a). Only 25% will go on to miscarry.

Inevitable miscarriage: Bleeding is usually heavier. Although the fetus may still be alive, the cervical os is open. Miscarriage is about to occur.

Incomplete miscarriage: Some fetal parts have been passed, but the os is usually open (Fig. 14.3b).

Complete miscarriage: All fetal tissue has been passed. Bleeding has diminished, the uterus is no longer enlarged and the cervical os is closed.

Septic miscarriage: The contents of the uterus are infected, causing endometritis [→ p.74]. Vaginal loss is offensive and the uterus is tender. A fever can be absent. If pelvic infection occurs there is abdominal pain and peritonism.

Missed miscarriage: The fetus has not developed or died *in utero*, but this is not recognized until bleeding occurs or ultrasound scan is performed. The uterus is smaller than expected from the dates and the os is closed (Fig. 14.3c).

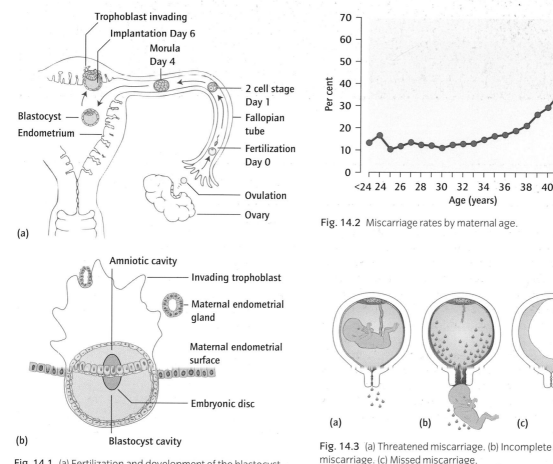

Fig. 14.1 (a) Fertilization and development of the blastocyst. (b) Implantation: day 6.

Fig. 14.2 Miscarriage rates by maternal age.

Fig. 14.3 (a) Threatened miscarriage. (b) Incomplete miscarriage. (c) Missed miscarriage.

Aetiology of sporadic miscarriage

Isolated non-recurring chromosomal abnormalities account for >60% of 'one-off' or sporadic miscarriages. However, if three or more miscarriages occur, then the rarer causes are more likely [→ p.117]. Exercise, intercourse and emotional trauma do not cause miscarriage.

Clinical features

History: Bleeding is usual unless a missed miscarriage is found incidentally at ultrasound examination. Pain from uterine contractions can cause confusion with an ectopic pregnancy.

Examination: Uterine size and the state of the cervical os are dependent on the type of miscarriage. Tenderness is unusual. Speculum examination may not be necessary following bimanual examination.

Investigations

Early pregnancy assessment units (EPAU) should be available at least 5 days per week and easily accessible by GPs. EPAU's streamline management, reduce costs and numbers and duration of admissions. A history is taken, examination performed, and *urine pregnancy test, ultrasound scan* and *blood tests* performed as indicated. An *ultrasound scan* will show if a fetus is in the uterus and if it is viable (Fig. 14.4), and it may detect retained fetal

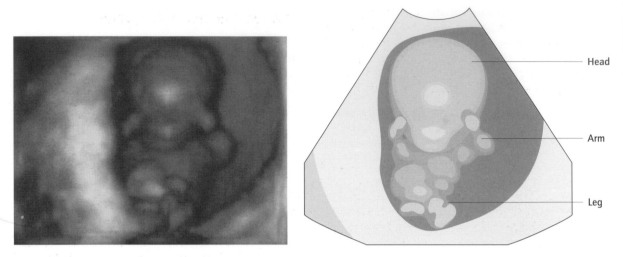

Fig. 14.4 Three-dimensional image of live fetus at 11 weeks' gestation.

tissue (products). If there is any doubt, the scan should be repeated a week later as non-viable pregnancies can be confused with a very early pregnancy, especially where the date of the last menstrual period is uncertain or periods irregular. Ultrasound does not always allow visualization of an ectopic pregnancy, but if a fetus is seen in the uterus, coexistent ectopic pregnancy (hetero-topic pregnancy) is extremely unlikely unless concep-tion followed *in vitro* fertilization (IVF) treatment with the replacement of multiple embryos. *HCG* levels in the blood normally increase by >66% in 48 h with a viable intrauterine pregnancy. This helps differentiate between ectopic and viable intrauterine pregnancies when no intrauterine gestation sac is visible on scan. The *full blood count* (FBC) and *rhesus group* should also be checked.

Management

Admission is necessary if ectopic pregnancy is suspected, if the miscarriage is inevitable or septic, or if the patient's social circumstances warrant it.
Resuscitation is occasionally required as bleeding can be heavy. Products of conception in the cervical os cause pain, bleeding and vasovagal shock and are removed via a speculum using polyp forceps. Intramuscular *ergomet-rine* will reduce bleeding by contracting the uterus, but is only used if the fetus is non-viable. If there is a fever, swabs for bacterial culture are taken and intravenous antibiotics are given. *Anti-D* is given to women who are rhesus negative if the uterus is instrumented or if there is bleeding after 12 weeks' gestation. This reduces the risk of iso-immunization leading to possible rhesus disease in future pregnancies [→ p.187].

Viable intrauterine pregnancy (threatened miscarriage)

Ninety per cent of women in whom fetal heart activity is detected at 8 weeks will not miscarry. Bed rest or hormone treatment with progesterone or hCG do not prevent miscarriage.

Non-viable intrauterine pregnancy

Options include *expectant*, *medical* or *surgical manage-ment* (*BMJ* 2006; **332**: 1235–40).
Expectant management can be continued as long as the woman is willing and there are no signs of infection. Success of expectant management increases with length of follow-up. It is successful within 2–6 weeks in >80% of women with incomplete miscarriage and in 30–70% of women with missed miscarriage. A large intact sac is associated with lower success rates.
Medical management is with prostaglandin (oral, sub-lingual or vaginal) sometimes preceded by the oral antiprogesterone mifepristone. Medical management is successful in >80% of women with incomplete miscar-riage (similar to expectant management) and 40–90% of women with missed miscarriage.

Surgical management: Evacuation of retained products of conception (ERPC) under anaesthetic using vacuum aspiration. Evacuation is suitable if the woman prefers it, if there is heavy bleeding, or signs of infection (perform under antibiotic cover). Success rates are >95% for both incomplete and missed miscarriage. Tissue is examined histologically to exclude molar pregnancy.

Complications

Vaginal bleeding with *expectant* or *medical* management can be heavy and painful so women must have 24 h direct access to an emergency gynaecological service for advice/treatment. Risks of *expectant* and *medical* management include the need for surgical evacuation (10–40%). Infection rates are similar (3%) between *expectant, medical or surgical* management. If infection becomes systemic, endotoxic shock occasionally ensues, with hypotension, renal failure, adult respiratory distress syndrome and disseminated intravascular coagulation. Surgical evacuation can partially remove the endometrium causing Asherman's syndrome [→ p.17] or perforate the uterus (<1%). Long-term conception rates do not differ between the management options. Surgical management is more expensive.

Counselling after miscarriage

Patients should be told that the miscarriage was not the result of anything they did or did not do and could not have been prevented. Reassurance as to the high chance of successful further pregnancies is important. Referral to a support group may be useful (www.miscarriageas-sociation.org.uk). Because miscarriage is so common, further investigation is usually reserved for women who have had three miscarriages.

Recurrent miscarriage

Definition and epidemiology

Recurrent miscarriage is when three or more miscarriages occur in succession; 1% of couples are affected. The chance of miscarriage in a fourth pregnancy is still only 40%, but a recurring cause is more likely and investigations and support should be arranged (*Lancet* 2006; **368**: 601).

Causes and their management

Whilst investigation may reveal a possible cause, few treatments are of proven value. These patients are often extremely distressed and support is vital. Serial ultrasound scans are used in early pregnancy for reassurance. In later pregnancy, 'high-risk' monitoring is important because late pregnancy complications are more common.

Antiphospholipid antibodies can cause recurrent miscarriage (*Lancet* 2003; **361**: 901). Thrombosis in the utero-placental circulation is likely to be the mechanism. Treatment is with aspirin and low-dose low molecular weight heparin.

Chromosomal defects are found in 4% of couples. Parental karyotyping is therefore necessary and translocations may be found leading to chromosomally imbalanced sperm or oocytes.

Anatomical factors: Uterine abnormalities are diagnosed with ultrasound or hysterosalpingogram. They are more common with late miscarriage. Many, however, are incidental findings and surgical treatment could lead to uterine weakness or adhesion formation. Cervical incompetence [→ p.192] is a recurrent cause of late (>16 weeks) miscarriage as well as preterm labour.

Infection: This is not a cause of recurrent early miscarriage but is implicated in preterm labour and late (>16 week) miscarriage, where treatment of bacterial vaginosis reduces the incidence of fetal loss [→ p.193].

Others: Obesity, smoking, PCOS and higher maternal age have been implicated.

Investigation of recurrent miscarriage
Antiphospholipid antibody screen (repeat at 6 weeks if positive)
Karyotyping of both parents
Pelvic ultrasound

Unwanted pregnancy and therapeutic abortion

Definition

Induced abortion or termination of pregnancy (TOP) is a very common gynaecological procedure. The World Health Organization (WHO) estimates that about 25%

of all pregnancies end in an induced abortion: approximately 50 million world-wide. Legislation about abortion varies throughout the world, can vary within different states of an individual country and is illegal in some countries. The upper time limit for legal induced abortion also varies. In countries where abortion is legal, the large majority of abortions (typically >90%) occur before the end of 12 weeks' gestation. The statutory grounds for termination of pregnancy in England are detailed in the box. The legal time limit for abortion is 24 weeks for clauses C and D. However, abortions after 24 weeks are allowed if there is grave risk to the life of the woman, evidence of severe fetal abnormality or risk of grave physical and mental injury to the woman.

Statutory grounds for termination of pregnancy in England

A The continuance of the pregnancy would involve risk to the life of the pregnant woman greater than if the pregnancy were terminated

B The termination is necessary to prevent grave permanent injury to the physical or mental health of the pregnant woman

C The pregnancy has *not* exceeded its 24th week and that the continuance of the pregnancy would involve risk, greater than if the pregnancy were terminated, of injury to the physical or mental health of the pregnant woman

D The pregnancy has *not* exceeded its 24th week and that the continuance of the pregnancy would involve risk, greater than if the pregnancy were terminated, of injury to the physical or mental health of any existing child(ren) of the family of the pregnant woman

E There is a substantial risk that if the child were born it would suffer from such physical or mental abnormalities as to be seriously handicapped

---

Methods of abortion

The method of TOP available depends on the gestation of the pregnancy and the woman's choice. The procedures offered also vary from one centre to another. Blood tests should be taken for haemoglobin, blood group and rhesus status and testing for haemoglobinopathies as indicated. Rhesus negative women should receive anti-D within 72 h of TOP. Women are usually screened for *Chlamydia*. Contraception should be discussed at the initial consultation. It can be administered at the time of surgical TOP and most methods can be safely used following medical TOP, either initiated on the day of misoprostol administration (oral pills, condoms, injectables, implants) or following the next menstrual cycle (intra-uterine device or sterilization).

Surgical methods

Suction curettage is usually used between 7 and 13 weeks. Before 7 weeks, failure rates are higher than with medical abortion. Above 13 weeks, surgical abortion by *dilatation and evacuation* (D&E), preceded by cervical preparation, is safe and effective when undertaken by appropriately skilled, experienced practitioners but medical methods are usually employed. Antibiotic cover is used for surgical abortion.

Medical methods

The antiprogesterone *mifepristone*, plus *prostaglandin* (misoprostol or gemeprost, prostaglandin E1 analogues) 36–48 h later, is the most effective method of abortion at gestations of less than 7 weeks and is also used in the 7–9 weeks' gestation band. For mid-trimester abortion (13–24 weeks' gestation) medical abortion with mifepristone followed by prostaglandin is usual. Beyond 22 weeks, feticide is performed first to prevent live birth, using KCl into the umbilical vein or fetal heart. Such later terminations are usually only performed where a fetal abnormality is present.

Selective abortion

This is occasionally performed with high-order multiple pregnancies [→ p.221] to reduce the risk, particularly, of preterm birth, or where a fetus of a multiple pregnancy is abnormal [→ p.221].

Complications of therapeutic abortion

Complications of TOP include haemorrhage (1 in 1000 overall, greater risk with later gestations), infection (up to 10% of cases and reduced by screening and prophylactic antibiotics), uterine perforation (1–4 in 1000), cervical trauma at the time of surgical abortion (no greater than 1 in 100) and failure (2.3 with 1000 surgical and 1–14 with 1000 medical abortion depending on the regimen used and the experience of the centre). Induced abortion is not associated with an increased risk in breast cancer. There are no proven associations between induced abortion and subsequent ectopic pregnancy, placenta praevia or infertility. Psychological sequelae are common but may also reflect underlying problems before the termination.

'Unsafe abortion' is defined as a procedure for terminating an unwanted pregnancy either by persons lacking the necessary skills or in an environment lacking the minimal medical standards or both. Unsafe abortion accounts for approximately 70 000 deaths worldwide per annum (www.who.int/reproductive-health/unsafe_abortion/index.html).

Ectopic pregnancy

Definition and epidemiology

An ectopic pregnancy is when the embryo implants outside the uterine cavity and occurs in 1 in 60–100 pregnancies. Three to four women die per year in the UK due to ruptured ectopic pregnancy and it is the fifth most common cause of maternal death. The mortality rate per ectopic pregnancy is 1 in 2000 (www.cemach.org.uk/publications). It is more common with advanced maternal age and lower socioeconomic class.

Pathology and sites of ectopic pregnancy

The most common site is in the fallopian tube (95%), although implantation can occur in the cornu, the cervix, the ovary and the abdominal cavity (Fig. 14.5). The thin-walled tube is unable to sustain trophoblastic invasion: it bleeds into its lumen or may rupture, when intraperito-

neal blood loss can be catastrophic. The ectopic can also be naturally aborted either within the tube or extruded through the fimbrial end.

Aetiology

No cause is evident with many, but any factor which damages the tube can cause the fertilized oocyte to be caught. Commonly, this is pelvic inflammatory disease, usually from sexually transmitted infection [→ p.75]. Assisted conception and pelvic, particularly tubal, surgery are additional risks as is having had a previous ectopic and being a smoker. An ectopic pregnancy must be urgently excluded in a woman who conceives despite having a copper-IUD in place (the coil prevents most intrauterine pregnancies but not those destined to implant in the tube).

Clinical features

The diagnosis is often missed. Abnormal vaginal bleeding, abdominal pain or collapse in any woman of reproductive age should all arouse suspicion and a urine pregnancy test should be performed. Increasing numbers of women are now diagnosed early and when asymptomatic, because of routine ultrasound.

History: Usually, lower abdominal pain is followed by scanty, dark vaginal bleeding. One may, however, be present without the other. The pain is variable in quality, often initially colicky as the tube tries to extrude the sac and then constant. Syncopal episodes and shoulder-tip pain suggest intraperitoneal blood loss. The 'classic' presentation of collapse with abdominal pain accounts for <25%. Amenorrhoea of 4–10 weeks is usual, but the patient may be unaware that she is pregnant and may interpret a vaginal bleed as a period.

Examination: Tachycardia suggests blood loss, and hypotension and collapse occur only *in extremis*. There is usually abdominal and often rebound tenderness. On pelvic examination, movement of the uterus may cause pain (cervical excitation) and either adnexum may be tender. The uterus is smaller than expected from the gestation and the cervical os is closed.

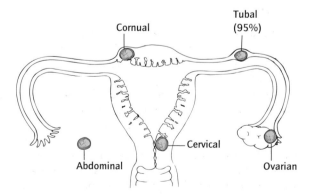

Cornual

Tubal (95%)

Abdominal

Cervical

Ovarian

Fig. 14.5 Sites of ectopic pregnancy.

Investigations

A pregnancy test (urine hCG) *must* be performed on all

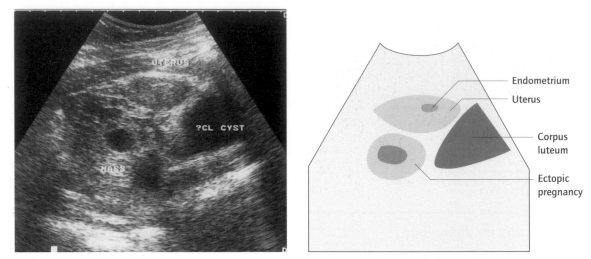

Fig. 14.6. Ultrasound of ectopic pregnancy. It is unusual to visualize the ectopic pregnancy with ultrasound.

women of reproductive age who present with pain, bleeding or collapse whatever the medical specialty to which the woman presents. It is almost always invariably positive with an ectopic pregnancy. Modern urine pregnancy tests are very sensitive and are positive even before the day of the missed period.

Ultrasound (preferably transvaginal) does not always visualize an ectopic pregnancy (Fig. 14.6), but it should detect an intrauterine pregnancy. If the latter is not present, the gestation is either too early (<5 weeks) or there has been a complete miscarriage, or the pregnancy is elsewhere, i.e. ectopic. In the adnexae a blood clot may be seen, 'free fluid' (i.e. blood), or a gestation sac with or without a fetus within. The probe may elicit tenderness.

Quantitative serum hCG is useful if the uterus is empty. If the maternal level is >1000 IU/mL then, if an intrauterine pregnancy is present, it will normally be visible on transvaginal ultrasound. If the level is lower than this, but rises by more than 66% in 48 h, an earlier but intrauterine pregnancy is likely. Declining or slower rising levels ('plateauing') suggest an ectopic or non-viable intrauterine pregnancy. Caution is still required as, particularly with assisted conception, an intrauterine and an ectopic pregnancy can occasionally coexist (heterotopic pregnancy).

Laparoscopy is the most sensitive investigation, but it is invasive. The combination of hCG and ultrasound allows for fewer 'negative' laparoscopies.

Management of the symptomatic suspected ectopic pregnancy
Nil by mouth
Full blood count (FBC) and cross-match blood
Pregnancy test
Ultrasound
Laparoscopy or consider medical management if criteria met
Intravenous access

Management

Where symptoms are present, the patient should be admitted. Intravenous access is inserted and blood is cross-matched. Anti-D is given if the patient is rhesus-negative.

Acute presentations

If the patient is haemodynamically unstable expedient resuscitation and surgery is required. Laparoscopy may be suitable for experienced operators but laparotomy is often performed. The affected tube is removed (salpingectomy) (Fig. 14.7).

Subacute presentations

Surgical management: Laparoscopy is standard and is

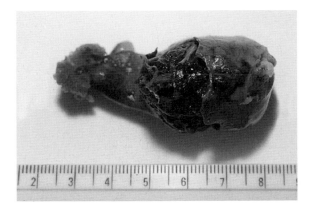

Fig. 14.7 The ectopic pregnancy (in Fig. 14.6) removed by salpingectomy.

preferable to laparotomy because recovery is faster and subsequent fertility rates are equivalent or better. At laparoscopy, the ectopic is either removed from the tube (salpingostomy) or a salpingectomy is performed. If salpingostomy is performed there is both a 10% chance that repeat surgery for persisting ectopic is required (detected by failure of serum hCG to fall on follow-up) and an increased risk of repeat ectopic since the damaged tube remains. Whether to perform a salpingostomy or salpingectomy should be discussed with the woman prior to surgery. If the contralateral tube is damaged then salpingostomy may allow for future spontaneous conception (and possibly ectopic) whereas salpingectomy will require IVF. If the contralateral tube appears normal then the subsequent intrauterine pregnancy rates are similar between salpingostomy or salpingectomy.

Medical management: If the ectopic is unruptured with no cardiac activity, and an hCG level <3000 IU/mL, systemic single-dose methotrexate can also be used, without recourse to laparoscopy. Serial hCG levels are subsequently monitored to confirm that all trophoblastic tissue has gone: a second dose (15% of women) or surgery (10%) may be required. Outcomes with systemic methotrexate are equivalent to laparoscopic salpingostomy (*Cochrane* 2007: CD000324).

Conservative management: If the ectopic is small and unruptured, or if the location of the pregnancy is not clear (not visualized in the uterus or adnexae) and hCG levels are low (<1000 IU/mL) and declining, careful observation may suffice as rupture is unlikely.

Complications

Women treated with salpingostomy or medical or conservative management must have serial hCG measurements until <20 IU/mL to confirm ectopic resolution. They must have clear information on warning signs and be within easy access to the hospital treating them. Particular support must be given to patients with ectopic pregnancy, who have not only 'lost their baby' through a life-threatening condition but have also undergone surgery and had their fertility reduced. Seventy per cent of women will subsequently have a successful pregnancy and up to 10% will have another ectopic pregnancy. Patient support groups are useful (www.ectopic.org.uk).

Hyperemesis gravidarum

Definition and epidemiology

Hyperemesis gravidarum is when nausea and vomiting in early pregnancy are so severe as to cause severe dehydration, weight loss or electrolyte disturbance. This occurs in only 1 in 750 women. However, vomiting in pregnancy is a common cause of hospital admission, but most patients are only mildly dehydrated and therefore have 'moderate' nausea and vomiting of pregnancy (NVP). It seldom persists beyond 14 weeks and is more common in multiparous women.

Nausea and vomiting of pregnancy (NVP)	
Mild NVP	Nausea and occasional morning vomiting 50% of pregnant women No treatment required
Moderate NVP	More persistent vomiting 5% of pregnant women Often admitted to hospital
Severe NVP	Hyperemesis gravidarum

Management

Predisposing conditions, particularly urinary infection and multiple or molar pregnancy, are excluded. Intravenous rehydration is given, with antiemetics and thia-

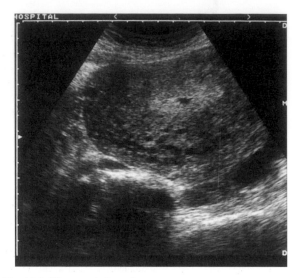
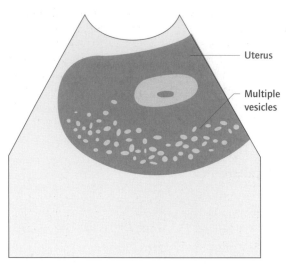

Uterus

Multiple
vesicles

Fig. 14.8 Ultrasound of a molar pregnancy.

mine (to prevent neurological complications of vitamin depletion such as Wernicke's encephalopathy). Steroids have been used in severe cases. Psychological support is essential, particularly as many of these women have social or emotional problems.

Gestational trophoblastic neoplasia

Definitions, pathology and epidemiology

In this, trophoblastic tissue, which is the part of the blastocyst that normally invades the endometrium, proliferates in a more aggressive way than is normal. HCG is usually secreted in excess. Proliferation can be localized and non-invasive: this is called a *hydatidiform mole*. *Hydatidiform mole* can be subdivided into *complete* and *partial* mole based on genetic and histopathological features. A *complete mole* is entirely paternal in origin, usually when one sperm fertilizes an empty oocyte and undergoes mitosis. The result is diploid tissue, usually 46 XX. There is no fetal tissue, merely a proliferation of swollen chorionic villi. A *partial mole* is usually triploid, derived from two sperms entering one oocyte. There is variable evidence of a fetus.

Alternatively, the proliferation may have characteristics of malignant tissue: if invasion is only present locally within the uterus, this is an *invasive mole*; if metastasis occurs, it is a *choriocarcinoma*. Molar pregnancy is uncommon, accounting for 1 in 500–1000 pregnancies, and is more common at the extremes of reproductive age and in Asians.

Clinical features

History: Vaginal bleeding is usual and may be heavy. Severe vomiting may occur. The condition may be detected on routine ultrasound.
Examination: The uterus is often large. Early pre-eclampsia and hyperthyroidism may occur.

Investigations

Ultrasound characteristically shows a 'snowstorm' appearance of the swollen villi with *complete moles* (Fig. 14.8), but the diagnosis can only be confirmed histologically. Serum hCG levels may be very high.

Management and follow-up

The trophoblastic tissue is removed by suction curettage (ERPC) and the diagnosis confirmed histologically.

Bleeding is often heavy. Thereafter, serial blood or urine hCG levels are taken: persistent or rising levels are suggestive of malignancy. Women with a molar pregnancy should be registered with a supraregional centre (London, Sheffield and Dundee) who will guide management and follow-up. Pregnancy and the combined oral contraceptive are avoided until hCG levels are normal because they may increase the need for chemotherapy.

Complications

Recurrence of molar pregnancy occurs in about 1 in 60 subsequent pregnancies (*BJOG* 2003; **110**: 22). After every future pregnancy further hCG samples are required to exclude disease recurrence.

Malignant trophoblastic disease, as an *invasive mole* or *choriocarcinoma*, follows 15% of *complete moles* and 0.5% of *partial moles*. However, molar pregnancy precedes only 50% of malignancies, because malignancy can also follow miscarriages and normal pregnancies, usually presenting as persistent vaginal bleeding. The diagnosis of malignancy is made from persistently elevated or rising hCG levels, persistent vaginal bleeding or evidence of blood-borne metastasis, commonly to the lungs. The tumour is highly malignant, but is normally very sensitive to chemotherapy.

Patients are scored into 'low-risk' and 'high-risk' categories according to prognostic variables. Low-risk patients receive methotrexate with folic acid, whereas higher risk patients receive combination chemotherapy. Five-year survival rates approach 100%.

Further reading

Rai R, Regan L. Recurrent miscarriage. *Lancet* 2006; **368**: 601–11.

Royal College of Obstetricians and Gynaecologists. The investigation and treatment of couples with recurrent miscarriage. RCOG Guideline No. 17(B). 2003. http://www.rcog.org.uk

Royal College of Obstetricians and Gynaecologists. The management of tubal pregnancy. RCOG Guideline No. 21. 2004. http://www.rcog.org.uk

Royal College of Obstetricians and Gynaecologists. The management of early pregnancy loss. RCOG Guideline No. 25. 2006. http://www.rcog.org.uk

Sagili H, Divers M. Modern management of miscarriage. *The Obstetrician and Gynaecologist* 2007; **9**: 102–108. http://www.rcog.org.uk/togonline

Verberg MF, Gillott DJ, Al-Fardan N, Grudzinskas JG. Hyperemesis gravidarum, a literature review. *Human Reproduction Update* 2005; **11**: 527–39.

Spontaneous Miscarriage at a Glance	
Definition	Expulsion or death of the fetus before 24 weeks
Epidemiology	15% of recognized pregnancies
Aetiology	Increasing maternal age. >50% chromosomal abnormalities, usually sporadic. Recurrent miscarriage also associated with antiphospholipid antibodies, uterine abnormalities, and parental chromosome abnormalities
Pathology	Products can be retained and cause haemorrhage and/or infection
Features	Heavy vaginal bleeding, often with pain. Cervix may be open. Little tenderness
Investigations	Ultrasound to confirm intrauterine site and fetal viability
Management	Anti-D if rhesus negative Evacuation of retained products of conception (ERPC) if heavy bleeding or infection Expectant or medical management an alternative for incomplete or missed miscarriage
Complications	Haemorrhage and infection, and of surgery

Ectopic Pregnancy at a Glance

Definition	Embryo implants outside the uterus
Epidemiology	1% + of pregnancies in UK
Aetiology	Idiopathic, tubal damage from pelvic inflammatory disease or surgery
Pathology	95% in fallopian tube. Occasionally cornu, cervix, ovary, abdomen Tubal implantation can lead to tubal rupture and intraperitoneal bleeding
Features	At 4–10 weeks of amenorrhoea Acute: Collapse with abdominal pain and bleeding, patient shocked Subacute: Abdominal pain, scanty dark per vaginum (PV) loss. Lower abdominal tenderness, cervical excitation, adnexal tenderness usual Incidental: Detected at ultrasound
Investigations	Pregnancy test and transvaginal ultrasound, human chorionic gonadotrophin (hCG) Laparoscopy to confirm and treat unless diagnosis certain and medical management proposed
Management	Surgical: To stop/prevent bleeding: salpingectomy/salpingostomy Medical: Methotrexate if criteria met
Complications	Haemorrhage can be fatal; repeat ectopic, subfertility

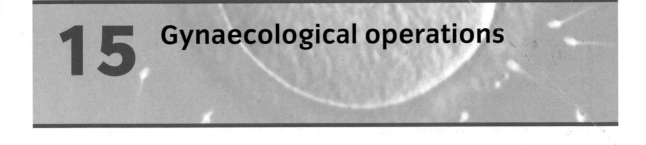

15 Gynaecological operations

There are three main routes to gain access to the pelvic organs:

1 The abdominal route involves opening the abdominal wall through a lower transverse ('Pfannenstiel') or, occasionally, a vertical mid-line incision.

2 The vaginal route is used both to inspect and operate on the inside of the uterus and for vaginal and pelvic surgery.

3 Laparoscopic surgery, using a video-monitor via a laparoscope with a camera attached; this and the instruments are inserted through small incisions ('ports') in the abdominal wall.

Endoscopy and endoscopic surgery

Diagnostic hysteroscopy

The uterine cavity is inspected with a rigid or flexible hysteroscope passed through the cervical canal. The cavity is distended using carbon dioxide or saline (Fig. 15.1). This can be performed without general anaesthesia. It is used as an adjunct to endometrial biopsy [→ p.12] or if menstrual problems do not respond to medical treatment.

Hysteroscopic surgery

An operating hysteroscope is used in which small instruments are passed down a parallel channel [→ p.14]. Using cutting diathermy and glycine irrigation fluid the endometrium (transcervical resection of endometrium [TCRE]) or intracavity fibroids (transcervical resection of fibroid [TCRF]) and polyps are removed. If a uterine septum is present this can be resected up to the fundus of

the cavity. The complications of uterine perforation and fluid overload are unusual with experienced surgeons. With TCRE and/or TCRF most patients have a significant reduction in blood loss. TCRE is best used with bleeding that is heavy but regular and not painful, in women approaching the menopause. Sterility is not ensured so sometimes a laparoscopic tubal sterilization is performed at the same time. Endometrial roller-ball diathermy, laser ablation or heating with an intrauterine hot balloon or microwave probe produce similar effects and may be safer but, because no specimen is produced, prior biopsies are essential.

Diagnostic laparoscopy

The peritoneal cavity is insufflated with carbon dioxide after carefully passing a small hollow Veress needle through the abdominal wall. This enables a sharp trocar to be inserted through the umbilicus with less risk of damaging organs or major blood vessels. A laparoscope is then passed down the trocar to enable visualization of the pelvis (Fig. 15.1). Laparoscopy is used to assess macroscopic pelvic disease in the management of pelvic pain and dysmenorrhoea, infertility (when dye is passed through the cervix to assess tubal patency: 'lap and dye'), suspected ectopic pregnancy and pelvic masses.

Laparoscopic surgery

Instruments to grasp or cut tissue are inserted through separate ports in the abdominal wall. Laparoscopic surgery is commonly performed to sterilize, to remove adhesions or areas of endometriosis, or remove an ectopic pregnancy. Virtually every gynaecological operation has now been performed laparoscopically. The advantages are better visualization of tissues, less tissue handling, less infection, reduced hospital stay and faster postoperative recovery with less pain. However, serious visceral damage has occurred in less experienced hands and/or with more complicated and extensive surgery.

Obstetrics and Gynaecology, 3rd edition. By Lawrence Impey and Tim Child. Published 2008 by Blackwell Publishing, ISBN: 978-1-4051-6095-7.

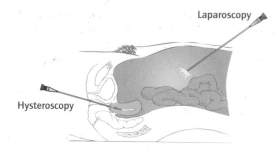

Fig. 15.1 Gynaecological endoscopy.

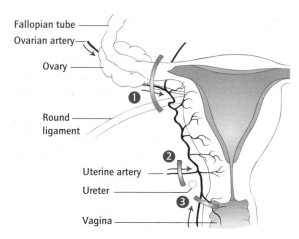

Fig. 15.2 Hysterectomy. (1) Blood: the anastomosis between uterine and ovarian arteries. If the ovaries are removed the ovarian artery and vein are ligated instead. Ligament: the round ligament. (2) Blood: the main uterine artery. Ligament: the cardinal ligament. The bladder is first dissected off the cervix and upper vagina, to prevent injury to it or to the ureters, which are close. (3) Blood: the cervico-vaginal branches of the uterine artery supplying the cervix and upper vagina. Ligament: the uterosacral ligament.

Hysterectomy

This is the most common major gynaecological operation (Fig. 15.2). The ovaries can also be removed (bilat-eral salpingo-oöphorectomy [BSO]). Hysterectomy is most commonly performed for menstrual disorders, fibroids, endometriosis, chronic pelvic inflammatory disease and prolapse; the treatment of pelvic malignancies also includes hysterectomy. Advances in medical management, e.g. of abnormal uterine bleeding (such as the intrauterine system [IUS]; [→ p.13]) should make the operation rarer and should be tried before this last resort.

Types of hysterectomy

Total abdominal hysterectomy (TAH) is removal of the uterus and cervix through an abdominal incision. The steps are performed from above, and therefore in the order 1, 2, 3 shown in Fig. 15.2. Specific indications include malignancy (ovarian and endometrial, in conjunction with a full laparotomy), a very large or immobile uterus and when abdominal inspection is required. In a subtotal hysterectomy, the cervix is retained and step 3 (Fig. 15.2) is omitted. This reduces the risk of damaging the ureters or bladder since less extensive dissection is required. However, the patient will need to continue with regular cervical smears (so it is inappropriate if there is a history of abnormal smears) and some will continue to have menstrual spotting from small amounts of endometrium remaining in the cervical canal.

Vaginal hysterectomy (VH) is removal of the cervix and uterus after incising the vagina from below, and therefore in the order 3, 2, 1 (Fig. 15.2). The vaginal vault is closed after hysterectomy is complete. The specific indication is uterine prolapse, but absence of prolapse and moderate enlargement are not contraindications in experienced hands. VH has a lower morbidity and quicker recovery than abdominal hysterectomy.

Laparoscopic hysterectomy can involve steps 1 and 2 (Fig. 15.2) from above with laparoscopic instruments, with step 3 completed vaginally (*laparoscopically assisted vaginal hysterectomy* [LAVH]), or be performed completely from above with the vault closed with laparoscopic sutures (*total laparoscopic hysterectomy* [TLH]). This is an alternative to TAH not VH, since if there is sufficient prolapse the latter operation is cheaper with similar recovery times. A subtotal hysterectomy can be performed laparoscopically and the uterine body removed from the peritoneal cavity with a morcellator instrument.

Wertheim's (radical) hysterectomy [→ p.36] involves removal of the parametrium, the upper third of the vagina and the pelvic lymph nodes. The usual indication is Stage 1a(ii)–2a *cervical carcinoma*. Occasionally, radical hysterectomy is performed vaginally (Schauta's radical hysterectomy).

Complications of hysterectomy	
Mortality:	1 in 10 000
Immediate:	Haemorrhage, bladder or ureteric injury
Postoperative:	Venous thromboembolism (use prophylactic low-molecular-weight heparin [LMWH]), pain, retention and infection of urine, wound and chest infection (use prophylactic antibiotics), pelvic haematoma
Long term:	Prolapse, genuine stress incontinence, premature menopause, pain and psychosexual problems

Other common gynaecological operations

Dilatation and curettage (D&C)

The cervix is dilated with steel rods (Hegar dilators) of

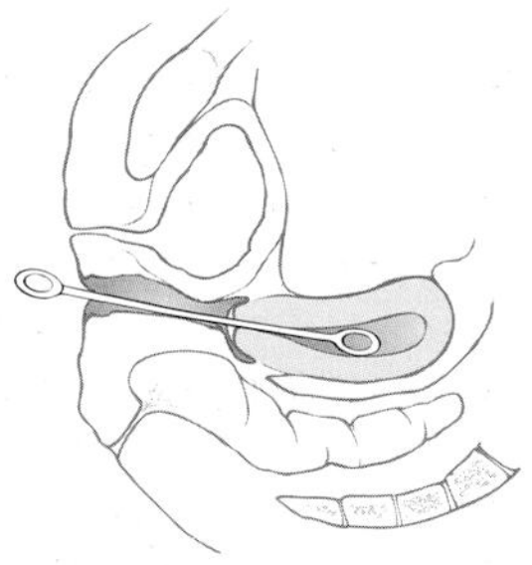

Fig. 15.3 Dilatation and curettage (D&C).

increasing size; the endometrium is then curetted to biopsy it (Fig. 15.3). This is a diagnostic procedure and inferior to hysteroscopy because the cavity is not inspected. It is now not commonly performed.

Evacuation of retained products of conception (ERPC)

The cervix is dilated and a retained non-viable fetus or placental tissue is removed using a suction curette. Surgical therapeutic abortion before 12 weeks' gestation uses a similar method.

Operations for cervical intraepithelial neoplasia

Large loop excision of the transformation zone (LLETZ) [→ p.34]: This involves using cutting diathermy, under local anesthetic, to remove the transformation zone of the cervix where cervical intraepithelial neoplasia (CIN) is present.

Cone biopsy [→ p.36]: This removes the transformation zone and much of the endocervix by making a circular cut with a scalpel or loop diathermy in the cervix. It is used to stage apparently early cervical carcinoma and is sufficient treatment for Stage 1a(i) disease. A general or epidural/spinal anesthetic is required. The cervix can be left 'incompetent' and a cervical suture [→ p.192] may be needed for future pregnancies.

Operations for prolapse [→ p.54]

'Repair' operations: An anterior repair (cystocoele) involves excision of prolapsed vaginal wall and plication of the bladder base and fascia. The vagina is then closed. A posterior repair (rectocoele) is similar, the levator ani muscle on either side being plicated between rectum and vagina. These operations are often performed together, or with a vaginal hysterectomy for uterine prolapse. Specific complications include retention of urine and overtightening of the vagina—it is important to ascertain if the patient is sexually active.

Sacrohysteropexy is used for prolapse of the uterus without removing it. The uterus and cervix are attached to the sacrum using a bifurcated non-absorbable mesh. This can be as an open or laparoscopic procedure.

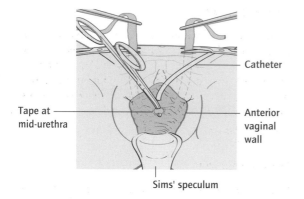

Fig. 15.4 Tension-free vaginal tape (TVT). The mid-urethra and bladder neck are supported by the tape.

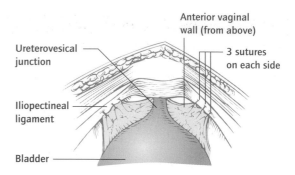

Fig. 15.5 The Burch colosuspension.

Sacrocolpopexy is used where for prolapse of the vaginal vault after hysterectomy: the mesh is attached to the vaginal vault. This can be open or laparoscopic.

Sacrospinous fixation, using a vaginal approach, is also used for vault prolapse. It is less effective than sacrocolpopexy.

Operations for genuine stress incontinence [→ p.63]

The principle is to elevate the bladder neck to allow it to be compressed when abdominal pressure rises [→ p.61].

Tension-free vaginal tape (TVT): The tape, made of polypropylene mesh, is approximately 1 cm wide and fixed to a trocar at each end. A small 3-cm vertical incision is made on the anterior vaginal wall over the mid-urethral section. After lateral dissection, the tape is introduced vaginally with the trocars entering the retropubic space. The trocars are brought out through small transverse suprapubic incisions with the tape in position without tension and the vaginal skin is closed over (Fig. 15.4). A cystoscopy is performed to ensure that the bladder has not been perforated. If the tape has been over-tightened postoperative urinary retention will persist. Rarely, the tension needs to be released by cutting the tape.

Trans-obturator tape (TOT): A variation of the TVT in which the tape is passed through the obturator canal.

Burch colposuspension involves dissection through an abdominal incision in the extraperitoneal space over the bladder and anterior vaginal wall (Fig. 15.5). The vaginal wall on either side of the bladder neck is hitched up to the iliopectineal ligament on either side of the symphysis pubis with non-absorbable sutures. The operation is usually performed now for failed tape procedures.

Operations for fibroids (see Chapter 3)

Myomectomy can be performed through the cervix (TCRF) or abdominally (laparoscopic or open approach). Risks include adhesion formation, uterine rupture during labour and peroperative haemorrhage requiring blood transfusion and, rarely, hysterectomy.

Uterine artery embolization is an alternative to hysterectomy for women with fibroids who do not wish to preserve fertility.

Precautions in major gynaecological surgery

Thromboembolism

The combined oral contraceptive is usually stopped 4 weeks prior to major abdominal surgery. If HRT [→ p.111] is not stopped, low molecular weight heparin (LMWH) must be used. All women should be mobilized early, given thromboembolic disease stockings (TEDS) and kept hydrated; LMWH is given according to risk assessment (see box below).

Thromboprophylaxis in gynaecological surgery	
Low risk:	Minor surgery or major surgery <30 min, no risk factors
Moderate risk:	*Consider* antiembolus stockings and/or subcutaneous heparin for: Surgery >30 min, obesity, gross varicose veins, current infection, prior immobility, major current illness
High risk:	*Use* LMWH prophylaxis for 5 days or until mobile for: Cancer surgery, prolonged surgery, history of deep vein thrombosis/thrombophilia, ≥3 of moderate risk factors above

Infection

Prophylactic antibiotics are used for major abdominal or vaginal surgery.

Urinary tract

Routine catheterization is performed before most operations. An indwelling transurethral catheter (e.g. Foley catheter) is left overnight after major vaginal and abdominal procedures. Following surgery for genuine stress incontinence a suprapubic catheter is often used so that the ability to pass urine urethrally can be assessed before catheter removal.

Further reading

Baggish MS, Karam MM. *Atlas of Pelvic Anatomy and Gynecologic Surgery*, 2nd edn. Philadelphia: Saunders, 2006.

http://www.websurg.com/index.php (Free online surgical site with video tutorials and demonstrations)

Obstetrics section

16 The history and examination in obstetrics

The obstetric patient is usually a healthy woman undergoing a normal life event. The history and examination are to enable the doctor or midwife to safeguard both mother and fetus during this event, and are different from other specialities. Nevertheless, the student still needs to develop a consistent system of history-taking and examination to obtain the necessary information.

The obstetric history

Personal details

Ask her name, age, occupation, gestation and parity.

Presenting complaint/present circumstances

If she is an in-patient, why is she in hospital? Common reasons for admission are hypertension, pain, antepartum haemorrhage, unstable lie and possible ruptured membranes. If the pregnancy has hitherto been uncomplicated, say so.

History of present pregnancy

Dates: What was the first day of her last menstrual period (LMP)? What was the length of her menstrual cycle and was it regular? How many weeks' gestation is she? (If a woman is at 38 weeks' gestation, it is actually 36 weeks since conception.) To estimate the expected day of delivery (EDD), subtract 3 months from the date of the LMP, add 7 days and 1 year (Nägle's rule). In practice, this can be quickly calculated using an obstetric 'wheel'

Obstetrics and Gynaecology, 3rd edition. By Lawrence Impey and Tim Child. Published 2008 by Blackwell Publishing, ISBN: 978-1-4051-6095-7.

(Fig. 16.1). If a cycle is > 28 days, the EDD will be later and needs to be adjusted: the number of days by which the cycle is longer than 28 is added to the date calculated using Nägle's rule. The reverse applies if the cycle is shorter than 28 days. If a woman has recently stopped the combined oral contraceptive, her cycles can be anovulatory and LMP is less useful.

Estimation of gestational age (Fig. 16.2)

From last menstrual period (LMP), allowing for cycle length
Ultrasound scan:
1 Measurement of crown–rump length between 7 and 14 weeks (if > 1-week difference between LMP date and scan, use scan date).
2 Biparietal diameter or femur length between 14 and 20 weeks if no early scan and LMP unknown.
Measurements to calculate gestational age are of little use beyond 20 weeks.

Complications of pregnancy: Has there been any bleeding or hypertension, diabetes, anaemia, urine infections, concerns about fetal growth, or other problems? Ask if she has been admitted to hospital in the pregnancy?
Tests: What tests have been performed (e.g. ultrasound scan, blood tests, prenatal diagnostic tests [→ p.149]).

Past obstetric history

Take details of past pregnancies in chronological order. Ask what was the mode and gestation of delivery and, if operative, why. Ask the birth weight and sex of the baby, and if the mother or the baby had any complications.
Parity: This is the number of times a woman has delivered potentially viable babies (in UK law this is defined as beyond 24 completed weeks). A woman who has had three term pregnancies is 'para 3', even if she is now in her fourth pregnancy. A suffix denotes the number of pregnancies that have miscarried (or been terminated)

before 24 weeks; for example, if the same woman had had two prior miscarriages at 12 weeks, she would be described as 'para 3 + 2'. A nulliparous woman has never delivered a potentially live baby, although she may have had miscarriages or abortions; a multiparous woman has delivered at least one baby at 24 completed weeks or more.

Gravidity: This describes the number of times a woman has been pregnant. The woman above would be gravida 6, encompassing her three term deliveries, two miscarriages and the present pregnancy. The use of the term gravid is less descriptive and is best avoided.

Nulliparity and multiparity
Nulliparous: Has delivered no live/potentially live babies
Multiparous: Has delivered live/potentially live (>24 week) babies

Symptoms of pregnancy
Amenorrhoea
Urinary frequency
Nausea ± vomiting
Breast tenderness

Other history

Past gynaecological history: This should be brief. Ask about intermenstrual and postcoital bleeding (IMB and PCB). Ask for the date of the last cervical smear and if one has ever been abnormal. Ask about prior contraception and any difficulty in conceiving.

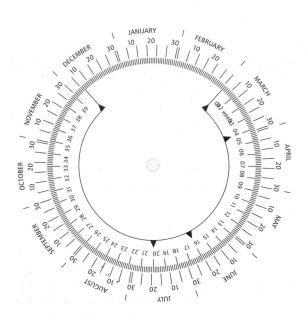

Fig. 16.1 The obstetric 'wheel'.

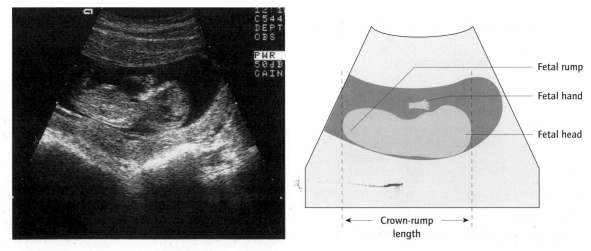

Fig. 16.2 Measurement of crown–rump length (12-week fetus).

Past medical history: Ask about operations, however distant. Ask about heart disease, hypertension, diabetes, anaemia, jaundice and epilepsy. If you elicit no history, ask 'Have you ever been in hospital?'

Past pychiatric history: Ask if she has ever consulted a psychiatrist or been treated for psychiatric disease. This is important because psychiatric illness is an important cause of postnatal problems including maternal death.

Systems review: Ask the usual cardiovascular, respiratory, abdominal and neurological questions.

Drugs: Does she take any regular medication? Did she take preconceptual folic acid?

Family history: Is there a family history of twins, of diabetes, hypertension, pre-eclampsia, autoimmune disease, venous thromboembolic disease or thrombophilia, or of any inherited disorder?

Personal/social history: Does she smoke? Does she drink alcohol? If either, how much? Ask, sensitively, about other drugs. Is she in a married or stable relationship and, if not, is there support at home? Where does she live, and what sort of accommodation is it?

Allergies: Ask specifically about penicillin and latex.

Other questions

Now ask: 'Is there anything else you think I ought to know?' The patient may be knowledgeable about her condition and this gives her the opportunity to help you if you have not discovered all the important facts.

Presenting the history

Start by summing up the important points, including important facts about any presenting complaint:
This is . . . aged . . ., who is . . . weeks into her . . . pregnancy and has been admitted to hospital because of . . .

Example: This is Mrs X, aged 30 years, who is 38 weeks into her previously uncomplicated second pregnancy and has been admitted to hospital because of a painless antepartum haemorrhage.

N.B. You have demonstrated your understanding by mentioning the absence of pain, an important factor in the differential diagnosis of antepartum haemorrhage.

Now go through the history in some detail.

Then sum up again, in one sentence, including any important findings in the history.

Obstetric history: specific essential questions

Gestation and certainty
If in-patient, presenting complaint/reason for admission
Complications of the pregnancy
Parity and details of previous pregnancies
Gynaecological questions: intermenstrual bleeding (IMB), postcoital bleeding (PCB) and date of last cervical smear
Relevant past medical history
Relevant family history

Why routinely palpate the abdomen?

<24 weeks: To check dates, twins
>24 weeks: To assess well-being by assessing size and liquor
>36 weeks: To check lie, presentation and engagement

The obstetric examination

General examination

General appearance, weight, height, temperature, oedema of the ankles and sacrum, and possible anaemia are assessed. At the booking visit, the chest, breasts, cardiovascular system and legs are also examined. The *blood pressure* and *urinalysis* tests should be performed together so that they are not forgotten (Fig. 16.3). The patient lies comfortably with her back semi-prone at 45°. Diastolic blood pressure is recorded as Korotkoff V (when the sound disappears). If the blood pressure is raised or if there is proteinuria, examine elsewhere also [→ p.168] (e.g. for epigastric tenderness).

Abdominal examination

The patient should now lie as flat as is comfortable, discreetly exposed from just below the breasts to the symphysis pubis. In later pregnancy, the semi-prone position or left lateral tilt will avoid aortocaval compression [→ p.231].

The uterus is normally palpable abdominally at 12–14 weeks. By 20 weeks the fundus is usually at the level of the umbilicus. Before 20 weeks a uterus that is larger than expected is probably due to the gestation being incorrect, but could also be due to the presence of a full bladder, multiple pregnancy, uterine fibroids [→ p.21] or a pelvic mass.

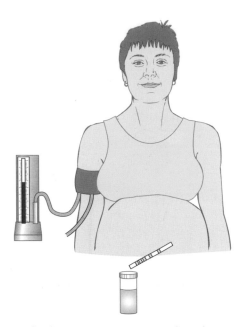

Fig. 16.3 Blood pressure measurement and urinalysis are essential.

Inspect

Look at the size of the pregnant uterus and look for striae, the linea nigra and scars, particularly in the suprapubic area (Fig. 16.4). Fetal movements are often visible in later pregnancy.

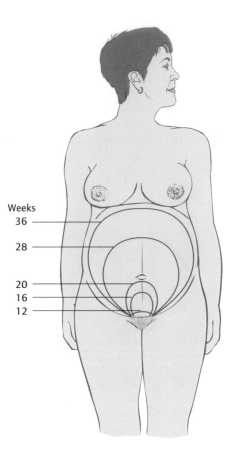

Fig. 16.4 Abdominal palpation of uterine size.

Palpation

This is purposeful and firm, but must be gentle. As you palpate ask yourself the reasons why you are doing it:
1 Is the fetus adequately grown?
2 Is the liquor volume normal?
3 Is the lie longitudinal?
4 Is the presentation cephalic and, if so, is it engaged?
   Palpation can be considered as consisting of three steps (Figs 16.5–16.7):
Step 1: Find the fundus using the fingers and ulnar border of the left hand. *Measure the distance to the symphysis pubis* with a tape measure (Fig. 16.5). After 24 weeks, the symphysis–fundal height in centimetres approximately corresponds to the gestation ± 2 cm. This is the best clinical test for detecting the 'small for dates' fetus [→ p.208], but the sensitivity is only 70%. Also look for tenderness or uterine irritability.

Step 2: Next, facing the mother, use both hands to palpate down the fetus towards the pelvis (Fig. 16.6). Use 'dipping' movements to *palpate fetal parts* and *estimate the liquor volume*. Imagine an irregular potato in a small plastic bag containing water. Pressing on the outside of the bag will allow palpation of the potato, and the feel of the water is exactly how liquor feels. If none is present, the contents are easy to feel: if fluid volume is excessive (polyhydramnios), the bag will be tense and the fingers will need to dip in far to feel anything. Try to ascertain what you are feeling: the head is hard and, if free, can be gently 'bounced' or balloted between two hands, whereas the breech is softer, less easy to define and cannot be balloted.

The lie refers to the relationship between the fetus and the long axis of the uterus. If longitudinal, the head and

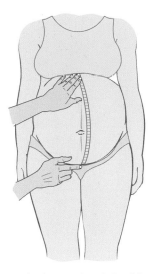

Fig. 16.5 Abdominal palpation. Step 1: Fundal palpation and measurement of symphysis–fundal height.

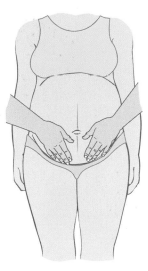

Fig. 16.7 Abdominal palpation. Step 3: Examination of presentation.

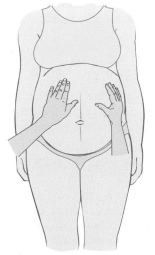

Fig. 16.6 Abdominal palpation. Step 2: Examination of fetal parts.

Common causes of polyhydramnios
Diabetes/gestational diabetes
Fetal abnormality
Idiopathic

Step 3: Turn to face the pelvis and press the fingers of both hands firmly down just above the symphysis pubis to assess the *presentation*: the fetal part that occupies the lower segment or pelvis (Fig. 16.7). With a longitudinal lie (Fig. 16.8), it is the head, or occasionally the buttocks. *Engagement of the head* (Fig. 16.10) occurs when the widest diameter descends into the pelvis: descent is described as 'fifths palpable'. If only two-fifths of the head is palpable abdominally, then more than half has entered the pelvis and so the head must be engaged. If more than two-fifths of the head is palpable, it is not engaged. If you are still unsure of the presentation, grasp the presenting fetal part between the thumb and index finger of the examining hand (Pawlik's grip). This can be uncomfortable for the patient and is seldom necessary.

Attempting to determine the *position* or *attitude* of the fetus is not a useful part of antenatal palpation of the abdomen. Where a woman has complained of pain or antepartum haemorrhage it is important to look for

buttocks are palpable at each end (Fig. 16.8). If transverse, the fetus is lying across the uterus and the pelvis will be empty (Fig. 16.9). If oblique, the head or buttocks are palpable in one of the iliac fossae.

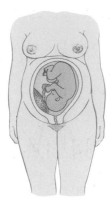

Fig. 16.8 Longitudinal lie (cephalic presentation in this instance).

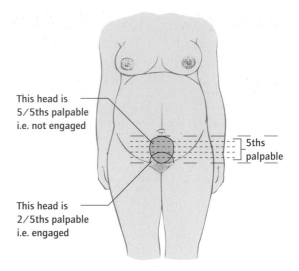

This head is 5/5ths palpable i.e. not engaged

This head is 2/5ths palpable i.e. engaged

5ths palpable

Fig. 16.10 Engagement of the fetal head.

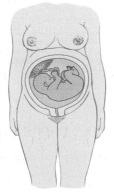

Fig. 16.9 Transverse lie.

areas of tenderness and uterine irritability (it contracts when palpated).

Auscultate

Listening over the anterior shoulder (usually palpable between the head and the umbilicus), the fetal heart should be heard with a Pinard's stethoscope. Place this flat over the shoulder, press it on the abdomen with your ear, keeping both hands free and time the heart rate with your watch. It should be 110–160 beats/minute.

Vaginal examination is not a useful part of routine antenatal examination, unless labour is suspected or is to be induced and is therefore described in the chapters on labour.

Other features of relevance

Consider examination of fundi, reflexes, temperature, epigastrium, legs, chest, etc. if clinically indicated from history or other examination findings.

Abdominal findings in pregnancy	
Uterine size:	Fundus palpable at 12–14 weeks At umbilicus at 20 weeks At xiphoid sternum at 36 weeks Fundal height increases approx. 1 cm/week after 24 weeks
Presentation:	Breech in 30% at 28 weeks Breech in 3% after 37 weeks
Engagement:	Usual in nulliparous after 37 weeks Multiparous often not engaged

The postnatal history and examination

History

Ascertain the name and age of the mother and the number of days since delivery.
Delivery: Ask about the gestation and mode of delivery, and if instrumental or Caesarean, ask why. Ask about the mode of onset (e.g. spontaneous or induced), length of labour, analgesia and any procedures in labour (e.g. fetal blood sampling). Was there excessive blood loss?
Infant: Ask about the infant's sex, birth weight and Apgar scores, cord pH if taken, and mode and success of feeding. Was vitamin K given?
History of puerperium so far: Ask about lochia (volume, any odour), have her bowels opened yet, is she passing urine normally, or is there difficulty, leaking or dysuria? Does she have pain, particularly in the perineum?
Plans for the puerperium: What contraception does she intend to use? (Progesterone-only contraception is suitable for breastfeeding mothers; the combined pill can be started at 4–6 weeks if bottle feeding.) What help is available at home?
History of pregnancy and obstetric history: This should be brief, but ask about her parity and major antenatal complications, e.g. pre-eclampsia, diabetes.
Social/personal history: Consider home conditions for the neonate.

Apgar scoring

Sign	0	1	2
Heart rate	Absent	<100	>100
Respiratory effort	Absent	Weak, irregular	Strong cry
Muscle tone	Absent	Limb flexion	Active motion
Colour	All blue/pale	Extremities blue	All pink
Reflex irritability (stimulate foot)	No response	Grimace	Cry

Total score out of 10, at 1 and 5 min
1-min Apgar gives indication of need for resuscitation, but has little prognostic value
5-min Apgar correlates very vaguely with subsequent neurological outcome

Presenting the postnatal history

Summarize her labour, delivery, and her and the neonate's current health:
Mrs X, aged . . . had a . . . delivery . . . (if not normal, state indication, i.e. for . . .) days ago and delivered a . . . (sex) infant, weighing . . . kilograms, with Apgar of . . . and . . . labour was . . . (mode of onset) at . . . weeks' gestation and lasted . . . hours. This was her . . . pregnancy, which . . . (state any major complications). She is currently . . . (brief assessment of her health: blood pressure, anaemia, uterine involution), is . . . (bottle or breast) feeding and plans to use . . . as contraception.

Example: Mrs X, aged 32 years, had a ventouse delivery for prolonged second stage 2 days ago and delivered a girl weighing 3.7 kg. Labour was spontaneous at 40 weeks' gestation and lasted 9 h. This was her first pregnancy and was uncomplicated. She is well, afebrile, her blood pressure is 120/80 mmHg, her uterus is well contracted, she is breastfeeding and plans to use the progesterone-only pill.

Management/discharge plans. Mention anti-D and rubella vaccination if relevant.

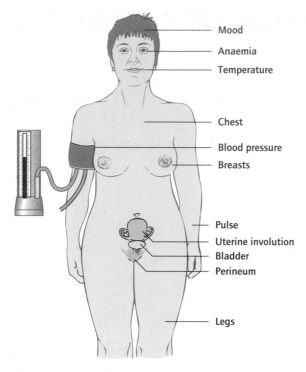

Mood
Anaemia
Temperature

Chest

Blood pressure
Breasts

Pulse
Uterine involution
Bladder
Perineum

Legs

Fig. 16.11 Postnatal examination.

Examination

General examination: Assess mood and appearance, temperature, pulse, blood pressure, possible anaemia. Also examine chest, breasts, any wound or intravenous site and legs if fever or tachycardia (Fig. 16.11).

Abdominal examination: Look for uterine involution and a palpable bladder. Examine the perineum if there is discomfort.

Basic neonatal assessment

History. Review the family history, antenatal course, labour course and delivery method and if resuscitation was required. Review birth weight, birth weight centile and weight gain/loss.

Examination. Examine the neonate in the presence of his/her mother. Undress the baby fully. Handle gently and wrap the neonate up after examination.

Neonatal examination	
General:	Colour (pallor/jaundice/cyanosis), features (dysmorphism/evidence of trauma/birthmarks/any abnormalities), posture, behaviour and feeding movement (abnormal or restricted), respiration
Measure:	Heart rate, temperature, head measurements, weight
Examine:	Look for primitive reflexes (grasp, Moro, rooting) Inspect back and spine with baby prone Heart, check all pulses equal (e.g. radiofemoral delay) Abdomen, genitalia (undescended testes/hernias/ambiguous genitalia), anus Look and examine for congenital dislocation of the hip and talipes

Investigations: Serum bilirubin (SBR) if jaundiced. Day 7: Guthrie (phenylketonuria, thyroid)

Obstetric History at a Glance

Personal details	Name, age, occupation, gestation, parity
Presenting complaint or present circumstances	
History of present pregnancy	Dates: Last menstrual period (LMP), cycle length, calculate expected day of delivery (EDD) and check present gestation Complications: Specific complications, hospital admissions Tests done: e.g. ultrasound scan, prenatal diagnosis, booking bloods [→ p.143]
Obstetric history	Past pregnancies: year, gestation, mode of delivery, complications, birth weight, ante/intra/postpartum complications
Gynaecological history	Intermenstrual bleeding (IMB), postcoital bleeding (PCB), last cervical smear, contraception, subfertility
Medical history	Operations; major illnesses, particularly diabetes, hypertension, psychiatric illness
Systems review	
Drugs	
Personal	Smoking and alcohol, drugs of abuse
Social	Stable relationship, finances, accommodation
Allergies	
Is there anything else you think I should know?	

Obstetric Examination at a Glance

General	Appearance, weight, oedema (full examination at booking), blood pressure, urinalysis
Abdomen	Inspect: Size, scars, fetal movements Palpate: Measure symphysis–fundal height, lie and presentation, liquor volume, engagement of presenting part Listen: Fetal heart over anterior shoulder
Vaginal examination	Not usually indicated antenatally
Other features	If relevant

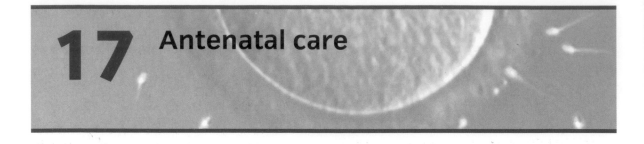

17 Antenatal care

Pregnancy and childbirth are physiological events; most women are healthy and few need medical intervention. The main purpose of antenatal care is to identify mothers who do need medical attention. Some are identifiable at the booking visit, but most show no indication of the problems that can develop in pregnancy or labour.

The success of pregnancy care and the recognition that few pregnancies need intervention is now reflected in the UK by attempts to return to more natural labour and community-based care. The hospital-based, consultant-led system has been criticized as lacking in continuity of care and emphasizing the abnormal. Pressure from consumer groups has led to government support for more community-based care, and choice for women as to who is responsible for their care and where they deliver. These decisions are usually made early in the pregnancy but, because most problems are unpredictable at booking, they need to be constantly re-evaluated as the pregnancy proceeds.

The aims of antenatal care

1 Detect and manage pre-existing maternal disorders that may affect pregnancy outcome.
2 Prevent or detect and manage maternal complications of pregnancy.
3 Prevent or detect and manage fetal complications of pregnancy.
4 Detect congenital fetal problems, if requested by the patient.
5 Plan, with the mother, the circumstances of delivery to ensure maximum safety for the mother and baby, and maximum maternal satisfaction.
6 Provide education and advice regarding lifestyle and 'minor' conditions of pregnancy.

Obstetrics and Gynaecology, 3rd edition. By Lawrence Impey and Tim Child. Published 2008 by Blackwell Publishing, ISBN: 978-1-4051-6095-7.

Preconceptual care and counselling

Many of the aims of antenatal care could be better fulfilled before conception. *Previous pregnancies* may have been traumatic and the implications of another can be discussed. The *health check* is better performed before conception and hitherto undetected problems such as cervical smear abnormalities can be treated. *Rubella status* can be checked so that immunization can occur before pregnancy. Health in women with chronic disease can be optimized; for instance, strict preconceptual *glucose control in diabetics* reduces the incidence of congenital abnormalities. *Medication* can be optimized for pregnancy: for instance, certain antiepileptics, e.g. lamotrigine are safer than others, e.g. sodium valproate. Routine preconceptual administration of 0.4 mg/day *folic acid* reduces the chance of neural tube defects (*Lancet* 1991; **338**: 132). Advice regarding *smoking, alcohol* and *drugs* [→ p.183] can be given. The woman should be encouraged to record the *dates of menstruation* so calculation of gestation is easier.

The booking visit

The first appointment should be at 9–11 weeks' gestation. The most important purpose is to screen for possible complications that may arise in pregnancy, labour and the puerperium. 'Risk' is therefore assessed, using the history and examination and the investigations that are a standard feature of the booking visit. As discussed in Chapter 25, the benefits of this remain limited. Decisions about the type and frequency of antenatal care, as well as decisions about delivery, can be made in conjunction with the parents. These must be constantly re-evaluated as the pregnancy proceeds. At the same time, the gestation of the pregnancy is checked, appropriate prenatal screening is discussed and a general health check is accompanied by health advice.

History

Age: Women below the age of 17 years and above the age of 35 years have an increased risk of obstetric and medical complications in pregnancy. Chromosomal trisomies are more common with advancing maternal age.

History of present pregnancy: The accuracy of the last menstrual period is checked and the gestation adjusted for cycle length. The need for a dating ultrasound may be identified.

Past obstetric history: Many *obstetric disorders* have a small but significant recurrence rate. These include preterm labour, the small-for-dates and the 'growth-restricted' fetus [→ p.203], stillbirth, antepartum and postpartum haemorrhage, some congenital anomalies, rhesus disease, pre-eclampsia and gestational diabetes. Women with a history of preterm labour should be considered for cervical cerclage, or at least cervical ultrasound [→ p.192] and screening for bacterial vaginosis [→ p.193]. The *mode of delivery* of previous pregnancies will affect that of the current one: with one previous Caesarean section, vaginal delivery is often attempted, but if more than one Caesarean has occurred, it is usual in the UK to perform an elective Caesarean.

Past gynaecological history: A history of subfertility increases perinatal risk; if fertility drugs or assisted conception have also been used, the likelihood of a multiple pregnancy is also increased. Women with previous uterine surgery (e.g. myomectomy) are usually delivered by elective Caesarean section. A cervical smear history is taken.

Past medical history: Women with a history of hypertension, diabetes, autoimmune disease, haemoglobinopathy, thromboembolic disease, cardiac or renal disease, or other serious illnesses are at an increased risk of pregnancy problems and usually need input from the appropriate specialist.

Drugs: Drugs that are contraindicated in pregnancy should be changed to those considered to be safe. Ideally, this should have occurred at a preconceptual counselling visit.

Family history: Gestational diabetes is more common if a first degree relative is diabetic. Hypertension, thromboembolic and autoimmune disease, and pre-eclampsia are also familial.

Personal/social history: Smoking, alcohol and drug abuse are sought.

Examination

General health and nutritional status are assessed: many pregnancy complications are more common in women weighing >100 kg. A baseline blood pressure enables comparison if hypertension occurs in later pregnancy. If pre-existing hypertension is found, the risk of subsequent pre-eclampsia is increased. Incidental disease such as breast carcinoma may occasionally be detected.

Abdominal examination before the third trimester is limited. Once the uterus is palpable (about 12 weeks), the fetal heart can be auscultated with an electronic monitor. A uterus that is palpable before 12 weeks suggests multiple pregnancy. Routine vaginal examination and clinical assessment of pelvic capacity are inappropriate at this stage. If a smear has not been performed for 3 years it is usually done 3 months postnatally.

Booking visit investigations

Ultrasound scan

Ultrasound between 11 and 13 weeks should be offered. This confirms gestation and viability, usually provides considerable maternal reassurance, and will diagnose multiple pregnancy. It can also be used in screening for chromosomal abnormalities: nuchal translucency [→ p.149], in conjunction with blood levels of human chorionic gonadotrophin beta-subunit (β-hCG) and pregnancy-associated plasma protein A (PAPPA), as the 'combined test' [→ p.152]. The availability of screening for chromosomal abnormalities with a sensitivity of 75% for a false positive rate of 3% (achieved by the combined test) is now required in the UK.

Blood tests

A *full blood count* (FBC) check identifies pre-existing anaemia.

Serum antibodies (e.g. anti-D) identify those at risk of intrauterine isoimmunization [→ p.187].

Blood glucose levels, particularly if both fasting and postprandial, help identify pre-existing and gestational diabetics [→ p.174]. This is, probably incorrectly, not currently recommended.

Blood tests for syphilis are still routine because of the serious implications for the fetus.

Rubella immunity [→ p.159] is checked: vaccination, if required, will be offered postnatally.

Human immunodeficiency virus (HIV) and *hepatitis B* counselling and screening is offered [→ p.161].

Haemoglobin electrophoresis is performed in women at risk of the *sickle-cell anaemias* or *thalassaemias* [→ p.184]. The former is common in Afro-Caribbean women, the latter in Mediterranean and Asian women. The partner can be tested if the woman is found to be a carrier, to identify women who should be offered prenatal diagnosis.

Other tests

Screening for infections implicated in preterm labour (e.g. *Chlamydia*, bacterial vaginosis [→ p.191]) could be performed at this stage, in women at increased risk.

Urine microscopy and culture are performed because asymptomatic bacteriuria in pregnancy commonly (20%) leads to pyelonephritis.

Urinalysis for *glucose*, *protein* and *nitrites* screen for underlying diabetes, renal disease and infection, respectively.

Booking investigations
Urine culture
Full blood count (FBC)
Antibody screen
Glucose
Serological tests for syphilis
Rubella immunoglobulin G
Offer human immunodeficiency virus (HIV) and hepatitis B
Ultrasound scan
Screening for chromosomal abnormalities
Consider: Haemoglobin electrophoresis, cervix/vaginal swabs

Health promotion and advice

Medications are generally avoided in the first trimester, but teratogenicity is rare. Regular medication should ideally be adjusted preconceptually.

Diet in pregnancy should be well balanced, with a daily energy intake of about 2500 calories.

Folic acid supplementation, with 0.4 mg/day folic acid, should continue until at least 12 weeks. *Vitamin D* supplementation is given to women who receive little expo-

sure to sunlight. Iron supplementation is commonplace but should not be routine.

Coitus is not contraindicated in pregnancy, except when the placenta is known to be praevia or the membranes have ruptured.

Alcohol is best avoided; if taken a maximum of 1 unit/day is recommended [→ p.183].

Smoking advice is given. Effective interventions include advice, group sessions and behavioural therapy.

Avoidance of infection: Listeriosis [→ p.163] is avoided by drinking only pasteurized or UHT milk, by avoiding soft and blue cheeses, paté and uncooked or partially cooked ready prepared food. Salmonella is avoided by cooking eggs or poultry well.

A dental check-up is advised.

Exercise in pregnancy is advised: swimming is ideal; heavy contact sports are avoided.

Travel: Most airlines will only carry women at <34–36 weeks. The risk of venous thromboembolism [→ p.180] is reduced by adequate hydration and compression stockings, but if additional risk factors are present, low-dose aspirin or even fragmin may be used. Vaccination and insurance issues should be discussed. When driving, a seatbelt should be worn, above and below the 'bump'.

Preparation for birth

Antenatal classes should educate women and their partners about pregnancy and labour. Knowledge and understanding help alleviate fear and pain, and allows women to have more control and make choices about their antepartum and intrapartum care. In addition, intrapartum techniques of posture, breathing and pushing can be taught (Fig. 17.1).

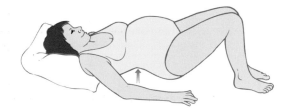

Fig. 17.1 Pelvic tilt at antenatal classes.

Planning pregnancy care

At the end of the booking visit, the doctor or midwife can advise the woman of the most appropriate type of antenatal care, and a plan for visit frequency, extra surveillance or intervention is made. A choice can be made between two care options:

Community care: A core team of midwives is responsible for all antepartum and intrapartum care, usually with a general practitioner. Women can be referred to the hospital for advice or for pregnancy care later in the pregnancy if complications occur.

Consultant-led care: Visits are shared by a consultant obstetrician-led team, with the community midwives and often general practitioner. The degree of obstetric involvement will depend on the pregnancy risk and the occurrence of complications.

Later pregnancy screening

Ultrasound for structural abnormalities

An ultrasound examination should be offered at 20 weeks. This 'anomaly scan' enables detection of most structural fetal abnormalities [→ p.149], although reported success rates vary widely.

Ultrasound screening for risk assessment

Doppler of the uterine arteries [→ p.205] at 23 weeks can be used as a screening test for intrauterine growth restriction and pre-eclampsia (*AmJOG* 2006; **195**: 330). Its use is imperfect, expensive and not routine. Nevertheless, it is far more effective at predicting major pregnancy complications than the medical or obstetric history. This could make the test cost effective in comparison to the current system, and, in the future, pregnancy risk assessment is likely to involve its routine use.

Continuing antenatal care

Frequency of antenatal visits

The woman is seen at decreasing intervals through the pregnancy because complications are more common later in the pregnancy. The frequency with which she is seen is dependent on the likelihood of complications and on the apparent fetal and maternal health as assessed in subsequent visits. NICE recommends an antenatal appointment schedule (Fig. 17.2) for uncomplicated pregnancies of 10 appointments for nulliparous and 7 for multiparous women. More frequent visits are appropriate for many 'high-risk' pregnancies. Less intensive

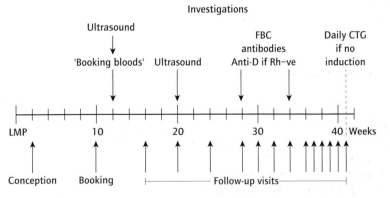

Fig. 17.2 Basic antenatal care in nulliparous women.

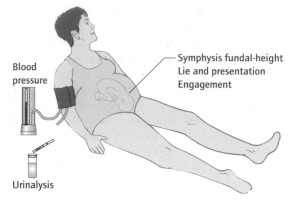

Fig. 17.3 Obstetric examination at antenatal visits in the late third trimester.

care is often less well accepted by women and health carers alike.

Conduct of antenatal visits (Fig. 17.3)

At each visit, the history is briefly reviewed. The woman is asked about her physical and mental state and given the opportunity to ask questions. She is normally weighed, although this is of little use unless gross oedema is found. The blood pressure is taken and the urine is checked for protein, glucose, leucocytes and nitrites. Urine culture is performed if the latter are detected. The abdomen is examined in the normal manner, but presentation is variable and unimportant until 36 weeks. Listening to the fetal heart is reassuring. A reassessment of pregnancy risk is taken.

The following is the basic antenatal schedule as recommended by NICE, and more intensive surveillance is appropriate for pregnancies at risk of, or who develop, complications:

16 weeks: The results of screening tests for chromosomal abnormalities and booking blood tests should specifically be reviewed. If screening for chromosomal abnormalities was missed, an alternative 'triple test' [→ p.152] is offered.

20 weeks: The anomaly scan is performed. A repeat scan is arranged at 36 weeks if the placenta is low.

25 weeks (recommended for nulliparous women only): Serial measurements of fundal height can be plotted on a customized growth chart (*Obstet Gynecol* 1999; **94**: 591) to help identify the baby that is pathologically small and

should be referred for ultrasound assessment [→ p.206].

28 weeks: Fundal height is measured. The FBC and antibodies are checked. Glucose levels can again be tested. Anti-D is given to rhesus-negative women.

31 weeks (nulliparous women only): Fundal height is measured. The blood tests from 28 weeks are reviewed.

34 weeks: Fundal height is measured. The full blood count and antibodies are checked again. Anti-D is again given to rhesus-negative women.

36, 38 and 40 weeks: Fundal height is measured and the fetal lie and presentation is checked. Referral for external cephalic version (ECV) [→ p.213] is offered if the presentation is breech. Pelvic examination is inappropriate unless induction is contemplated or there is suspicion of obstruction (and placenta praevia is excluded).

41 weeks: Fundal height is measured and the fetal lie and presentation is checked. Membrane sweeping [→ p.251] is offered, as is induction of labour before 42 weeks. If induction of labour is not performed, particularly close surveillance is indicated [→ p.210].

Conduct of antenatal visits	
History:	Physical and mental health Fetal movements
Examination:	Blood pressure and urinalysis Symphisis–fundal height Lie and presentation of fetus Engagement of presenting part Fetal heart auscultation
Management:	Offer advice Reassess pregnancy risk

'Minor' conditions of pregnancy

Itching is common in pregnancy. The sclerae are checked for jaundice, and liver function tests and bile acids are assessed. Although rare, liver complications in pregnancy [→ p.179] often present with itching.

Symphisis pubis dysfunction is common (*Eur J Obstet Gynecol Reprod Biol* 2002; **105**: 143) and causes varying degrees of discomfort in the pubic and sacroiliac joints. Physiotherapy, corsets, analgesics and even crutches may be used. Care with leg abduction is required. It is usually but not invariably cured after delivery.

Abdominal pain is universal to some degree in pregnancy; it is usually benign and unexplained. However, medical and surgical problems are no less common in pregnancy, and may have a worse prognosis, particularly appendicitis and pancreatitis. Urinary tract infections and fibroids [→ p.21] can cause pain in pregnancy.

Heartburn affects 70% and is most marked in the supine position. Extra pillows are helpful; antacids are not contraindicated, ranitidine can be used in severe cases. Pre-eclampsia can present with epigastric pain.

Backache is almost universal and may cause sciatica. Most cases resolve after delivery. Physiotherapy, advice on posture and lifting, a firm mattress and a corset may all help.

Constipation is common and often exacerbated by oral iron. A high fibre intake is needed. Stool softeners are used if this fails.

Ankle oedema is common, worsens towards the end of pregnancy and is an unreliable sign of pre-eclampsia. However, a sudden increase in oedema warrants careful assessment and follow-up of blood pressure and urinalysis: if associated with pre-eclampsia, the sacrum, fingers and even the face are often affected. Benign oedema is helped by raising the foot of the bed at night; diuretics should not be given.

Leg cramps affect 30% of women. Treatments are generally unproven, but sodium chloride tablets, calcium salts or quinine may be safely tried.

Carpal tunnel syndrome is due to fluid retention compressing the median nerve. It is seldom severe and is usually temporary. Splints on the wrists may help.

Vaginitis due to candidiasis is common in pregnancy and more difficult to treat. There is an itchy, non-offensive, white–grey discharge associated with excoriation. Imidazole vaginal pessaries (e.g. clotrimazole) are used for symptomatic infection.

Tiredness is almost universal and is often incorrectly attributed to anaemia.

Further reading

Carroli G, Villar J, Piaggio G, *et al.* WHO Antenatal Care Trial Research Group. WHO systematic review of randomised controlled trials of routine antenatal care. *Lancet* 2001; **357**: 1565–70.

National Institute for Clinical Excellence (NICE). *Antenatal care: Routine care for the healthy pregnant woman.* Clinical Guideline No 6. October 2003.

Villar J, Carroli G, Khan-Neelofur D, Piaggio G, Gulmezoglu M. Patterns of routine antenatal care for low-risk pregnancy. *Cochrane Database System Review (Online: Update Software)* 2001; **4**: CD000934.

Physiological Changes in Pregnancy at a Glance	
Weight gain	10–15 kg
Genital tract	Uterus weight increase from 50 to 1000 g Muscle hypertrophy, increased blood flow and contractility Cervix softens, may start to efface in late third trimester
Blood	Blood volume: 50% increase Red cell mass: increase Haemoglobin: decrease (normal lower limit 10.5 g/dL) White blood cell count (WBC) increase
Cardiovascular system	Cardiac output: 40% increase Peripheral resistance: 50% reduction Blood pressure: small mid-pregnancy fall
Lungs	Tidal volume: 40% increase Respiratory rate: no change
Others	Renal blood flow: glomerular filtration rate 40% increase, so creatinine/urea decrease Reduced gut motility: delayed gastric emptying/constipation Thyroid enlargement

18 Congenital abnormalities and their identification

Congenital abnormalities affect 2% of pregnancies (1% major). They can be *structural deformities* (e.g. diaphragmatic hernia) or *chromosomal abnormalities* (most commonly trisomies, e.g. Down's syndrome) or *inherited diseases* (e.g. cystic fibrosis), or are the result of *intrauterine infection* (e.g. rubella) or *drug exposure* (e.g. antiepileptics).

Abnormalities account for about 25% of perinatal deaths and are a major cause of disability in later life. Prenatal identification of such abnormalities is important to prepare the parents, to allow delivery to be at an appropriate time and place, to prepare neonatal services and, in the case of severe disabilities, to enable the parents to terminate the pregnancy if they wish. The prognosis of some conditions can also be improved by treatment *in utero*. Parental attitudes vary with age, religion and social background: counselling must be non-directive. The parents must be given the facts to allow their choice to be informed. This applies to when an abnormality is found, or whether the abnormality should be sought in the first place. Screening for Down's syndrome, for instance, should only be performed if the parents would wish to know. The facts about, and implications of the available tests should be discussed at the booking visit.

The difference between screening and diagnostic tests

A screening test is available for all (women) and gives a measure of the risk of (the fetus) being affected by a particular disorder. The 'higher-risk' patient can then be offered a diagnostic test. A result might be: 'the risk of Down's syndrome in this pregnancy is 1 in 50'.

A diagnostic test is performed on women with a 'high risk' to confirm or refute the possibility, e.g. 'this fetus does not have Down's syndrome'.

Obstetrics and Gynaecology, 3rd edition. By Lawrence Impey and Tim Child. Published 2008 by Blackwell Publishing, ISBN: 978-1-4051-6095-7.

Screening and diagnostic tests

These aim to identify subjects at increased risk for a given condition. In pregnancy they are usually offered to all women. A good screening test is *cheap*, has a *high sensitivity* (i.e. does not miss affected individuals) and *specificity* (i.e. not many false positives) and is *safe*. There must also be an *acceptable diagnostic test* for the disorder for which it is screening and the implications of being affected by the *condition should be serious* enough to warrant the test. This diagnostic test must diagnose or refute the condition. Diagnostic tests are not always offered as a first line because they may be expensive or have significant complications. By performing diagnostic tests only in women identified as high risk the impact of these is minimized.

Terms describing screening tests

The *sensitivity* is the proportion of subjects with the condition classified by the test as screen positive for the condition. The *negative predictive value* (NPV) is the probability that a subject who is screen negative will not have the condition. The *specificity* is the proportion of subjects without the condition who are classified as screen negative.

The *screen positive rate* is the proportion of subjects who are classified as high risk by the test. The *positive predictive value* (PPV) is the probability that a subject who is screen positive will have the condition. In practice, the PPV is often low: most screen positives do not have the condition, and the screen positive rate is similar to the *false positive rate* (FPR), the number classified as high risk who do not nevertheless have the condition.

Performance of screening tests

The sensitivity and specificity are related. For instance, Down's syndrome [→ p.151] is more common in older mothers, so maternal age can be used alone as a screening test. The performance of the test will depend on what maternal age is considered 'screen positive'. Although age is a risk factor, most babies born with Down's syndrome will be to younger mothers because, although their individual risks are lower, they are more likely to be pregnant. If we were to call all women over 30 years screen positive, the test would detect most Down's babies, or have a high sensitivity and high NPV. However, at this age cut-off about half of the population would be classified as screen positive, so the test would have a low specificity and PPV, and a high false positive rate. Sensitivity is therefore quoted at a given screen positive rate, often 3 or 5%.

Integration of risk factors

It is clear that age alone is a poor screening test for Down's syndrome: with it and some other conditions there are several potential screening tests. If these tests are independent of each other, they can be 'integrated' or used together to create a more accurate overall single screening test. This is now the principle behind all Down's syndrome screening.

Methods of prenatal testing for congenital abnormalities

Maternal blood testing

As a screening test

Neural tube defects: Alpha fetoprotein (AFP) is a product of the fetal liver. When the fetus has an open neural tube defect (NTD), maternal levels are raised: this can be confirmed or refuted by ultrasound after 16 weeks. Raised levels in the absence of NTDs are also associated with other abnormalities such as gastroschisis [→ p.154]. They may also indicate a higher risk of third trimester complications (see Chapter 25). AFP is seldom used nowadays as ultrasound is more accurate.

Chromosomal abnormalities: The levels of several maternal blood markers are also altered where the fetus has a chromosomal abnormality such as Down's syndrome. These include human chorionic gonadotrophin beta-subunit (β-hCG), pregnancy-associated plasma protein A (PAPP-A), AFP, oestriol and inhibin A. The results of these can be integrated with other risk factors such as maternal age and ultrasound measurements (e.g. nuchal translucency) to screen for the trisomies 21 (Down's syndrome), 18 and 13.

As a diagnostic test

Prenatal diagnosis from the few fetal cells in the maternal circulation will revolutionize prenatal diagnosis in the future. Already, fetal gender can be determined this way (*J Obstet Gynaecol Res* 2007; **33**: 747).

Ultrasound

To confirm dates

Ultrasound is used to confirm the gestation, pregnancy site and exclude multiple pregnancy.

As a screening test for abnormalities

Ultrasound is the cornerstone of screening for trisomies. The nuchal translucency (the space between skin and soft tissue overlying the cervical spine) between 11 and 14 weeks is measured (Fig. 18.1) and the larger it is, the higher the risk. (Figs 18.2 & 18.3) A larger nuchal translucency also indicated a higher risk of structural, particularly cardiac abnormalities (*Ultrasound Obstet Gynecol* 2001; **18**: 9). In addition, 50% of fetuses with trisomies have structural abnormalities, e.g. exomphalos, which are visible at a 20-week ultrasound.

To aid other diagnostic tests

Amniocentesis and chorionic villus sampling (CVS) are performed under ultrasound vision.

As a diagnostic test

Structural abnormalities are usually diagnosed at 20 weeks at the 'anomaly scan'. Congenital malformations of all organs and systems are detectable. Up to 25% of abnormalities can actually be identified at 11–14 weeks at the time of nuchal translucency assessment. However, particularly with the heart, many remain undiagnosed even at 20 weeks, and this is related to operator experience. In addition, some abnormalities do not become evident until later either because they are not visible or because they develop with gestation. The development of increased liquor volume, polyhydramnios [→ p.157], in later pregnancy can be the result of a fetal abnormality and warrants a repeat detailed ultrasound examination.

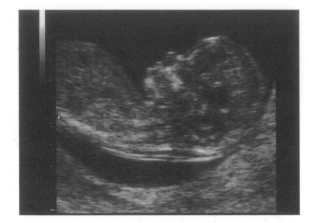

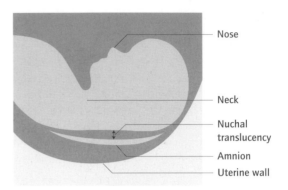

Fig. 18.1 Normal nuchal translucency.

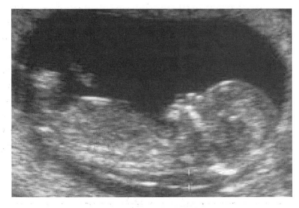

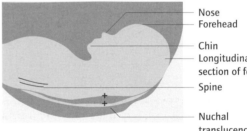

Fig. 18.2 Ultrasound of enlarged nuchal translucency.

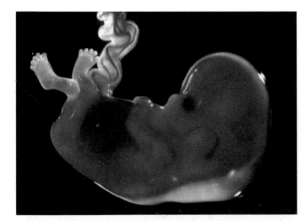

Fig. 18.3 Photograph of enlarged nuchal translucency.

Fetal magnetic resonance imaging

Magnetic resonance imaging (MRI) scanning of the fetus *in utero* is under evaluation but is increasingly used in the diagnosis of intracerebral lesions (*BJOG* 2004; **111**: 784) and is better at differentiating between different types of soft tissue, e.g. liver and lung. It may also have a role as an alternative to postmortem examination.

3-D/4-D ultrasound

3-D or real time 3-D (known as 4-D ultrasound) using a computer reconstructured 3-D ultrasound image can allow better evaluation of certain abnormalities, and is

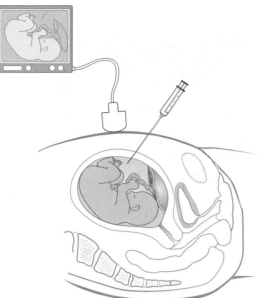

Fig. 18.4 Amniocentesis.

being intensively used. Whether it improves the diagnosis of, or outcome for most abnormalities remains to be seen. However, it does allow parents to see certain abnormalities (e.g. cleft lip) more clearly.

Amniocentesis

This is a diagnostic test, involving removal of amniotic fluid using a fine gauge needle under ultrasound guidance (Fig. 18.4). It is safest performed from 16 weeks' gestation, but it may be done later. This enables prenatal diagnosis of chromosomal abnormalities, some infections such as cytomegalovirus (CMV) and toxoplasmosis, and inherited disorders such as sickle-cell anaemia, thalassaemia and cystic fibrosis. One per cent of women miscarry after an amniocentesis (*Obstet Gynecol* 2006; **108**: 1067).

Chorionic villus sampling

This diagnostic test involves biopsy of the trophoblast, by passing a small needle through the abdominal wall or cervix and into the placenta, after 11 weeks (*Cochrane*

2000: CD000077). The test result is obtained faster than with amniocentesis and allows an abnormal fetus to be identified at a time when abortion, if requested, could be performed under general anaesthesia. The miscarriage rate is slightly higher than after amniocentesis, but this is because it is performed earlier, when spontaneous miscarriage is more common, and because it is a more difficult procedure. It is used to diagnose chromosomal problems and autosomal dominant and recessive conditions.

With both amniocentesis and CVS, fluorescence *in situ* hybridization (FISH) and polymerase chain reaction (PCR) can both be used to diagnose the most common abnormalities in less than 48 h.

Preimplantation genetic diagnosis

In vitro fertilization (IVF) [→ p.90] allows cell(s) from a developing embryo to be removed for genetic analysis before the embryo is transferred to the uterus (*Hum Reprod* 2003; **18**: 465). This allows selection, and therefore implantation, only of embryos that will not be affected by the disorder for which it is being tested. The technique is expensive and presents ethical dilemmas, but has been used in prenatal diagnosis of sex-linked disorders, trisomies, and both autosomal dominant and recessive conditions. It does require IVF, even in couples who are fertile.

Chromosomal abnormalities

These affect 6 per 1000 live births. As a cause of miscarriage, they are more common than this in early pregnancy. Most are trisomies.

Down's syndrome

Trisomy 21 is the most common chromosomal abnormality among live births. It is usually the result of random non-dysjunction at meiosis, although occasionally (6%) it arises as a result of a balanced chromosomal translocation in the parents. It is more common with advancing maternal age (Fig. 18.5). The affected infant has mental retardation, characteristic facies and often (50%) congenital cardiac disease. Other structural abnormalities may also be present. Unless the result of a balanced

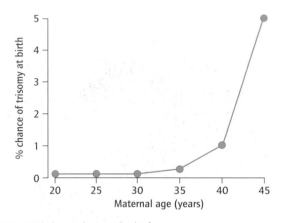

Fig. 18.5 Maternal age and risk of trisomies.

translocation, the recurrence risk is low and determined largely by maternal age.

Other chromosomal abnormalities

Trisomy 18 and *trisomy 13* are also more common with advanced maternal age. They are associated with major structural defects, and affected fetuses die *in utero* or more usually shortly after birth. Sex chromosome abnormalities include *Klinefelter's syndrome* (47 XXY). These males have normal intellect, small testes and are infertile. In *Turner's syndrome* (a single X chromosome only: X0), affected individuals are female, infertile but with normal intellect.

Risk factors for Down's syndrome	
History:	High maternal age
	Previous affected baby (risk increased 1%)
	Balanced parental translocation (rare)
Ultrasound:	Thickened nuchal translucency
	Some structural abnormalities
	Absent or shortened nasal bone
	Triscuspid regurgitation
Blood tests:	Low pregnancy-associated plasma protein A (PAPP-A) (1st trimester)
	High human chorionic gonadotrophin beta-subunit (β-hCG) (1st/2nd trimester)
	Low alpha fetoprotein (AFP) (1st/ 2nd trimester)
	Low oestriol (2nd trimester)
	High inhibin (2nd trimester)

Screening and diagnosis of chromosomal abnormalities

Amniocentesis and *CVS* are diagnostic tests for chromosomal abnormalities. Traditionally they have been offered to women over the age of about 35 years. However, younger women have more babies and therefore, despite a lower individual risk, account for more Down's syndrome pregnancies. These would go undetected without a screening programme for all consenting women.

In the UK, the National Screening Committee (www.nsc.nhs.uk) recommends that all pregnant women are offered a screening test for trisomies including Down's syndrome, which for the latter has a 75% sensitivity and ≤ 3% false positive rate. This can be achieved by integrating the risk from maternal age, with PAPP-A and β-hCG blood tests, and nuchal translucency measurement by ultrasound at 11–13 + 6 weeks in what is called the 'combined test'. The 'triple test', a blood test at 16 weeks which uses AFP, hCG and oestriol, is less accurate and does not meet these standards. It should be reserved for where screening is performed later than 14 weeks. It nevertheless remains in use where nuchal translucency scanning is not available because, not requiring a detailed ultrasound scan, it is less expensive.

A bewildering array of screening tests exist. Common currently available tests are outlined in the box below. These broadly are divided into three types; intimate knowledge of these is not required:
1 The risk at a nuchal translucency scan can be modified by other risk factors at this scan: markers include the presence or absence of the nasal bone (*Lancet* 2001; **358**: 1665), and tricuspid regurgitation (*Ultrasound Obstet Gynecol* 2005; **26**: 22). Less widely accepted and requiring considerable expertise, they may lead to better detection rates in the future.
2 A two-stage assessment combines the risk from the first trimester (with or without a nuchal scan) with blood tests in the second. This only allows a result to be given at 16 weeks.
3 Thirdly, and including the widely available triple test, are second trimester blood tests only.

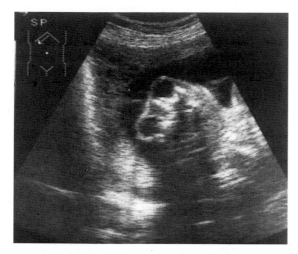
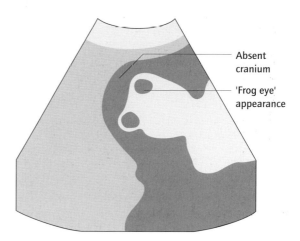

Absent
cranium

'Frog eye'
appearance

Fig. 18.6 Neural tube defect (NTD): anencephaly.

Common screening tests for Down's syndrome and chromosomal abnormalities							
Risk factor used	Age	NT scan	PAPP-A	β-hCG	β-hCG oestriol and AFP	Inhibin A	Sensitivity for FPR (approx.)
Gestation		(11–13 + 6)	(9–13 + 6)	(9–13 + 6)	(15–20)	(15–20)	
Test							
Age > 35 alone	+						40% for 15%
Combined	+	+	+	+			90% for 5%
Serum integrated	+		+		+	+	85% for 3%
Integrated	+	+	+		+	+	95% for 3%
Triple	+				+		85% for 9%
Quadruple	+				+	+	85% for 6%

AFP, alpha fetoprotein; β-hGC, human chorionic gonadotrophin beta; FPR, false positive rate; NT, nuchal translucency; PAPP-A, pregnancy-associated plasma protein A.

Structural abnormalities

Open neural tube defects (NTDs)

These are the result of failure of closure of the neural tube. Neural tissue is exposed, to varying degrees, and may degenerate. Less than 1 in 200 pregnancies are affected, and the incidence is declining. The type and severity of defect depends on its site and degree. The best known examples are *spina bifida* and *anencephaly* (Fig. 18.6): in the former, severe disability is common but not invariable; the latter is incompatible with life. Precon-

ceptual folic acid supplementation for 3 months (0.4 mg/day) reduces the incidence of NTDs and should be taken by all women considering pregnancy. NTDs recur in 1 in 10 pregnancies, but this risk is greatly reduced by higher dose folic acid (4 mg/day).

Screening and diagnosis of NTDs

AFP levels are elevated in pregnancies affected by open NTDs and this has been used as a screening test. The now almost routine use of *ultrasound* at 20 weeks, which may diagnose NTDs with a sensitivity of ~95%, has rendered screening almost redundant.

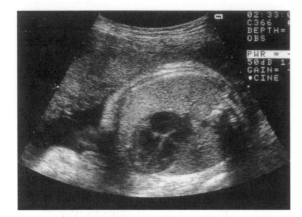

Placenta
Liquor
Abdominal wall
Lung tissue
Spine
A pulmonary vein
Left ventricle
Right ventricle

Fig. 18.7 Normal heart: transverse view of chest.

Cardiac anomalies

These occur in 1% of pregnancies. They are more common in women with congenital cardiac disease, diabetes and when previous offspring have been affected (overall recurrence risk 3%) and where other structural abnormalities or chromosomal disorders are present. In about half of major abnormalities the nuchal translucency was increased at the 11–14 week scan. Most are non-lethal; others may be correctable or partly correctable with surgery after birth. The most common are ventricular septal defects. Ultrasound can be used to detect and diagnose prenatal cardiac disease very accurately; in expert hands at the time of nuchal translucency measurement. Nevertheless, in practice, less than one-third of cases are diagnosed prenatally (Fig. 18.7).

Other structural abnormalities

Polyhydramnios (excessive amniotic fluid) [→ p.157] is common with many abnormalities. *Exomphalos* is characterized by partial extrusion of abdominal contents in a peritoneal sac. Fifty per cent of affected infants have a chromosomal problem and amniocentesis is offered. *Gastroschisis* (Fig. 18.8) is characterized by free loops of bowel in the amniotic cavity and is rarely associated with chromosomal defects. *Diaphragmatic hernias* occur when the abdominal contents herniate into the chest. Many neonates die because of associated anomalies or pulmonary hypoplasia. These disorders are all visible on ultrasound at 20 weeks and can be seen as early as 12 weeks.

Fetal hydrops (Fig. 18.9)

This occurs when extra fluid accumulates in two or more areas in the fetus. It occurs in 1 in 500 pregnancies and, because of its high mortality, is rarer in late pregnancy. It can be 'immune', in association with anaemia and haemolysis as a result of antibodies including rhesus disease [→ p.187]. Or it can be 'non-immune', secondary to another cause. There are five main categories of non-immune hydrops:

1 *Chromosomal abnormalities* such as trisomy 21 are most common in early pregnancy.

2 Many *structural abnormalities* (e.g. diaphragmatic hernia) can cause hydrops, the presence of which usually worsens the fetal prognosis.

3 Congenital *cardiac abnormalities* or *arrhythmias* may be present: the latter can be treated by maternal administration of antiarrhythmic.

4 Cardiac failure due to *anaemia* (e.g. parvovirus infection [→ p.160], feto–maternal haemorrhage or fetal alpha thalassaemia major) may also be responsible.

5 *Twin–twin transfusion syndrome* [→ p.218] in monochorionic twins causes hydrops in severe cases.

Investigation involves careful ultrasound assessment, including a specialist cardiac scan and assessment of the middle cerebral artery [→ p.189]. Maternal blood is taken for Kleihauer and parvovirus immunoglobulin M testing. Fetal blood sampling is performed if anaemia is suspected; it or amniocentesis are performed for karyotyping. The management and prognosis depends on the cause.

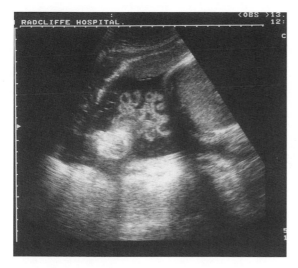

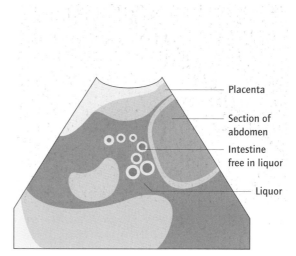

Placenta

Section of abdomen

Intestine free in liquor

Liquor

Fig. 18.8 Gastroschisis.

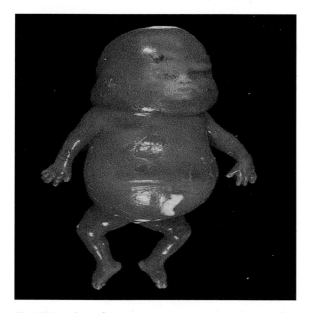

Fig. 18.9 Hydropic fetus.

Single gene disorders

Autosomal dominant conditions (e.g. neurofibromatosis) affect 1 in 150 live births. One affected parent has a 50% chance of passing on the condition.

Autosomal recessive genes (e.g. cystic fibrosis or sickle-cell disease) have different prevalences in different populations. If both parents are carriers, the neonate has a 1 in 4 chance of being affected by the disease, whilst half will be carriers. Detection of carrier status for most cystic fibrosis genes and for haemoglobinopathies is possible. Partners of women who have or are carriers of recessively inherited disease may be tested to see if they too are carriers. Prenatal diagnosis, usually with CVS, may then be offered.

Further reading

Bui TH, Blennow E, Nordenskjold M. Prenatal diagnosis: molecular genetics and cytogenetics. *Best Practice & Research. Clinical Obstetrics & Gynaecology* 2002; **16**: 629–43.

Gilbert RE, Augood C, Gupta R, *et al.* Screening for Down's syndrome: effects, safety, and cost effectiveness of first and second trimester strategies. *British Medical Journal* 2001; **323**: 423–5.

http://www.fetalmedicine.com

http://www.nsc.nhs.uk

Kurjak A, Hafner T, Kos M, Kupesic S, Stanojevic M. Three-dimensional sonography in prenatal diagnosis: a luxury or a necessity? *Journal of Perinatal Medicine* 2000; **28**: 194–209.

Nicolaides KH. First trimester screening for chromosomal abnormalities. *Semininars in Perinatology* 2005; **29**: 190–4.

Ultrasound at a Glance

Definition		3.5–7.0 MHz sound waves are passed into the body; the intensity of deflection from different tissues depends on their densities: this can be represented in 2-D form or computer reconstructed 3-D form
Gynaecology		Assessment of pelvic mass [→ p.287] and normal pelvic anatomy. 'Follicle tracking' in ovulation induction [→ p.85]. Endometrial cavity assessment in abnormal menstrual bleeding [→ p.12]
Obstetric	First trimester:	In exclusion of ectopic pregnancy [→ p.119], assessment of pregnancy viability, detection of retained products of conception after miscarriage. Estimation of gestational age (e.g. crown-rump length at 9–12 weeks). Detection of multiple pregnancy and determination of chorionicity [→ p.217]. Screening for chromosomal abnormalities (nuchal translucency) [→ p.149]. Diagnosis of structural abnormalities
	Second trimester:	Diagnosis of structural abnormalities [→ p.149]. Screening for chromosomal abnormalities. Help other diagnostic (e.g. amniocentesis) or therapeutic (e.g. transfusion [→ p.189]) techniques. Doppler for fetal assessment [→ p.206] or of uterine arteries [→ p.205]
	Third trimester:	Assessment of fetal growth [→ p.206]. As part of biophysical profile for fetal well-being [→ p.196]. Diagnosis of placenta praevia [→ p.196]. Determining presentation in difficult cases. Doppler for fetal assessment
	Benefits:	Aids diagnosis in gynaecology and first trimester. Maternal reassurance, screening for and detection of abnormalities. Reduction of perinatal mortality in high-risk pregnancy. Benefit in low-risk pregnancy mainly better diagnosis of abnormalities
	Safety:	Extremely safe. Possible small increase in left-handedness and lower birth weight

Prenatal Screening and Diagnosis of Congenital Abnormalities at a Glance

Booking	Counsel all regarding prenatal diagnosis options Check rubella immunity to identify need for postnatal immunization Check hepatitis B to allow immunoglobulin administration to neonate Check for syphilis infection and HIV status Arrange genetic counselling ± later chorionic villus sampling (CVS) or amniocentesis if risk of inherited disorder
9–12 weeks	Ultrasound scan to date pregnancy and identify twins: Advise regarding screening for chromosomal trisomies: with nuchal translucency and blood tests Counsel and offer CVS or amniocentesis if the risk is high
20 weeks	Routine anomaly ultrasound to detect structural abnormalities Counsel and consider amniocentesis if abnormalities found Offer cardiac scan if high risk
Later	Some abnormalities only visible in later pregnancy: ultrasound if polyhydramnios, breech, suspected intrauterine growth restriction (IUGR)

Polyhydramnios at a Glance

Definition	Liquor volume increased. Normal volume varies with gestation, but deepest liquor pool >10 cm generally considered abnormal
Epidemiology	1% of pregnancies
Aetiology	Idiopathic; maternal disorders (established and gestational diabetes, renal failure); twins (particularly twin–twin transfusion syndrome [→ p.218]); fetal anomaly (20%) (particularly upper gastrointestinal obstructions or inability to swallow, chest abnormalities, myotonic dystrophy)
Clinical features	Maternal discomfort. Large for dates, taut uterus, fetal parts difficult to palpate
Complications	Preterm labour; maternal discomfort, abnormal lie and malpresentation

Management

To diagnose fetal anomaly:	Detailed ultrasound screening
To diagnose diabetes:	Maternal blood glucose testing [→ p.174]
To reduce liquor:	If < 34 weeks and severe, amnioreduction [→ p.193], or use of non-steroidal anti-inflammatory drugs (NSAIDS) to reduce fetal urine output
	Consider steroids if < 34 weeks
Delivery:	Vaginal unless persistent unstable lie or other obstetric indication

19 Infections in pregnancy

Infections

These assume a particular importance in pregnancy in several ways:

- *Maternal illness* may be worse, as with varicella.
- *Maternal complications*, as with pre-eclampsia in HIV-positive women, may be more common.
- *Preterm labour* [→ p.190] is also associated with infection.
- *Vertical transmission* of otherwise fairly innocuous infections can cause miscarriage, can be teratogenic, as with rubella, or damage already developed organs. Or, as with human immunodeficiency virus (HIV) or hepatitis B, it can cause serious infection in the child. Vertical transmission occurs, or is most damaging, at different times in pregnancy with different infections.
- *Neurological damage* (in addition to the above effects) is more common in the presence of bacterial infection in both preterm and term babies.
- *Antibiotic* usage in pregnancy is occasionally limited by adverse effects to the fetus.

Cytomegalovirus

Pathology/epidemiology: Cytomegalovirus (CMV) is a herpesvirus that is transmitted by personal contact. About 35% of women in the UK are immune. Up to 1% of women develop CMV infection, usually subclinical, in pregnancy. CMV is a common cause of childhood handicap and deafness.

Fetal/neonatal effects: Vertical transmission to the fetus occurs in 40%. Approximately 10% of infected neonates are symptomatic at birth, with intrauterine growth restriction (IUGR) [→ p.203], pneumonia and throm-

Obstetrics and Gynaecology, 3rd edition. By Lawrence Impey and Tim Child. Published 2008 by Blackwell Publishing, ISBN: 978-1-4051-6095-7.

bocytopenia: most of these will develop severe neurological sequelae such as hearing, visual and mental impairment, or will die. The asymptomatic neonates are at risk (15%) of deafness.

Diagnosis: Ultrasound abnormalities such as intracranial or hepatic calcification are evident in only 20%, and most infections are diagnosed when CMV testing is specifically requested. CMV immunoglobulin M (IgM) remains positive for a long time after infection, which could predate the pregnancy: titres will rise and IgG avidity will be low with a recent infection. If maternal infection is confirmed, amniocentesis [→ p.151] at least 6 weeks after maternal infection will confirm or refute vertical transmission.

Management: Most infected neonates are still not seriously affected: close surveillance for ultrasound abnormalities, and fetal blood sampling at 32 weeks for fetal platelet levels, may help determine those at most risk for severe sequelae. There is no prenatal treatment, and termination may be offered. Because most maternal infections do not result in neonatal sequelae and amniocentesis involves risk, routine screening is not advised. Vaccination is not available.

Herpes simplex

Pathology/epidemiology: The type 2 deoxyribonucleic acid (DNA) virus is responsible for most genital herpes (Figs 19.1 & 19.2). Less than 5% of pregnant women have a history of prior infection, but many more have antibodies.

Fetal/neonatal effects: Herpes simplex is not teratogenic. Neonatal infection is rare, but has a high mortality. Vertical transmission occurs at vaginal delivery particularly if vesicles are present. This is most likely to follow recent primary maternal infection (risk 40%), because the fetus will not have passive immunity from maternal antibodies.

Diagnosis: This is usually clear clinically and swabs are of little use in pregnancy.

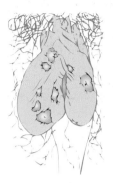

Fig. 19.1 Herpes simplex.

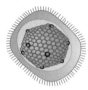

Herpes simplex virus (HSV)	Cold sores (type 1) Genital herpes (type 2)
Cytomegalovirus (CMV)	Cytomegalic inclusion disease in neonates

Fig. 19.2 Herpesvirus.

Management: Referral to a genitourinary clinic is indicated. Caesarean section is recommended for those delivering within 6 weeks of a primary attack, and those with genital lesions from primary infection at the time of delivery. The risk is very low in women with recurrent herpes who have vesicles present at the time of labour. Daily aciclovir in late pregnancy may reduce the frequency of recurrences at term (*Obstet Gynecol* 1996; **87**: 69). Exposed neonates are given aciclovir. Screening is of little benefit.

Rubella

Pathology/epidemiology: The rubella virus usually affects children and causes a mild febrile illness with a macular rash, which is often called 'German measles'. Congenital rubella is very rare in UK women because of widespread immunization: <10 affected neonates are born each year (*BMJ* 1999; **7186**: 769). Immunity is lifelong.

Fetal/neonatal effects: Maternal infection in early pregnancy frequently causes multiple fetal abnormalities, including deafness, cardiac disease, eye problems and mental retardation. The probability and severity of malformation decreases with advancing gestation: at 9 weeks the risk is 90%; after 16 weeks, the risk is very low.

Management/screening: If a non-immune woman develops rubella before 16 weeks' gestation, termination of pregnancy is offered. Screening remains routine at booking to identify those in need of vaccination after the end of pregnancy. Rubella vaccine is live and contraindicated in pregnancy, although harm has not been recorded.

Toxoplasmosis

Pathology/epidemiology: This is due to the protozoan parasite *Toxoplasma gondii*. It follows contact with cat faeces or soil, or eating infected meat. In the UK, 20% of adults have antibodies; infection in pregnancy occurs in 0.2% of women in the UK, but it is more common in mainland Europe.

Fetal/neonatal effects: Fetal infection follows in under half: this is more common as pregnancy progresses, but earlier infection is more likely to result in severe sequelae. These include mental retardation, convulsions, spasticities and visual impairment (<10 per year in the UK).

Diagnosis: Ultrasound may show hydrocephalus, but maternal infection is usually diagnosed after maternal testing for IgM is performed because of exposure or anxiety. False positives and negatives are common. Vertical transmission is diagnosed or excluded using amniocentesis performed after 20 weeks.

Management: Health education reduces the risk of maternal infection. Spiramycin is started as soon as maternal toxoplasmosis is diagnosed. If vertical transmission is subsequently confirmed, additional combination therapy is also used. Whilst this protocol probably improves the prognosis for the neonate, this remains debated (*BMJ* 1999; **318**: 1511). Screening is not recommended where the prevalence is low.

Herpes zoster

Pathology/epidemiology: Primary infection with this DNA herpesvirus causes chickenpox, a common childhood illness; reactivation of latent infection is shingles, which usually affects adults in one or two dermatomes. A woman who is not immune to zoster can develop chickenpox after exposure to chickenpox or shingles. Chickenpox in pregnancy is rare (0.05%), but can cause severe maternal illness.

Fetal/neonatal effects: Teratogenicity is a rare (1–2%) consequence of early pregnancy infection, which is immediately treated with oral aciclovir. Maternal infection in the 4 weeks preceding delivery can cause severe neonatal infection: this is most common (up to 50%) if delivery occurs within 5 days after or 2 days before maternal symptoms.

Management: Immunoglobulin is used to prevent, and aciclovir to treat infection. Therefore, pregnant women exposed to zoster are tested for immunity: immunoglobulin is recommended if they are non-immune, and aciclovir if infection occurs. In late pregnancy, neonates delivered 5 days after or 2 days before maternal infection are given immunoglobulin, closely monitored and given aciclovir if infection occurs. Vaccination is possible but not universal.

Infections suitable for screening
Syphilis
Hepatitis B
Rubella
Probably: *Chlamydia*
Bacterial vaginosis
β-haemolytic streptococcus

Teratogenic infections
Cytomegalovirus (CMV)
Rubella
Toxoplasmosis
Syphilis
Chickenpox

Parvovirus

Epidemiology: The B19 virus infects 0.25% of pregnant women, and more during epidemics; 50% of women are immune. A 'slapped cheek' appearance (erythema infectiosum) is classic but many have arthralgia or are asymptomatic. Infection is usually from children.

Neonatal/fetal effects: The virus suppresses fetal erythropoesis causing anaemia. Variable degrees of thrombocytoenia also occur. Fetal death occurs in 9% of pregnancies (*BJOG* 1998; **105**: 174), usually with infection before 20 weeks' gestation.

Diagnosis: Where maternal exposure or symptoms have occurred, positive maternal IgM testing will prompt fetal surveillance. Anaemia is detectable on ultrasound, initially as increased blood flow velocity in the fetal middle cerebral artery [→ p.189] and subsequently as oedema (fetal hydrops [→ p.154]) from cardiac failure. Or maternal testing may follow the identification of fetal hydrops. Spontaneous resolution of anaemia and hydrops occurs in about 50%.

Management: Mothers infected are scanned regularly to look for anaemia. Where hydrops is detected, *in utero* transfusion is given if this is severe. Survivors have an excellent prognosis although very severe disease has recently been associated with neurological damage (*Obstet Gynecol* 2007; **109**: 42).

Group B streptococcus

Pathology/epidemiology: The bacterium *Streptococcus agalactiae* is carried, without symptoms, by about 25% of pregnant women.

Neonatal effects: The fetus can be infected, normally during labour after the membranes have ruptured. This is most common with preterm labours, if labour is prolonged, or there is a maternal fever. Early onset neonatal group B streptococcus (GBS) sepsis [→ p.241] occurs in 1 in 500 neonates. It causes severe illness and has a mortality of 6% in term infants and 18% in preterm infants.

Management/screening: Known GBS carriers and those at high risk are given high dose intravenous penicillin throughout labour (*Cochrane* 2000: CD000115). This reduces neonatal infection by about 80%. Preventative strategies are based on risk factors either alone or in conjunction with *screening* (see box below) (RCOG Guideline 36, 2003: www.rcog.org.uk). The latter is more expensive and requires a greater use of antibiotics, but is more effective. This screening requires swabs from the vagina and rectum as near as possible to the time of delivery and a special culture medium.

Prevention of vertical transmission of group B streptococcus	
Strategy 1: Risk factors alone	*Strategy 2: Risk factors + screening*
No screening	Vaginal and rectal swab at 34–36 weeks
Treat with intravenous penicillin in labour if: Previous history Intrapartum fever >38°C Current preterm labour Rupture of the membranes >18 h	Treat with intravenous penicillin in labour if: Swabs positive, or any risk factor presents (except prolonged rupture of membranes)

Hepatitis B

Pathology/epidemiology: This is caused by a small DNA virus, transmitted by blood products or sexual activity. Infection resolves in 90% of adults, but in 10% persistent infection occurs. This infectious state is present in 1% of pregnant women in the West but in up to 25% of women in, or from, parts of Asia and Africa. The degree of infectivity depends on antibody status: individuals with the 'surface' antibody (HBsAb positive) are immunologically cured and of low infectivity to others and their fetus. Those with the surface antigen but not the antibody (HBsAg positive) and those with the E antigen (HBeAg positive) are more infectious.

Neonatal effects: Vertical transmission occurs at delivery. Importantly, 90% of infected neonates become chronic carriers, compared to only 10% of infected adults.

Management/screening: Neonatal immunization (*BMJ* 2006; **332**: 328) reduces the risk of infection by over 90%. Because high risk groups encompass only 50% of chronic carriers, maternal screening is routine in the UK. Known carriers should be handled with sensitive precautions for fear of infecting staff.

Human immunodeficiency virus

Epidemiology: The retroviruses that cause acquired immune deficiency syndrome (AIDS) have infected up to 1% of women in some inner city areas in the UK and over 1000 pregnancies a year occur in women known to be infected. In parts of Africa and Asia, rates of infection are 20%. Heterosexual transmission is now the most important route.

Maternal effects: Pregnancy does not hasten progression to AIDS. The incidence of pre-eclampsia is greater in HIV infected women, and this may be increased by antiretroviral therapy (*Lancet* 2002; **360**: 1152). Gestational diabetes may also be more common.

Neonatal/fetal effects: Stillbirth, pre-eclampsia, IUGR [→ p.203] and prematurity are more common. Congenital abnormalities are not, and antiretrovirals are not teratogenic, but folic acid antagonists (e.g. co-trimoxazole) are often prescribed to HIV infected women. The most important risk is of vertical transmission. This is mostly beyond 36 weeks, intrapartum or during breastfeeding (*Lancet* 1992; **339**: 1007). It occurs in 15% in the absence of preventative measures, and in up to 40% of breastfeeding women in Africa, although passively acquired antibodies in the neonate are universal because of transplacental transfer. Transmission is greater with low CD4 counts and high viral load (early and late stage disease), co-existent infection, premature delivery and during labour, particularly with ruptured membranes for more than 4 h. Twenty-five per cent of HIV infected neonates develop AIDS by 1 year and 40% will develop AIDS by 5 years.

Management/screening: HIV-positive women should be managed in conjunction with a physician and have regular CD4 and viral load tests. Prophylaxis against *Pneumocystic carinii* pneumonia (PCP) is given if the CD4 count is low. Drug toxicity is monitored with liver and renal function, haemoglobin and blood glucose testing. Genital tract infections such as *Chlamydia* should be sought.

Strategies to prevent vertical transmission unfortunately need to differ according to the social and economic circumstances of the population. This is because of the cost of medication and complications of obstetric intervention, and the benefits of breastfeeding in an under-resourced population. The 'ideal' policy is highly active antiretroviral therapy (HAART), currently including zidovudine, which reduces viraemia (Fig. 19.3) and maternal disease progression. This is continued throughout pregnancy and delivery, and the neonate is treated for the first 6 weeks. When women are not receiving prepregnancy treatment for their own health, therapy is

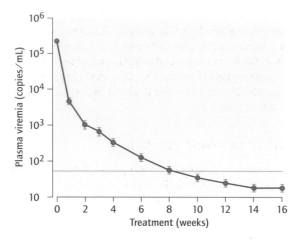

Fig. 19.3 Decline in human immunodeficiency virus (HIV) particles with highly active antiretroviral therapy (HAART).

usually started around 28 weeks: individual regimens vary. Caesarean section is performed and breastfeeding is avoided. This 'best' strategy reduces vertical transmission to <1%.

In under-resourced countries, nevirapine, as single doses in labour and to the neonate, greatly reduces vertical transmission in women delivering vaginally. Amniotomy [→ p.234] is deferred. Breastfeeding is still advised, but should be exclusive, limited to 6 months, and with antiviral prophylaxis: a policy of formula feeding under these conditions, whilst associated with a slightly lower vertical transmission rate than breastfeeding with zidovudine prophylaxis, is associated with a higher mortality (*JAMA* 2006; **296**: 794).

Vertical transmission still occurs, even in resourced countries, largely because of lack of knowledge of HIV status and because of poor access to health care. Screening in pregnancy is now routinely available.

Methods to prevent vertical transmission of human immunodeficiency virus (HIV)
Maternal antiretroviral therapy
Elective Caesarean section
Avoidance of breastfeeding
Neonatal antiretroviral therapy

Other important infections

Group A streptococcus

This remains an important cause of puerperal sepsis [→ p.269], particularly in developing countries.

Syphilis

This sexually transmitted disease due to *Treponema pallidum* is rare in the UK, although endemic in developing countries. Active disease in pregnancy usually causes miscarriage, severe congenital disease or stillbirth. Prompt treatment with benzylpenicillin is safe and will prevent, but not reverse, fetal damage. Therefore screening tests, such as the Venereal Disease Research Laboratories (VDRL) test, which are cheap and accurate, are still in routine use. False positives occur particularly with autoimmune disease and the diagnosis should be confirmed using *Treponema*-specific tests.

Mycobacterium tuberculosis

Worldwide, tuberculosis (TB) is very common, and its incidence in the UK is increasing because of immigration, HIV infection and travel. Tuberculin testing is safe; Bacille bilié de Calmette–Guérin (BCG) vaccination is live and contraindicated. Diagnosis in late pregnancy is associated with prematurity and IUGR [→ p.203], and TB is a significant cause of maternal mortality in the developing world. Treatment with first line drugs and additional vitamin B_6 is safe in pregnancy, but streptomycin is contraindicated. Congenital TB is very rare.

Hepatitis C

In the UK, infection is found in 0.5%, mostly from high-risk groups, particularly HIV infected women (30%). Most are asymptomatic. Vertical transmission occurs in 6%, is increased by concomitant HIV infection and a high viral load. Infected neonates are prone to chronic hepatitis. Most data suggest that elective Caesarean section does not reduce vertical transmission rates. Screening is restricted to high-risk groups.

Malaria

Although rare in the UK, malaria infection is very

common in developing countries: in sub-Saharan Africa 8% of infant mortality is attributed to it. Maternal complications, including severe anaemia are more frequent in pregnancy, and IUGR and stillbirth are more common. Congenital malaria complicates 1% of affected pregnancies. Drug usage is dictated by local sensitivity, but most falciparum malaria is resistant to chloroquine or mefloquine, and artemisin combination therapy (ACT) is increasingly used and appears safe (*Mal J* 2007; **6**: 15). Prevention of maternal and neonatal effects involves intermittent preventative treatment (IPT) of two doses at least a month apart, insecticide impregnated mosquito nets and appropriate drug treatment.

Listeriosis

Infection with the bacterium *Listeria monocytogenes*, a Gram-negative bacillus, can occur from consumption of pâtés, soft cheeses and prepacked meals, and causes a non-specific febrile illness. It is common in human faeces, but if bacteraemia occurs in pregnancy (0.01% of women) potentially fatal infection of the fetus may follow. The diagnosis is established from blood cultures. Screening is impractical. Prevention involves the avoidance of high-risk foods in pregnancy [→ p.144].

Chlamydia and gonorrhoea

Chlamydia trachomatis infection in pregnancy in the UK occurs in about 5% of women and *Neisseria gonorrhoeae* in 0.1%. Most women are asymptomatic. Although best known as causes of pelvic inflammatory disease and subfertility, both have been associated with preterm labour and with neonatal conjunctivitis. *Chlamydia* is treated with azithromycin or erythromycin; tetracyclines cause fetal tooth discoloration. Gonorrhoea is treated with cephalosporins as resistance to penicillin is common. *Screening* and treatment is worthwhile in developing countries, before termination of pregnancy and in single women with a history of preterm labour: treatment may reduce the incidence of preterm birth.

Bacterial vaginosis

This common overgrowth of normal vaginal lactobacilli by anaerobes such as *Gardnerella vaginalis* and *Myco-*plasma hominis* can be asymptomatic or cause an offensive vaginal discharge in women. Preterm labour and late miscarriage are more common. *Screening* and treatment (best with oral clindamycin) only reduces the risk of preterm birth if used before 20 weeks (*Cochrane* 2007: CD 000262) or in women with a history of preterm birth.

Other obstetric infections

- Urinary tract infections and pyelonephritis [→ p.180]
- Endometritis [→ p.74]
- Chorioamnionitis [→ p.191]

Further reading

Apgar BS, Greenberg G, Yen G. Prevention of group B streptococcal disease in the newborn. *American Family Physician* 2005; **71**: 903–10.

Brocklehurst P, Volmink J. Antiretrovirals for reducing the risk of mother-to-child transmission of HIV infection. *Cochrane Database of Systematic Reviews (Online: Update Software)* 2002; **2**: CD003510.

Ergaz Z, Ornoy A. Parvovirus B19 in pregnancy. *Reproductive Toxicology* 2006; **21**: 421–35.

Foster CJ, Lyall EG. HIV in pregnancy: evolution of clinical practice in the UK. *International Journal of STD & AIDS* 2006; **17**: 660–7.

http://www.aidsmap.com

Kourtis AP, Lee FK, Abrams EJ, Jamieson DJ, Bulterys M. Mother-to-child transmission of HIV-1: timing and implications for prevention. *Lancet Infectious Diseases* 2006; **6**: 726–32.

Lee C, Gong Y, Brok J, Boxall EH, Gluud C. Effect of hepatitis B immunisation in newborn infants of mothers positive for hepatitis B surface antigen: systematic review and meta-analysis. *British Medical Journal* 2006; **332**: 328–36.

Ormerod P. Tuberculosis in pregnancy and the puerperium. *Thorax* 2001; **56**: 494–9.

Ornoy A, Diav-Citrin O. Fetal effects of primary and secondary cytomegalovirus infection in pregnancy. *Reproductive Toxicology* 2006; **21**: 399–409.

Rorman E, Zamir CS, Rilkis I, Ben-David H. Congenital toxoplasmosis: prenatal aspects of *Toxoplasma gondii* infection. *Reproductive Toxicology* 2006; **21**: 458–72.

Watts DH. Treating HIV during pregnancy: an update on safety issues. *Drug Safety* 2006; **29**: 467–90.

HIV in Pregnancy at a Glance

Epidemiology	Approx. 1000 pregnancies/year in UK; >10 million worldwide
Maternal effects	Pre-eclampsia. Disease progression not faster
Fetal effects	Prematurity, intrauterine growth restriction (IUGR), stillbirth Vertical transmission: <1% with best prophylaxis, 15% with none, up to 40% if under-resourced area and breastfeeding. Increased by early/late disease, high CD4 or low viral load, prematurity, other infection, labour, long rupture of membranes, breastfeeding
Management	If resources available: combination therapy (continue or start at 28 weeks), elective Caesarean section, avoid breastfeeding, treat neonate for 6 weeks. Screen for other infections If poor resources: nevirapine during labour and for breastfeeding

Infections in Pregnancy at a Glance

Cytomegalovirus (CMV)	1% maternal infection rate, 40% vertical transmission. Maternal diagnosis from IgM, IgG avidity. Fetal diagnosis from amniocentesis at 20+ weeks. 10% of infected fetuses severely affected, deafness common. No treatment, screening or vaccination
Rubella	Most women immune, so rare. High percentage of fetuses affected if <16 weeks: termination of pregnancy (TOP) offered. Screening identifies those in need of postnatal immunization
Toxoplasmosis	0.2% maternal infection rate. Low percentage of fetuses permanently affected. Screening not routine in the UK. Maternal diagnosis from IgM; fetal from amniocentesis at 20+ weeks. Proven infection treated with spiramycin; fetal toxoplasmosis treated with combination therapy
Syphilis	Rare. Screening routine because treatment prevents congenital syphilis
Herpes simplex virus (HSV)	Common. Neonatal infection is rare but serious. High risk of neonatal herpes (therefore Caesarean is indicated) if primary infection within 6 weeks of delivery, or active vesicles at time of labour. Aciclovir used
Group B streptococcus	High maternal carrier rate; major cause of severe neonatal illness. Treatment with intrapartum penicillin of high-risk groups ± positive third trimester screen greatly reduces neonatal infection
Herpes zoster	Many immune. Severe maternal illness in pregnancy. Infection <20 weeks occasionally teratogenic. Infection just before delivery can cause severe neonatal infection, so immunoglobulin given to neonate
Hepatitis B	Carriage common in high-risk women. High transmission rate, high chronic disease rate and mortality in neonate. Universal screening identifies neonates in need of immunoglobulin
Hepatitis C	Mostly in high-risk (e.g. human immunodeficiency virus [HIV]) women: 6% vertical transmission
Chlamydia	5% in pregnancy. Neonatal conjunctivitis and preterm labour. Antibiotics may prevent latter, so screening probably worthwhile
Bacterial vaginosis	Common. Associated with preterm labour. Screening and treatment if previous preterm labour
Parvovirus	0.25%, more in epidemics. 9% excess fetal death, most with infection pre-20 weeks. Fetus develops anaemia and subsequent hydrops. If IgM positive, surveillance for anemia with middle cerebral artery Doppler and ultrasound. *In utero* transfusion if anaemia very severe

Obstetrics and Gynaecology, 3rd edition. By Lawrence Impey and Tim Child. Published 2008 by Blackwell Publishing, ISBN: 978-1-4051-6095-7.

20 Hypertensive disorders in pregnancy

Normal blood pressure changes in pregnancy

Blood pressure is dependent on systemic vascular resistance and cardiac output. It normally falls to a minimum level in the second trimester, by about 30/15 mmHg, because of reduced vascular resistance. This occurs in both normotensive and chronically hypertensive women. By term, the blood pressure again rises to prepregnant levels (Fig. 20.1). Hypertension due to pre-eclampsia is largely due to an increase in systemic vascular resistance. Protein excretion in normal pregnancy is increased, but in the absence of underlying renal disease is less than 0.3 g/24 h.

Classification of hypertensive disorders in pregnancy

The classification of these is diverse and often inconsistent. The definitions below are used because they are simple and best represent the pathological processes involved.

Pregnancy-induced hypertension

This is when the blood pressure rises above 140/90 mmHg. It can be due to either pre-eclampsia or transient hypertension. *Pre-eclampsia* is a disorder in which hypertension and proteinuria appear in the second half of pregnancy, usually with oedema. Eclampsia, or the occurrence of epileptiform seizures, is the most dramatic complication. Proteinuria is occasionally absent, e.g. in early disease, when it is not always distinguishable from *transient hypertension*. These patients without significant (<0.3 g/24 h) proteinuria are 'latent' hypertensives who commonly develop hypertension in later life.

Pre-existing or chronic hypertension

This is present when the diastolic blood pressure is more than 140/90 mmHg before pregnancy or before 20 weeks' gestation. This may be *essential hypertension*, or it may be *secondary* to renal or other disease. There may be pre-existing proteinuria because of renal disease. Patients with underlying hypertension are at an increased risk (sixfold) of developing 'superimposed' pre-eclampsia.

Classification of hypertension		
Pregnancy induced:	Pre-eclampsia	
	Transient	
Pre-existing:	Essential	
	Secondary	

Pre-eclampsia

Definitions and terminology

Pre-eclampsia is a multisystem disease that is usually manifest as hypertension and proteinuria. It is peculiar to pregnancy, of placental origin and cured only by delivery. Blood vessel endothelial cell damage, in association with an exaggerated maternal inflammatory response (*AmJOG* 1999; **180**: 499) leads to vasospasm, increased capillary permeability and clotting dysfunction (Fig. 20.2). These can affect all the maternal organs *to varying degrees* and account for all manifestations and complications. Increased vascular resistance accounts for the hypertension, increased vascular permeability for proteinuria, reduced placental blood flow for intrauter-

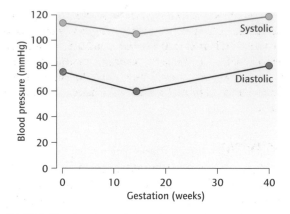

Fig. 20.1 Blood pressure changes in pregnancy.

ine growth restriction (IUGR) and reduced cerebral perfusion for eclampsia.

The multisystem nature of the disease explains why the clinical features are variable. Hypertension is just a sign rather than the disease itself, and is even occasionally absent until late stages; proteinuria is often absent in early disease. Although traditionally central to *establishing* the diagnosis, one or other of these features may nevertheless be absent in a woman who has pre-eclampsia (*BMJ* 1994; **309**: 1395). Furthermore, eclampsia, the most dramatic complication, is just one of many. Differing definitions confuse the issue: 'pregnancy-induced hypertension' encompasses 'transient hypertension', which, although often indistinguishable from mild pre-eclampsia on clinical grounds, is a different disease entity.

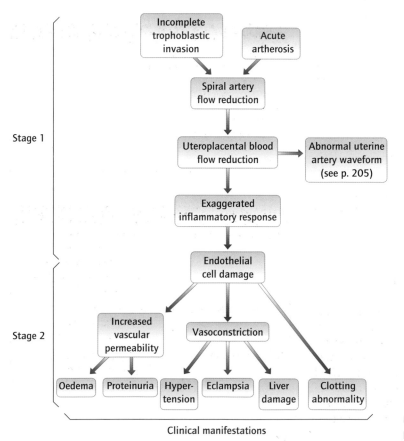

Fig. 20.2 Simplified pathogenesis of pre-eclampsia.

Establishing the diagnosis of pre-eclampsia
Blood pressure rises >140/90 mmHg *with* Proteinuria >0.3 g/24 h

Course and degrees of the disease

The disease is progressive, but variable and unpredictable. Hypertension *usually* precedes proteinuria, a relatively late sign. Some women develop life-threatening disease at 24 weeks; others merely develop mild hypertension at term. Although only partly reflecting the severity of disease, the degree of hypertension can be used to help assess it (see box below).

Epidemiology

Pre-eclampsia affects 6% of nulliparous women to varying degrees. It is less common in multiparous women unless additional risk factors are present.

Degrees of pre-eclampsia	
Classifications vary: the one below encompasses the principles and diversity of the disease	
Mild:	Proteinuria and hypertension <170/110 mmHg
Moderate:	Proteinuria and hypertension ≥170/110 mmHg
Severe:	Proteinuria and hypertension <32 weeks or with maternal complications

Pathophysiology

The mechanism is incompletely understood but it appears to be a two-stage process (Fig. 20.2):
1 *Stage 1 accounts for the development of the disease*, occurs before 20 weeks and causes no symptoms. In normal pregnancy, trophoblastic invasion of spiral arterioles leads to vasodilatation of vessel walls. In pre-eclampsia this invasion is incomplete. This impaired maternofetal trophoblast interaction may be caused by altered immune responses. In addition, spiral arterioles may contain atheromatous lesions. The result is decreased uteroplacental blood flow.

2 *Stage 2 is the manifestation of the disease*: The ischaemic placenta, probably via an exaggerated maternal inflammatory response, induces widespread endothelial cell damage, causing vasoconstriction, increased vascular permeability and clotting dysfunction. These cause the clinical manifestations of disease.

Aetiology

Predisposing factors (*BMJ* 2005; **330**: 565) include nulliparity, a previous or family history of pre-eclampsia, a new partner, long inter-pregnancy interval, obesity, polycystic ovary syndrome, extremes of maternal age (particularly older age), disorders characterized by microvascular disease (chronic hypertension, chronic renal disease, sickle-cell disease [→ p.184], diabetes, autoimmune disease, particularly antiphospholipid syndrome) and pregnancies with a large placenta (twins, molar pregnancy).

Principal risk factors for pre-eclampsia
Nulliparity Previous history, family history Older maternal age Chronic hypertension Diabetes Twin pregnancies Autoimmune disease Renal disease Obesity

Assessment of urinary protein		
1	Dipsticks (bedside): trace:	Seldom significant 1+ Possible significant proteinuria: quantify ≥2+ Significant proteinuria likely: quantify
2	Protein: creatinine ratio:	>30 mg/nmol Probable significant proteinuria
3	24 h collection:	>0.3 g/24 h Confirmed significant proteinuria

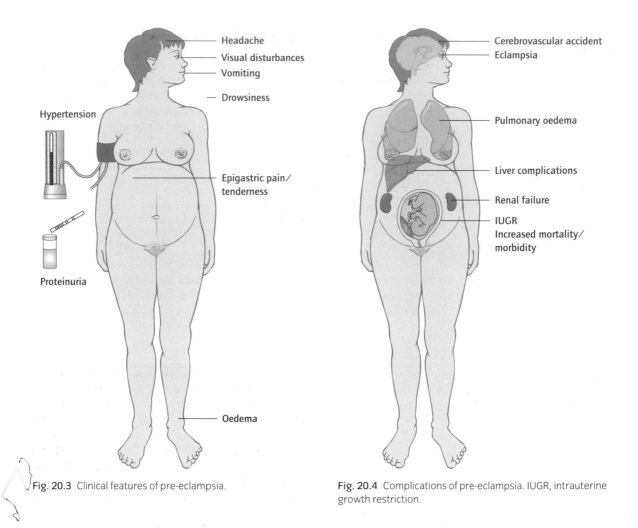

Fig. 20.3 Clinical features of pre-eclampsia.

Fig. 20.4 Complications of pre-eclampsia. IUGR, intrauterine growth restriction.

HELLP syndrome	
1 H (haemolysis):	Dark urine, raised lactic dehydrogenase (LDH), anaemia
2 EL (elevated liver enzymes):	Epigastric pain, liver failure, abnormal clotting
3 LP (low platelets):	Normally self-limiting

Clinical features

History. Pre-eclampsia is usually asymptomatic, but headache, drowsiness, visual disturbances, nausea/ vomiting or epigastric pain may occur at a late stage.

Examination. Hypertension is usually the first sign, but it is occasionally absent until the late stages. Oedema is found in most pregnancies but in pre-eclampsia may be massive, not postural or of sudden onset. The presence of epigastric tenderness is suggestive of impending complications. Urine testing for protein with dipsticks should be considered part of the clinical examination (Fig. 20.3).

Complications of pre-eclampsia (Fig. 20.4)

Maternal

Early onset disease tends to be more severe. The occurrence of any of the following complications, which may occur together, is an indication for delivery whatever the gestation. They may also occur postpartum as it takes at least 24 h for delivery to 'cure' the disease.

Eclampsia is grand mal seizures (0.05% of all pregnancies in UK), probably resulting from cerebrovascular vasospasm. Mortality can result from hypoxia and concomitant complications of severe disease. Treatment is with magnesium sulphate (*Lancet* 1995; **345**: 1455), and intensive surveillance for other complications.

Cerebrovascular haemorrhage results from a failure of cerebral blood flow autoregulation at mean arterial pressures above 140 mmHg. Treatment of blood pressure reaching 170/110 mmHg should prevent this.

Liver and coagulation problems: 'HELLP' syndrome consists of haemolysis (H), elevated liver enzymes (EL) and low platelet count (LP). Disseminated intravascular coagulation (DIC), liver failure and liver rupture may also occur. The woman typically experiences severe epigastric pain; occasionally this is the presenting feature of pre-eclampsia, and it may occur postnatally in a hitherto well woman. Haemolysis turns the urine dark. Treatment is supportive and includes magnesium sulphate prophylaxis against eclampsia. Intensive care therapy is required in severe cases. High dose steroids are often given although their benefits are debated (*AmJOG* 2005; **193**: 1591).

Renal failure is identified by careful fluid balance monitoring and creatinine measurement. Haemodialysis is required in severe cases.

Pulmonary oedema: The severe pre-eclamptic is particularly vulnerable to fluid overload. Pulmonary oedema is treated with oxygen and frusemide; assisted ventilation may be required. Adult respiratory distress syndrome (ARDS) may develop and is a common cause of maternal mortality associated with pre-eclampsia.

Fetal

Perinatal mortality and morbidity of the fetus is greatly increased.

In pregnancies affected before 36 weeks, the principal problem is IUGR. Preterm delivery is often required, although spontaneous preterm labour is also more common. IUGR results from the ischaemic placenta, which may contain areas of infarction.

At term, pre-eclampsia affects birth weight less but is nevertheless also associated with an increased morbidity and mortality. At all gestations there is an increased risk of placental abruption [→ p.198].

Complications of pre-eclampsia	
Maternal: (can cause maternal death)	Eclampsia Cerebrovascular accident (CVA) Haemolysis, elevated liver enzymes and low platelet count (HELLP) Disseminated intravascular coagulation (DIC) Liver failure Renal failure Pulmonary oedema
Fetal: (can cause fetal death)	Intrauterine growth restriction (IUGR) Preterm birth Placental abruption Hypoxia

Investigations

To confirm the diagnosis: If bedside dipstick urinalysis is positive, infection is excluded by urine culture, and the protein is quantified. Traditionally, a 24-h urine collection was performed. Nearly as good, and faster and cheaper, the protein : creatinine ratio on a single sample can also be used (*Acta Obstet Gynecol Scand* 2006; **85**: 1327). A level of 30 mg/nmol is equivalent to approximately 0.3 g/24 h protein excretion. Proteinuria may be absent in early disease and testing for proteinuria is repeated.

To monitor maternal complications: Blood tests often show elevation of the uric acid, although this predicts complications poorly (*BJOG* 2006; **113**: 369). The haemoglobin is often high as a result of haemoconcentration. A rapid fall in platelets due to platelet aggregation on damaged endothelium indicates impending HELLP or DIC. Liver function tests are initially normal, but a rise also suggests impending liver damage or HELLP. LDH levels rise with liver disease and haemolysis. Renal function is often mildly impaired; a rapidly rising creatinine suggests severe complications and renal failure.

To monitor fetal complications: An ultrasound scan helps estimate fetal weight at early gestations and is used to assess fetal growth. Umbilical artery Doppler [→ p.206] and if abnormal, daily cardiotocography (CTG) [→ p.207] are used to evaluate fetal well-being.

Screening and prevention

All pregnant women, especially those at high risk [→ p.205], have regular blood pressure and urinalysis checks. Screening tests are relatively inaccurate. The most commonly used is *uterine artery Doppler* [→ p.205] at 23 weeks' gestation. The sensitivity for pre-eclampsia at any stage in pregnancy is about 40% for a 5% screen positive rate [→ p.148]; for early onset or severe pre-eclampsia the figures are better (*Ultrasound Obstet Gynecol* 2001; **18**: 441). In the near future, integration of independent risks including uterine artery Doppler is likely to improve this screening further.

It has been recently found that a molecule called soluble fms-like tyrosine kinase 1 (sFlt-1), which binds to cells of blood vessels and can induce a pre-eclampsia-like syndrome in animal models, is greatly raised some weeks before pre-eclampsia is manifest. Similarly, molecules that bind sFlt-1, e.g. vascular endothelial growth factor (VEGF) and placental growth factor (PIGF), are found in lower levels. Use of assays of these may allow earlier detection of pre-eclampsia in the future (*NEJM* 2006; **355**: 992).

Low-dose aspirin modestly reduces the risk of pre-eclampsia in high-risk women (*BMJ* 2001; **322**: 329); vitamin C and E do not. (*Lancet* 2006; **367**: 1145).

Management

Assessment

Women with new hypertension greater than 140/90 mmHg are assessed in a 'day assessment unit' (*Cochrane* 2001: CD001803), where blood pressure is rechecked and investigations are performed. Patients without proteinuria and whose diastolic blood pressure is <170/110 mmHg are usually managed as out-patients. Their blood pressure and urinalysis are repeated twice weekly and ultrasound is performed fortnightly unless suggestive of fetal compromise [→ p.203].

Criteria for admission in pre-eclampsia or suspected pre-eclampsia

Symptoms
Proteinuria 2+ or more on dipstick; or >0.3 g/24 h on 24 h collection
Diastolic blood pressure ≥170/110 mmHg
Suspected fetal compromise

Admission

This is necessary with moderate or severe pre-eclampsia, or if fetal compromise is suspected. Patients with new proteinuria of 2+ or more should be admitted to hospital, whatever the blood pressure. Those without significant proteinuria on 24-h testing can be discharged. If there is 1+ proteinuria only, quantification and subsequent review 2 days later, but not admission, are usual.

Drugs in pre-eclampsia

Antihypertensives are given if the blood pressure reaches 170/110 mmHg. Methyldopa is best for maintenance, but causes drowsiness. Oral nifedipine is used for initial control, with intravenous labetalol as second line with severe hypertension. The aim is a pressure of about 140/90 mmHg. Antihypertensives do not change the course of pre-eclampsia, and are used with caution, but increase safety for the mother, reduce hospitalization and, provided monitoring remains intense, may allow prolongation of a pregnancy affected preterm.

Magnesium sulphate is used both for the treatment (*Lancet* 1995; **345**: 1455) and in severe disease, prevention (*Lancet* 2002; **359**: 1877) of eclampsia. An intravenous loading dose is followed by an intravenous infusion. This drug is not an anticonvulsant but, by increasing cerebral perfusion, probably treats the underlying pathology of eclampsia. Toxicity is severe, resulting in respiratory depression and hypotension, but is preceded by loss of patellar reflexes, which are tested regularly. The dose will need to be reduced or even stopped if renal impairment is present.

Steroids [→ p.194] are used to promote fetal pulmonary maturity if the gestation is <34 weeks.

Timing of delivery

Pre-eclampsia is progressive, unpredictable and cured only by delivery. As a general rule, one or more fetal or maternal complications are likely to occur within 2 weeks of the onset of proteinuria (*Lancet* 1993; **341**: 1451).

Mild hypertension without fetal compromise is monitored for deterioration. Induction of labour at term is wise.

Moderate or severe pre-eclampsia requires delivery if the gestation exceeds 34–36 weeks, after which time complications of prematurity are less of a problem. Hypertension reaching 170/110 mmHg must be controlled first. *Before 34 weeks*, conservative management may be appropriate (*AmJOG* 1994; **171**: 818), in a specialist unit with full neonatal care facilities, but the possible benefits of increasing fetal maturity must be weighed against the risks of disease complications. Steroids are given prophylactically, hypertension is treated and there is intensive maternal and fetal surveillance involving daily clinical assessment, CTG and fluid balance, and frequent blood testing. Clinical deterioration, either of the mother or the fetus, will prompt delivery.

Severe pre-eclampsia with complications or fetal distress requires delivery whatever the gestation.

Conduct of delivery

Before 34 weeks, Caesarean section is usual. After 34 weeks, labour can usually be induced with prostaglandins. Epidural analgesia helps reduce the blood pressure. The fetus is continuously monitored by CTG and the blood pressure and fluid balance are closely observed. Antihypertensives can be used in labour. Maternal pushing should be avoided if the blood pressure reaches 170/110 mmHg in the second stage, as it raises intracranial pressure and risks cerebral haemorrhage. Oxytocin rather than ergometrine is used in the third stage as the latter can increase the blood pressure.

Potential pitfalls in managing pre-eclampsia
Pre-eclampsia is unpredictable
Hypertension may be absent: beware of proteinuria
Epigastric pain is ominous and liver function testing is mandatory
Severe hypertension must be treated
Treatment of hypertension may disguise pre-eclampsia
Excessive fluid administration causes pulmonary oedema
Complications commonly arise after delivery

Postnatal care of the pre-eclamptic patient

Whilst delivery is the only cure for pre-eclampsia it often takes at least 24 h for severe disease to improve and it may worsen during this time.

Blood investigations: Liver enzymes, platelets and renal function are still monitored closely. Low platelet levels usually return to normal within a few days.

Fluid balance monitoring is essential: pulmonary oedema and respiratory failure may follow uncontrolled administration of intravenous fluid. If the urine output is low, central venous pressure (CVP) monitoring will guide management. If the CVP is high (suggesting overload), frusemide is given. If it is low, fluid but not albumin is given. If it is normal and oliguria persists, renal failure is likely, and a rising potassium level may dictate the need for dialysis.

The blood pressure is maintained at around 140/90 mmHg. The highest level tends to be reached about 5 days after birth, and continued admission until then is advised. Postnatal treatment is usually with a beta-blocker; second line drugs include nifedipine and angiotensin-converting enzyme (ACE) inhibitors, of which captopril is appropriate as it is safe when breastfeeding. Treatment may be needed for several weeks and communication with the GP and community midwives is essential.

Pre-existing hypertension in pregnancy

Definitions and epidemiology

This is diagnosed when the diastolic blood pressure exceeds 140/90 mmHg before 20 weeks. Patients with pregnancy-induced hypertension that is 'transient' also have an underlying predisposition to hypertension and may need treatment later in life. Underlying hypertension is present in about 5% of pregnancies. It is more common in older and obese women, and in women with a positive family history or who developed hypertension taking the combined oral contraceptive.

Aetiology

Essential or 'idiopathic' hypertension is the most common cause. Secondary hypertension is commonly associated with obesity, diabetes or renal disease such as polycystic disease, renal artery stenosis or chronic pyelonephritis. Other rarer causes are phaeochromocytoma, Cushing's syndrome, cardiac disease and coarctation of the aorta.

Clinical features

Hypertension increases in late pregnancy. Symptoms are often absent, although fundal changes, renal bruits and radiofemoral delay should be excluded in all hypertensives. Proteinuria in patients with renal disease is usually present at booking.

Complications

The principal dangers are worsening hypertension and pre-eclampsia, the risk of which is increased sixfold; in the absence of these, perinatal mortality is only marginally increased.

Investigations

To identify secondary hypertension: Phaeochromocytoma is excluded by performing at least two 24-h urine collections for vanillylmandelic acid (VMA). This is worthwhile because the maternal mortality of this condition is very high.

To look for coexistent disease: Renal function is assessed and a renal ultrasound is performed.

To identify pre-eclampsia (see below): Quantification of any proteinuria at booking and a uric acid level allow for comparison in later pregnancy.

Management

Hypertension: Ideally, prepregnancy medication will be changed: ACE inhibitors are teratogenic and affect fetal urine production; beta-blockers are associated with slightly reduced birth weight and used rarely. Methyldopa is normally used, with nifedipine as a second line agent. Medication may not be required in the second trimester because of the physiological fall in blood pressure.

Risk of pre-eclampsia: The pregnancy is treated as 'high risk'. Screening using uterine artery Doppler and additional antenatal visits are usual. Pre-eclampsia is suggested by a rise in uric acid levels or worsening hypertension and confirmed by the finding of significant proteinuria for the first time after 20 weeks.

Delivery is usually undertaken by 40 weeks, although the benefits of this are debated.

Further reading

Borzychowski AM, Sargent IL, Redman CW. Inflammation and pre-eclampsia. *Seminars in Fetal Neonatal Medicine* 2006; **11**: 309–16.

Duley L. Pre-eclampsia and hypertension. *Clinical Evidence* 2005; **14**: 1776–90.

Frishman WH, Schlocker SJ, Awad K, Tejani N. Pathophysiology and medical management of systemic hypertension in pregnancy. *Cardiology in Review* 2005; **13**: 274–84.

http://www.doorbar.co.uk/apec.html for information on pre-eclampsia.

Milne F, Redman C, Walker J, *et al.* The pre-eclampsia community guideline (PRECOG): how to screen for and detect onset of pre-eclampsia in the community. *British Medical Journal* 2005; **330**: 576–80.

Redman CW, Sargent IL. Latest advances in understanding pre-eclampsia. *Science* 2005; **308**: 1592–4.

The management of severe pre-eclampsia/eclampsia. RCGOG Green Top Guideline 10 (A) March 2006. http://www.rcog.org.uk/resources/Public/pdf/management_pre_eclampsia_mar06.pdf.

Pre-eclampsia at a Glance

Definition	Multisystem disease unique to pregnancy that usually manifests as hypertension (blood pressure [BP] >140/90 mmHg) after 20 weeks with proteinuria that is due to:	
Pathology	Endothelial cell damage and vasospasm, which can affect the fetus and almost all maternal organs. It is of placental origin and cured only by delivery	
Degrees	Mild:	Proteinuria and BP <170/110 mmHg
	Moderate:	Proteinuria and BP ≥170/110 mmHg
	Severe:	Proteinuria and hypertension before 32 weeks or with maternal complications
Epidemiology	6%	
Aetiology	Nulliparity, previous/family history, older age, obesity, pre-existing hypertension, diabetes, autoimmune disease, multiple pregnancy	
Features	None until late stage, then headache, epigastric pain, visual disturbances	
Complications	Maternal:	Eclampsia, cerebrovascular accidents (CVAs), liver/renal failure, haemolysis, elevated liver enzymes and low platelet count (HELLP), disseminated intravascular coagulation (DIC), pulmonary oedema
	Fetal:	Intrauterine growth restriction (IUGR), fetal morbidity and mortality
Investigations	To confirm diagnosis:	Mid-stream urine (MSU) and urine protein measurement
	To monitor:	Watch BP, serial full blood count (FBC), urea and electrolytes (U&E), liver function tests (LFTs) and fetal surveillance
Screening	Observation of high-risk pregnancies. Uterine artery Doppler. sFlt-1 and vascular endothelial growth factor (VEGF)	
Prevention	Aspirin has limited role	
Management	Investigate if BP >140/90 mmHg; admit if proteinuria 2+ or moderate/severe disease	
	Antihypertensives if BP reaches 170/110 mmHg; steroids if moderate/severe at <34 weeks	
	Delivery:	Deliver after 34–36 weeks if possible
		Deliver if maternal complications whatever the gestation
	Magnesium sulphate if eclampsia; consider prophylactic use in severe disease	
	Postnatally, watch BP, urine output, blood tests: FBC, U&E, LFTs	

Other medical disorders in pregnancy

Diabetes and gestational diabetes

Physiology

Glucose tolerance decreases in pregnancy due to altered carbohydrate metabolism and the antagonistic effects of human placental lactogen, progesterone and cortisol. Pregnancy is 'diabetogenic': women without diabetes but with impaired or potentially impaired glucose tolerance often 'deteriorate' enough to be classified as diabetic in pregnancy (Fig. 21.1). They are called 'gestational diabetics' and have a high chance of developing subsequent overt diabetes. Definitions of gestational diabetes are artificial and even variable, and so the incidence of gestational diabetes varies accordingly.

The kidneys of non-pregnant women start to excrete glucose at a threshold level of 11 mmol/L. In pregnancy this varies more but often decreases, so glycosuria may occur at physiological blood glucose concentrations. Raised fetal blood glucose levels induce fetal hyperinsulinaemia, causing fetal fat deposition and excessive growth (macrosomia).

Definition and epidemiology

Pre-existing diabetes (whether type I or II) affects 0.1–0.3% of pregnant women. Increasing amounts of insulin will be required in these pregnancies to maintain normoglycaemia.

Gestational diabetes describes the development of significant glucose intolerance in pregnancy that disappears after the end of pregnancy. Definitions vary, but the most practical definition is when a glucose level in pregnancy is >9.0 mmol 2 h after a 75-g glucose load. This definition encompasses 2% of pregnant women. Risk

Obstetrics and Gynaecology, 3rd edition. By Lawrence Impey and Tim Child. Published 2008 by Blackwell Publishing, ISBN: 978-1-4051-6095-7.

factors are a previous history of gestational diabetes, a fetus >4 kg, a previous unexplained stillbirth, a family history of diabetes, weight >100 kg or polycystic ovary syndrome (PCOS) [→ p.82]. In pregnancy, the presence of polyhydramnios or persistent glycosuria also indicates increased risk.

Diabetes in pregnancy	
Pre-existing diabetes (<0.3%):	Insulin requirements increase in pregnancy
Gestational diabetes (2%):	Glucose levels rise temporarily to diabetic level

Fetal complications (Fig. 21.2)

Complications are related to glucose levels, so gestational diabetics are usually less affected than established diabetics. Type I and II diabetics are similarly affected. *Congenital abnormalities* (particularly neural tube and cardiac defects) are 3–4 times more common in established diabetics, and are related to periconceptual glucose control. *Preterm labour*, natural or induced, occurs in 10% of established diabetics, and *fetal lung maturity* at any given gestation is less than with non-diabetic pregnancies. *Birthweight* is increased as fetal pancreatic islet cell hyperplasia leads to hyperinsulinaemia and fat deposition. This leads to increased urine output and *polyhydramnios* (increased liquor) [→ p.157] is common. As the fetus tends to be larger, *dystocia* and *birth trauma* (particularly shoulder dystocia) are more common. *Fetal compromise*, *fetal distress* in labour and *sudden fetal death* are more common, and related particularly to poor third trimester glucose control.

Maternal complications (Fig. 21.3)

Insulin requirements normally increase considerably by the end of pregnancy. *Ketoacidosis* is rare, but *hypogly-*

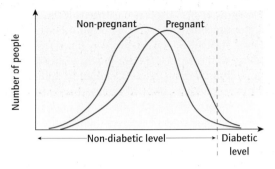

Fig. 21.1 Distribution of glucose tolerance in the non-pregnant and pregnant population.

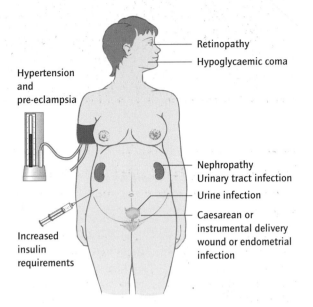

Fig. 21.3 Maternal complications of diabetes.

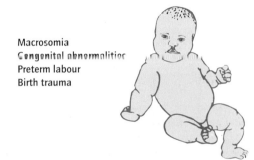

Macrosomia
Congenital abnormalities
Preterm labour
Birth trauma

Fig. 21.2 Fetal complications of diabetes.

caemia may result from attempts to achieve optimum glucose control. *Urinary tract infection* and *wound or endometrial infection* after delivery are more common. Pre-existing *hypertension* is detected in up to 25% of overt diabetics and *pre-eclampsia* is more common. Pre-existing *ischaemic heart disease* often worsens. *Caesarean or instrumental delivery* is more likely because of fetal compromise and increased fetal size. Diabetic *nephropathy* (5–10%) is associated with poorer fetal outcomes but does not usually deteriorate. Diabetic *retinopathy* often deteriorates and may need to be treated in pregnancy.

Detection and screening for gestational diabetes
Step 1: **Screening the general population**   Perform 'timed' glucose level. If >6 mmol/L when preprandial or >2 h after a meal, or >7 mmol/L <2 h after a meal, go to Step 2   If at high risk of gestational diabetes (history), undergo Step 2 at 20 and 30 weeks routinely
Step 2: **Diagnostic testing**   Perform glucose tolerance test with a 75-g oral glucose load. If abnormal (2-h level >9.0 mmol/L), gestational diabetes is diagnosed. Start on a high-fibre, low-carbohydrate diet, and after a few days proceed to Step 3
Step 3: **Assessing need for insulin**   Perform 'glucose series' measuring several levels in a day. If preprandial glucose levels are consistently >6 mmol/L, insulin therapy is started. If not, diet may be adequate

Risk factors for gestational diabetes
Previous history of gestational diabetes
Previous fetus >4 kg
Previous unexplained stillbirth
First-degree relative with diabetes
Polyhydramnios
Persistent glycosuria
Weight >100 kg or body mass index (BMI) >30
Polycystic ovary syndrome (PCOS)

Detection of and screening for gestational diabetes

Treatment of gestational diabetes improves both fetal and maternal outcomes (*NEJM* 2005; **352**: 2477). Therefore, universal screening is wise (*Diabetes Metab* 2006; **32**: 140), although this is not currently universally recommended. In women with PCOS, antenatal metformin reduces the risk of gestational diabetes (*Hum Reprod* 2002; **17**: 2858).

Management of diabetes in pregnancy

Precise glucose control and fetal monitoring for evidence of compromise are the cornerstones of management. Antenatal care is consultant-based, with delivery in a unit with neonatal intensive care facilities. A multidisciplinary approach involving an obstetrician, midwife, GP, dietitian and a physician is necessary (Fig. 21.4). The key member, however, is the woman, who has day-to-day control of her diabetes and needs to be educated about optimizing control. If she is not motivated, normoglycaemia will not be achieved.

Preconceptual care: Insulin-dependent diabetic women wishing to undergo pregnancy should have their renal function, blood pressure and retinae assessed. Glucose control is optimized, and folic acid 5 mg/day is prescribed. Optimal control reduces the risk of congenital abnormalities and preterm labour (*Diabetes Care* 2006; **29**: 1744). Methyldopa is used if antihypertensives are required. Unfortunately, prepregnancy assessment seldom happens.

Monitoring and treating the diabetes: Glucose levels are checked by the patient several times daily before and after food with a home 'glucometer'. The ideal is levels consistently between 4 and 6 mmol/L: this is usually achieved by a combination of one night-time-long/intermediate-acting and three preprandial short-acting insulin injections. Doses will usually need to be progressively increased as the pregnancy advances. Oral hypoglycaemic agents are seldom used in women with established diabetes. High concentrations of glycosylated haemoglobin (HbA1c) reflect poor prior control: the aim is for a level less than 7%. Visits occur fortnightly up to 34 weeks and weekly thereafter.

Monitoring the fetus: In addition to a dating scan or nuchal translucency scan [→ p.149] and a 20-week anomaly scan to detect abnormalities, a specialist cardiac scan is indicated. Serial ultrasound examinations monitor fetal growth and liquor volume. Even where glucose control has been good, macrosomia and polyhydramnios can occur (Fig. 21.5). Umbilical artery Doppler is not useful unless pre-eclampsia or intrauterine growth restriction (IUGR) develop.

Timing and mode of delivery: Evidence is limited (*Cochrane* 2001: CD001997). The *gestational diabetic* with good glucose control can be managed in the normal manner. The *pre-existing diabetic* normally undergoes delivery at 39 weeks, or earlier if glucose control has been poor. Birth trauma is more likely and, although prediction is imprecise, elective Caesarean section is often wise where the estimated fetal weight exceeds 4 kg or where the abdominal circumference exceeds the head circumference, as the risk of shoulder dystocia is greater [→ p.262]. During labour, glucose levels are maintained with a 'sliding scale' of insulin and a 10% dextrose infusion.

The neonate commonly develops hypoglycaemia because it has become 'accustomed to' hyperglycaemia and its

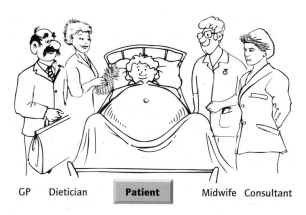

GP   Dietician   **Patient**   Midwife   Consultant

Fig. 21.4 The multidisciplinary approach to diabetes in pregnancy in 2008.

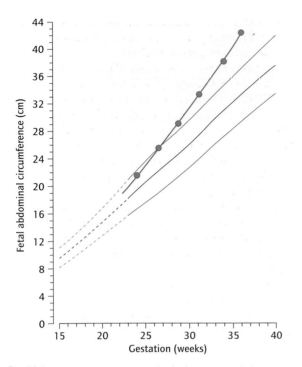

Fig. 21.5 Accelerated fetal growth of a fetus with a diabetic mother.

insulin levels are high. Respiratory distress syndrome occasionally occurs, even after 38 weeks. A careful examination is made to reveal hitherto undetected congenital abnormalities. Breastfeeding is strongly advised.

The puerperium and postnatal period: In the pre-existing diabetic, insulin can be rapidly changed to prepregnant doses. In the gestational diabetic, insulin is discontinued, but a glucose tolerance test should be performed at 3 months: 50% will be diagnosed as diabetic within the next 10 years.

Management of diabetes

Preconceptual glucose control
Assessment of maternal diabetic complications
Patient education and team involvement
Glucose monitoring and insulin adjustment
Anomaly and cardiac ultrasound and fetal surveillance
Delivery by 39 weeks

Cardiac disease

In pregnancy there is a 40% increase in cardiac output, due to both an increase in stroke volume and heart rate, and a 40% increase in blood volume. There is also a 50% reduction in systemic vascular resistance: blood pressure often drops in the second trimester, but is usually normal by term. The increased blood flow produces a flow (ejection systolic) murmur in 90% of pregnant women. The electrocardiogram (ECG) is altered during pregnancy: a left axis shift and inverted T-waves are common.

Epidemiology

Cardiac disease affects 0.3% of pregnant women. The incidence is increasing as more women with congenital disease are reaching reproductive age. The maternal risk is dependent on the cardiac status and most encounter no problems. However, acquired and uncorrected congenital disease mean that it is a major cause of maternal mortality, usually as a result of cardiac failure. Increased cardiac output acts as an 'exercise test' with which the heart may be unable to cope. This usually manifests before 24 weeks or in labour, but decompensation may also occur with blood loss or fluid overload. The latter can occur in the early puerperium, as uterine involution 'squeezes' a large 'fluid load' into the circulation.

Principles of management

Patients with significant disease are seen in conjunction with a *cardiologist*. Those with severe decompensated disease are advised against pregnancy. *Cardiac assessment*, particularly echocardiography, is needed. Fetal cardiac anomalies are more common (3%) and are best detected on *ultrasound* at 20 weeks' gestation. *Hypertension* should be treated. *Thromboprophylaxis* is required, depending on the lesion. Regular checks for anaemia are made. In labour, the *left lateral position* is encouraged to avoid aortocaval compression [→ p.231] and attention is paid to *fluid balance*. *Elective forceps* delivery helps avoid the additional stress of pushing in severe cases. *Antibiotics* in labour are recommended except for most except repaired patent ductus arteriosus (PDA) or mitral valve prolapse, to protect against endocarditis.

Types of cardiac disease and their management

Mild abnormalities such as mitral valve prolapse, PDA, ventricular septal defects (VSD) or atrial septal defects (ASD) do not usually cause complications.

Pulmonary hypertension (e.g. Eisenmenger's syndrome): Because of a high maternal mortality (40%) pregnancy is contraindicated and usually terminated.

Aortic stenosis: Severe disease (e.g. small valve area or large gradient) should be corrected before pregnancy and causes an inability to increase cardiac output when required. Beta-blockade is often used. Epidural analgesia is contraindicated in the most severe cases. Thromboprophylaxis is required for replaced aortic valves.

Mitral valve disease: This should be treated before pregnancy. In the rare, severe cases of stenosis, heart failure may develop late in the pregnancy; beta-blockade is used. Artificial metal valves are particularly prone to thrombosis and warfarin is often continued, despite its fetal risks.

Myocardial infarction is unusual in women of reproductive age; mortality is greater at later gestations.

Peripartum cardiomyopathy is a rare (1 in 3000) cause of heart failure specific to pregnancy. It develops in the last month or first 6 months after pregnancy and in the absence of a recognizable cause. It is frequently diagnosed late. It is a cause of maternal death (approx 15%) and in more than 50% of cases leads to permanent left ventricular dysfunction. Treatment is supportive, with diuretics and angiotensin-converting enzyme (ACE) inhibitors. There is a significant recurrence rate in subsequent pregnancies.

Respiratory disease

Tidal volume increases by 40% in pregnancy, although there is no change in respiratory rate. Asthma is common in pregnancy. Pregnancy has a variable effect on the disease: drugs should not be withheld, because they are generally safe and because a severe asthma attack is potentially lethal to mother and fetus. Well-controlled asthma has little detrimental effect on perinatal outcome. Women on long-term steroids require an increased dose in labour because the chronically suppressed adrenal cortex is unable to produce adequate steroids for the stress of labour.

Epilepsy

Epilepsy affects 0.5% of pregnant women. Seizure control can deteriorate in pregnancy, and epilepsy is a significant cause of maternal death. Therefore, antiepileptic treatment is continued. However, the risk of congenital abnormalities (e.g. neural tube defects [NTDs]) is increased (4% overall), and this is largely due to drug therapy. The risks are dose-dependent, higher with multiple drug usage and higher with certain drugs (e.g. sodium valproate). The fetus has a 3% risk of developing epilepsy.

Preconceptual assessment is ideal: management involves seizure control with as few drugs as possible at the lowest dose, together with folic acid (5 mg/day) supplementation. Ideally, sodium valproate should be avoided because it is associated with a higher rate of congenital abnormalities and with lower intelligence (*Neurol* 2005; **64**: 938) in children. However, preconception advice is rarely sought and fears of recurrence of seizures and losing the driving licence often prevent drug changes. Therefore, all women of reproductive age are best managed as if they are contemplating pregnancy. Carbamazepine and lamotrigine (*Epilepsia* 2002; **43**: 1161) are safest. In women without complete seizure control, doses may need to be increased, but the benefits of routine drug level monitoring remain debated. Folic acid 5 mg is continued throughout pregnancy and from 36 weeks, 10 mg vitamin K is given orally.

The anomaly scan and a specialist cardiac scan are important to exclude fetal abnormalities.

Thyroid disease in pregnancy

Thyroid status does not alter in pregnancy, although iodine clearance is increased. Goitre is more common. Fetal thyroxine production starts at 12 weeks; before, it is dependent on maternal thyroxine. Maternal thyroid-stimulating hormone (TSH) is increased in early pregnancy.

Hypothyroidism

This affects 1% of pregnant women. In the UK, most cases of hypothyroidism are due to Hashimoto's thyroiditis or thyroid surgery, but hypothyroidism is common where dietary iodine is deficient. Untreated disease is rare as anovulation is usual but is associated with a high perinatal mortality. Hypothyroidism is associated with intellectual impairment in childhood and this is related to the severity of the deficiency (*J Med Screen* 2001; **8**: 18). It is also associated with a slightly increased risk of pre-eclampsia, particularly if antithyroid antibodies are present. In euthyroid women the risk is probably not increased. Therefore adequate replacement is important: this is maintained and may need to be increased: 6-weekly assessments of TSH are performed.

Hyperthyroidism

This affects 0.2% of pregnant women and is usually due to Graves' disease. Untreated disease is rare as anovulation is usual. Inadequately treated disease increases perinatal mortality. Antithyroid antibodies also cross the placenta: rarely, this causes neonatal thyrotoxicosis and goitre. For the mother, thyrotoxicosis may improve in late pregnancy but poorly controlled disease risks a 'thyroid storm' whereby the mother gets acute symptoms and heart failure, usually near or at delivery. Symptoms may be confused with those of pregnancy. Hyperthyroidism is treated with propylthiouracil. This crosses the placenta and can occasionally cause neonatal hypothyroidism: the lowest possible dose is used and thyroid function is tested monthly. Graves' disease often worsens postpartum.

Postpartum thyroiditis

This is common (5–10%) and can cause postnatal depression. Risk factors include antithyroid antibodies and type I diabetes. In affected patients, there is a transient and usually subclinical hyperthyroidism, usually about 3 months postpartum, followed after about 4 months by hypothyroidism. This is permanent in 20%.

Liver disease

Acute fatty liver

This is a very rare (1 in 9000) condition that may be part of the spectrum of pre-eclampsia. Acute hepatorenal failure, disseminated intravascular coagulation (DIC) and hypoglycaemia lead to a high maternal and fetal mortality. There is extensive fatty change in the liver. Malaise, vomiting, jaundice and vague epigastric pain are early features, while thirst may occur weeks earlier. Early diagnosis and prompt delivery are essential, although correction of clotting defects and hypoglycaemia are needed first. Treatment is then supportive, with further dextrose, blood products, careful fluid balance and, occasionally, dialysis. The recurrence rate is very low.

Intrahepatic cholestasis of pregnancy

This is due to abnormal sensitivity to the cholestatic effects of oestrogens. It occurs in 0.7% of pregnant women in the West, is familial and tends to recur. It is associated with an increased risk of sudden stillbirth, and also preterm delivery. The risk of stillbirth (0.5–1%) is difficult to predict, but is due to the toxic effects of bile salts, possibly by precipitating fetal arrhythmia. Pruritus of the hands and feet is usual; serum bile acids and usually, liver enzymes are raised. Ursodeoxycholic acid (UDCA) helps relieve itching and may reduce the obstetric risks. Because ultrasound and cardiotocography predict adverse outcomes poorly, induction of labour around 38 weeks is usually advised. Nevertheless, evidence is lacking and the benefits of UDCA and induction remain debated. Because there is an increased maternal and fetal tendency to haemorrhage, vitamin K 10 mg/day is given from 36 weeks.

Thrombophilias and the antiphospholipid syndrome

Antiphospholipid syndrome

This is when the lupus anticoagulant and/or anticardiolipin antibodies occur (measured on two occasions at least 3 months apart) in association with adverse pregnancy complications, but in the absence of the other clinical manifestations of lupus. Recurrent miscarriage [→ p.117], IUGR and early pre-eclampsia are common, and the fetal loss rate is high. Placental thrombosis appears to be responsible. Low levels of these antibodies are also present in nearly 2% of all pregnant women and therefore treatment, normally with aspirin and low-molecular-weight heparin (LMWH) (*BMJ* 1997; **314**: 253) is restricted to those with the *syndrome*. The pregnancy is managed as 'high risk', with serial ultrasound and elective induction of labour at least by term. Postnatal anticoagulation is also recommended to prevent venous thromboembolism.

Other prothrombotic disorders

In addition to the risk of venous thromboembolism, *activated protein C resistance*, the *prothrombin gene variant*, *protein S and C deficiency or antithrombin III deficiency* are more common in women with recurrent pregnancy loss (*Lancet* 2003; **361**: 901), early pre-eclampsia, placental abruption and IUGR. The *Factor V Leyden gene* appears less serious. A family or personal history of venous thrombosis is also common (*BJOG* 2003; **110**: 462). Indeed, many thrombophilias have been associated with an increased risk of cerebral palsy (*Ann Neurol* 1998; **44**: 665). *Hyperhomocysteinaemia* is also associated with increased pregnancy loss and pre-eclampsia. Treatment is usually with high dose folic acid. Women with prothrombotic tendencies and an adverse pregnancy history are usually treated as for antiphospholipid syndrome, although the effectiveness of this is less proven. Postnatal anticoagulation is recommended.

Systemic lupus erythematosus

Systemic lupus erythematosus (SLE) affects 0.1–0.2% of pregnant women. In absence of the lupus anticoagulant or anticardiolipin antibodies (see above), the risks to the pregnancy are largely confined to those of associated hypertension or renal disease. Maternal symptoms often relapse after delivery.

Renal disease

In pregnancy, the glomerular filtration rate increases 40%, causing urea and creatinine levels to decrease.

Chronic renal disease

This affects 0.2% of pregnant women. Fetal and maternal complications are dependent on the degree of hypertension and renal impairment: and pregnancy is inadvisable if the creatinine level is >200 µmol/L. Renal function often deteriorates late in the pregnancy: this is more common in severe disease and can lead to a permanent deterioration. Rejection of renal transplants is not more common; immunosuppressive therapy, e.g. ciclosporin, must continue. Proteinuria can cause diagnostic confusion with pre-eclampsia, which is more common, but will usually have been present before 20 weeks. Fetal complications include pre-eclampsia, IUGR and preterm delivery. Management involves serial ultrasounds to assess fetal growth, measurement of renal function, screening for urinary infection (which may exacerbate renal disease) and control of hypertension. Vaginal delivery is usually appropriate.

Urinary infection

Urine infection is associated with preterm labour, anaemia and increased perinatal morbidity and mortality. *Asymptomatic bacteriuria* affects 5% of women, but in pregnancy is more likely (20%) to lead to pyelonephritis (Fig. 21.6). The urine should be cultured at the booking visit, and asymptomatic bacteriuria is treated. Subsequently, culture is performed if leucocytes, nitrites or protein are detected on routine urinalysis. *Pyelonephritis* affects 1–2% of women, causing loin pain, rigors, vomiting and a fever. This requires treatment with intravenous antibiotics. *Escherichia coli* accounts for 75% and is often resistant to amoxicillin.

Venous thromboembolic disease

Pregnancy is prothrombotic and the incidence of venous thromboembolism (VTE) is increased sixfold. Blood clotting factors are increased, fibrinolytic activity is reduced and blood flow is altered by mechanical obstruction and immobility. Women with inherited prothrombotic conditions and those with a family or personal history are particularly prone to thromboses.

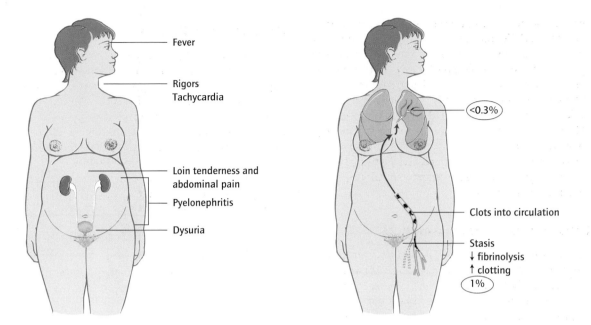

Fig. 21.6 Clinical features of pyelonephritis.

Fig. 21.7 Venous thromboembolism in pregnancy.

Pulmonary embolus

This is an important cause of maternal death [→ p.275] in developed countries. Embolism occurs in <0.3%, with a mortality of 1–3% (Fig. 21.7). Diagnosis is as in the non-pregnant woman using computed tomography (CT) or with perfusion ± ventilation (VQ) scanning. The ECG changes of a pulmonary embolus can be normal in pregnancy.

Deep vein thrombosis

Deep vein thrombosis (DVT) occurs in about 1% of pregnant women. Thromboses are more often iliofemoral and on the left. Although D-dimers are frequently raised in pregnancy, a normal level means thromboembolism is unlikely. Doppler examination of the leg and/or a venogram are used.

With both conditions, clinical signs may be absent, and many women with a pulmonary embolus are not diagnosed before death. A thrombophilia screen is performed before treatment. VTE is treated with subcutaneous LMWH as maintenance therapy because this is associated with a lower risk of osteoporosis and thrombocytopenia than heparin. LMWH doses are adjusted according to the anti-Factor Xa level. If possible, treatment is stopped shortly before labour, but is restarted and continued into the puerperium. Warfarin is teratogenic, may cause fetal bleeding and is seldom used antenatally.

Thromboprophylaxis

General measures include maintenance of hydration and mobilization. *Antenatal prophylaxis* with LMWH is restricted to women at very high risk, such as a previous thrombosis. *Postpartum prophylaxis* with LMWH or warfarin is usually continued for 6 weeks and is used more often: 50% of the mortality occurs at this time. LMWH is given to women with a previous or strong family history, a known prothrombotic tendency, and those who have had a Caesarean section *and* have three or more moderate risk factors (age >35 years, high parity, obesity, gross varicose veins, infection, pre-eclampsia, immobility or major current illness).

Risk factors for thromboembolism	
Pre-existing:	*Pregnancy:*
Previous VTE	Caesarean section
Thrombophilia	Prolonged labour
Family history of VTE	Severe haemorrhage
Increased age/ parity	Hyperemesis
Maternal illness	Immobility
Obesity	

Mental illness in pregnancy

Psychiatric illness in pregnancy is now recognized as a major risk factor for maternal death, particularly suicide. Whilst not more common during pregnancy, it is frequently not recorded. Prenatal treatment is continued or stopped after consideration of the risks of drug therapy versus that of the illness.

Bipolar affective disorder

This affects up to 1% of women. A family history is common. Episodes of depression or mania, sometimes with psychotic symptoms are typical, and may present for the first time postnatally. Lithium is frequently used and is associated with a slightly increased rate of cardiac abnormalities; however, discontinuation risks relapse. In women well or at low risk of relapse, it is usually stopped; in those unwell or at high risk it may be continued: monthly monitoring of levels is advised because of increased excretion during pregnancy. There is a high risk of maternal suicide and postnatal medication is important.

Depression

This is particularly common postnatally [→ p.269], but up to 3% of women conceive taking antidepressants (*BJOG* 2007; **114**: 1055). In general, selective serotonin reuptake inhibitors (SSRIs), usually fluoxetine, are preferable to tricyclic antidepressants, which are highly toxic in overdose. Paroxetine may cause cardiac defects and is not advised.

Anxiety disorders

These are common and variable. Cognitive–behaviour therapy is preferable to drugs such as benzodiazepines.

Schizophrenia

Up to 1% of women require medication for this. Therapy is usually continued because of the ramifications of the illness, but clozapine and olanzapine are usually avoided.

'Recreational' drugs in pregnancy

Illegal drugs

Women abusing drugs in pregnancy are often vulnerable personally and socially. They are at increased risk of other illnesses such as sexually transmitted infections (STIs), HIV and hepatitis C, and are at increased risk of maternal death. Pregnancy care should be multidisciplinary, include social support, and involvement of social workers may be indicated. Depending on the drugs taken the fetus may be at increased risk of congenital abnormalities; the pregnancy should be considered high risk, particularly of IUGR and preterm delivery.

Opiates: These are not teratogenic, but their use is associated with preterm delivery, IUGR, stillbirth, developmental delay and sudden infant death syndrome (SIDS). Methadone maintenance, without use of street drugs is advised; withdrawal of methadone is not. Some neonates experience severe withdrawal symptoms and convulsions.

Cocaine is probably teratogenic and can cause childhood intellectual impairment, but is particularly associated with IUGR and placental abruption, as well as preterm delivery, stillbirth and SIDS. Proper counselling concerning risks, social support and pregnancy monitoring are required.

Ecstasy is teratogenic, with an increased risk of cardiac defects and probably gastroschisis. Pregnancy complications are probably similar to cocaine and counselling and social support are required.

Benzodiazepines have been associated with facial clefts, and cause neonatal hypotonia as well as withdrawal symptoms.

Cannabis: Abuse of other drugs makes attribution of risk difficult but cannabis may cause IUGR and affect later childhood development.

Legal drugs

Alcohol: *Alcohol use in pregnancy.* In the West, about 50% of women drink no alcohol at all in pregnancy; about 10% admit to drinking more 3 units per week. Below this level, there is no consistent evidence of harm, although there is conflicting evidence regarding childhood development and best advice is to avoid alcohol altogether. At higher levels, the incidence of IUGR and birth defects increase.

Alcohol abuse in pregnancy greatly increases these risks and is associated with the *fetal alcohol syndrome*. The incidence in North America is 0.6 per 1000, and affected individuals have confirmed alcohol exposure (>18 units per day), facial abnormalities, IUGR and a small or abnormal brain, with developmental delay. *Alcohol spectrum disorders* (incidence 9 per 1000) encompass lesser variants of the syndrome. Advice and social support are required; ultrasound may not detect the syndrome, but is used to monitor fetal growth.

Tobacco: Smoking in pregnancy is related to social class: approximately one-third of women smoke during pregnancy and one-tenth of pregnancies are exposed to environmental smoke (*BMC Public Health* 2007; **16**: 81). Smoking is probably not teratogenic, but is associated, in a dose–response manner, with an increased risk of miscarriage, IUGR, preterm birth, placental abruption, stillbirth and SIDS. Pre-eclampsia is less common but more severe if it occurs. It is also associated with a wide variety of childhood illnesses. Women should be encouraged to stop, or at least cut down their smoking; nicotine replacement therapy is preferable to smoking. The pregnancy should be considered high risk.

Anaemias

The 40% increase in blood volume in pregnancy is relatively greater than the increase in red cell mass. The result is a net fall in haemoglobin concentration, such that 10.4 g/dL should be considered the lower limit of normal. More iron and folic acid are required in preg-

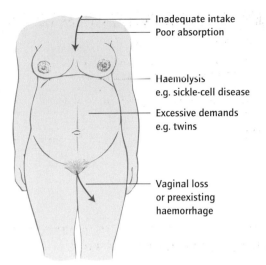

Fig. 21.8 Anaemia in pregnancy.

nancy because of the increase in red cell mass, uterine growth and fetal requirements and iron absorption increases (Fig. 21.8). A high haemoglobin level is actually associated with an increased risk of pregnancy complications such as preterm delivery and IUGR (*AmJOG* 2005; **193**: 220), possibly because it reflects low blood volume, as found in pre-eclampsia, and because of its association with smoking.

Iron deficiency anaemia

This affects 10% of pregnant women. Symptoms are usually absent unless the haemoglobin is <9 g/dL, and the fetus is unaffected unless severe anaemia is present. Folic acid deficiency may coexist. The blood film shows reduced mean cell volume and mean cell haemoglobin (Fig. 21.9). Ferritin levels are reduced. Treatment is with oral iron, achieving an increase of up to 0.8 g/dL per week, but can cause gastrointestinal upset. In severe cases, intravenous iron works more quickly (*BJOG* 2006; **113**: 1248) and may prevent the need for blood transfusion; intramuscular iron is seldom used.

Folic acid deficiency anaemia

This is rarer but often is missed. The mean cell volume is usually increased, neutrophils are hypersegmented and

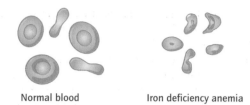

Normal blood   Iron deficiency anemia

Fig. 21.9 Picture of blood film of iron deficiency anaemia.

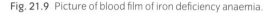

red cell folic acid is low. Folic acid deficiency should always be considered (measure red cell folic acid) if anaemia is present without marked microcytosis. Treatment is with oral folic acid.

Prophylaxis against anaemia

Routine iron supplements reduce the incidence of anaemia without affecting perinatal outcome (*Cochrane* 2000: CD001135). Postnatal blood transfusion may be required less frequently. However, iron is often poorly tolerated, particularly during the first trimester. Routine supplementation is not necessary: all women are given dietary advice, and the haemoglobin is checked at booking and at 28 and 34 weeks. Iron or folic acid are then given if the haemoglobin drops below 10.4 g/dL. Because routine preconceptual folic acid supplements (0.4 mg) reduce the incidence of neural tube defects (NTDs), these are recommended to all women. In those with epilepsy or a previous history of an NTD, a higher dose (5 mg) is used.

Dietary advice to avoid anaemia	
Food rich in iron:	Meat, particularly kidney and liver, eggs, green vegetables
Food rich in folic acid:	Lightly cooked or raw green vegetables, fish
Guinness is not recommended in pregnancy	

Haemoglobinopathies

The adult haemoglobin molecule (HbA) is made of two α chains and two β chains, bound together in a tetramer.

Fetal haemoglobin (HbF), which is normally gradually replaced by the adult type after birth, is made of two α chains and two γ chains.

Sickle-cell disease

This recessive disorder is due to abnormal β-chain formation (called an S chain) in the haemoglobin molecule. The result is an abnormal haemoglobin molecule made of two α chains bound to two S chains. Sickle S is found in people of Afro-Caribbean origin, and of those in the UK, 10% are heterozygotes or 'carriers'. Haemoglobin electrophoresis is routinely performed in all pregnant women who are not of northern European origin. The partners of heterozygotes are also tested: if positive, prenatal diagnosis is offered [→ p.155].

Homozygotes have only HbS, and many have been affected with 'crises' of chest pain and a fever, and chronic haemolytic anaemia all their life. In pregnancy, maternal complications include more frequent crises (35%), pre-eclampsia, thrombosis and infections. Fetal complications are miscarriage, IUGR [→ p.203], preterm labour and death. Regular exchange blood transfusions, screening for infection and maintenance of hydration are needed. Folic acid supplements are given; iron is avoided because of overload.

Heterozygotes have 35% HbS and usually have no problems, but may develop 'crises' under extreme conditions.

Thalassaemias

Alpha thalassaemia results from impaired synthesis of the α chain in the haemoglobin molecule. It occurs largely in people of South-East Asian origin. Four genes are responsible for α chain synthesis. Individuals with four gene deletions die *in utero*. Heterozygous individuals have one or two gene deletions, are usually anaemic, and require folic acid and iron supplementation.

Beta thalassaemia results from impaired β-chain synthesis. It occurs largely in people of South-East Asian and Mediterranean origin. Homozygous individuals are usually affected by iron overload and pregnancy is unusual, but folic acid *without* oral iron is needed. Heterozygous women have a chronic anaemia, which can worsen during pregnancy.

Prenatal diagnosis using chorionic villus sampling (CVS) [→ p.151] by mutation analysis from polymerase chain reaction (PCR) amplified deoxyribonucleic acid (DNA) must be offered if the partner is heterozygous for either the β or α form.

Further reading

ACOG Committee on Obstetrics. ACOG Practice Bulletin No. 78: Hemoglobinopathies in pregnancy. *Obstetrics and Gynecology* 2007; **109**: 229–37.

Adab N, Tudur SC, Vinten J, Williamson P, Winterbottom J. Common antiepileptic drugs in pregnancy in women with epilepsy. *Cochrane Database Systems Review* 2004; **3**: CD004848.

Alcohol Consumption and the Outcomes of Pregnancy. RCOG Statement 2006. http://www.rcog.org.uk/resources/Public/pdf/alcohol_pregnancy_rcog_statement5a.pdf.

Casey BM, Leveno KJ. Thyroid disease in pregnancy. *Obstetrics and Gynecology* 2006; **108**: 1283–92.

Empson M, Lassere M, Craig J, Scott J. Prevention of recurrent miscarriage for women with antiphospholipid antibody or lupus anticoagulant. *Cochrane Database Systems Review* 2005; **2**: CD002859.

http://www.cemach.org.uk/publications/CEMACHDiabetesOctober2005.pdf

Källén B. The safety of antidepressant drugs during pregnancy. *Expert Opinion on Drug Safety* 2007; **6**: 357–70.

Kuczkowski KM. The effects of drug abuse on pregnancy. *Current Opinion in Obstetrics and Gynecology* 2007; **19**: 578–85.

Macintosh MC, Fleming KM, Bailey JA, *et al.* Perinatal mortality and congenital anomalies in babies of women with type 1 or type 2 diabetes in England, Wales, and Northern Ireland: population based study. *British Medical Journal* 2006; **333**: 177. Epub 2006 June 16.

Pena-Rosas JP, Viteri FE. Effects of routine oral iron supplementation with or without folic acid for women during pregnancy. *Cochrane Database of Systematic Reviews* 2006; **3**: CD004736.

Sliwa K, Fett J, Elkayam U. Peripartum cardiomyopathy. *Lancet* 2006; **368**: 687–93.

Stratta P, Canavese C, Quaglia M. Pregnancy in patients with kidney disease. *Journal of Nephrology* 2006; **19**: 135–43.

Tincani A, Bompane D, Danieli E, Doria A. Pregnancy, lupus and antiphospholipid syndrome (Hughes syndrome). *Lupus* 2006; **15**: 156–60.

Uebing A, Steer PJ, Yentis SM, Gatzoulis MA. Pregnancy and congenital heart disease. *British Medical Journal* 2006; **332**: 401–6.

Diabetes in Pregnancy and Gestational Diabetes at a Glance

Definitions/Epidemiology	Pre-existing diabetes: 0.1–0.3% Gestational diabetes: impaired glucose tolerance in pregnancy 2% of women
Aetiology	Gestational diabetes: worsening glucose tolerance in pregnancy in susceptible women Risk factors: family or previous history, polycystic ovary syndrome (PCOS), previous large baby/unexplained stillbirth, weight >100 kg, persistent glycosuria, polyhydramnios
Complications	Related to glucose control; rarer in gestational diabetes Fetal: Congenital abnormalities, preterm labour, birth trauma, fetal death Maternal: Increased insulin requirements, hypoglycaemia, worsening retinopathy, pre-eclampsia, infections, operative delivery, rarely ketoacidosis
Management	Preconceptual glucose stabilization; patient education/involvement Increase insulin to achieve 'tight' control; reduce post-delivery Anomaly and cardiac ultrasound, then close fetal surveillance Induction/lower segment Caesarean section (LSCS) by 39 weeks unless well-controlled gestational diabetes

Thrombophilia in Pregnancy at a Glance

Main types	Antiphospholipid syndrome, protein S and C deficiency, activated protein C resistance and Factor V Leyden, prothrombin gene variant, antithrombin III deficiency, hyperhomocysteinaemia
Complications	Venous thromboembolism, miscarriage, preterm delivery, pre-eclampsia, placental abruption, intrauterine growth restriction (IUGR), fetal death
Management	Individualized: high-risk pregnancy care. Aspirin and low-molecular-weight heparin (LMWH) usually only if adverse previous obstetric history. Postnatal LMWH to prevent venous thromboembolism

Anaemia in Pregnancy at a Glance

Iron deficiency	10% of women. Mean cell volume (MCV), mean cell haemoglobin concentration (MCHC) and ferritin reduced Prophylaxis: disputed. Treat if haemoglobin (Hb) <10.4
Folic acid deficiency	Rarer, MCV often raised. Red cell folate reduced Prophylaxis: routine in early pregnancy and preconceptually High dose if epileptic or previous neural tube defect (NTD)
Sickle-cell disease	10% of Afro-Caribbeans in the UK carry gene Increased perinatal mortality, thrombosis, sickle crises Management: exchange transfusions, folic acid, avoid precipitating factors for crises. Avoid iron Test partner and offer prenatal diagnosis if carrier
Thalassaemias	Alpha: South-East Asian origin. Beta: Mediterranean origin as well Management: Give folic acid, avoid iron (beta thalassaemia). May need transfusions Test partner and offer prenatal diagnosis if carrier

Red blood cell isoimmunization

Definition

Red blood cell isoimmunization occurs when the mother mounts an immune response against antigens on fetal red cells that enter her circulation. The resulting antibodies then cross the placenta and cause fetal red blood cell destruction.

Pathophysiology

Blood groups: Blood is classified according to its ABO and rhesus genotype. The rhesus system consists of three linked gene pairs; one allele of each pair is dominant to the other: *C/c*, *D/d* and *E/e*. An individual inherits one allele of each pair from each parent in a Mendelian fashion. The most significant in isoimmunization is the *D* gene. As *D* is dominant to *d*, only individuals who are *DD* or *Dd* (i.e. homozygous or heterozygous) express the D antigen and are 'D rhesus positive' (Fig. 22.1). Individuals homozygous for the recessive *d* (*dd*) are 'D rhesus negative', and their immune system will recognize the D antigen as foreign if they are exposed to it.

Sensitization: Small amounts of fetal blood cross the placenta and enter the maternal circulation during uncomplicated pregnancies and particularly at sensitizing events such as delivery, placental abruption and amniocentesis [→ p.151]. If the fetus is 'D rhesus positive' and the mother is 'D rhesus negative', the mother will mount an immune response (sensitization), creating anti-D antibodies. Immunity is permanent, and if the mother's immune system is again exposed to the antigen, large numbers of antibodies are rapidly created. They can cross the placenta and bind to fetal red blood cells, which are then destroyed in the fetal reticuloendothelial system (Fig. 22.2). This can cause haemolytic anaemia and ultimately death, and is called rhesus haemolytic disease. A similar immune response can be mounted against other red blood cell antigens): the most important antibodies are anti-c and anti-Kell (a non-rhesus antibody), particularly after blood transfusion.

Potentially sensitizing events
Termination of pregnancy or evacuation of retained products of conception (ERPC) after miscarriage
Ectopic pregnancy
Vaginal bleeding < 12 weeks, or if heavy
External cephalic version
Invasive uterine procedure, e.g. amniocentesis or chorionic villus sampling (CVS)
Intrauterine death
Delivery

Prevention: using anti-D

Production of maternal anti-D can be prevented by the administration of exogenous anti-D to the mother. This 'mops up' fetal red cells that have crossed the placenta, by binding to their antigens, thereby preventing recognition by the mother's immune system. Anti-D (500 IU) should be given to all women who are rhesus negative at 28 and 34 weeks (*Cochrane* 2000: CD000020): this alone will reduce the rate of isoimmunization in a first pregnancy from 1.5% to 0.2%. Anti-D is also given within 72 h of any sensitizing event, although some benefit is gained within 9 days, and if the neonate is found to be rhesus positive after delivery. A Kleihauer test, to assess the number of fetal cells in the maternal circulation, is usually performed postnatally to detect larger fetomaternal haemorrhages that require larger doses of anti-D to 'mop up'. Anti-D is unnecessary if the neonate is rhesus negative; its status is therefore routinely checked at birth. It is still usually given even if the partner is known to be rhesus negative because of the possibility of non-paternity but this issue must be handled with care. It is pointless if maternal anti-D is already present, as sensitization has already occurred.

Obstetrics and Gynaecology, 3rd edition. By Lawrence Impey and Tim Child. Published 2008 by Blackwell Publishing, ISBN: 978-1-4051-6095-7.

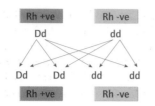

Rh +ve   Rh -ve
Dd   dd

Dd   Dd   dd   dd
Rh +ve   Rh -ve

Fig. 22.1 Mendelian inheritance of *D/d* gene pair.

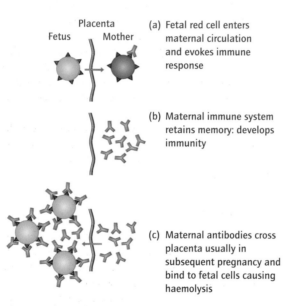

Placenta
Fetus   Mother

(a) Fetal red cell enters maternal circulation and evokes immune response

(b) Maternal immune system retains memory: develops immunity

(c) Maternal antibodies cross placenta usually in subsequent pregnancy and bind to fetal cells causing haemolysis

Fig. 22.2 The mechanism of red cell isoimmunization.

Prevention of rhesus disease

Booking and 34 weeks: Check all women for antibodies

Rhesus-negative women: Give anti-D at 28 and 34 weeks, after any bleeding or potentially sensitizing event, and after delivery if neonate is rhesus positive

---

Epidemiology

Fifteen per cent of Caucasian women, but fewer African or Asian women, are D rhesus negative. In the absence of prophylaxis, many will develop anti-D antibodies. The use of anti-D, smaller family size, and good management of isoimmunization has resulted in perinatal deaths attributable to rhesus disease becoming extremely rare. Currently only 1.7% of D rhesus negative women have been sensitized in the UK, mostly as a result of omitted or inadequate anti-D.

Aetiology of isoimmunization

Anti-D: Although now rare, D rhesus isoimmunization still occurs because of omitted and inadequate doses of prophylactic anti-D. If both parents are known to be D rhesus negative, the fetus must be rhesus negative also and therefore will be unaffected.

Other antibodies: Anti-c, anti-E and anti-Kell now account for as many cases of fetal anaemia, largely because of the decline in anti-D rhesus disease. Many other rare antibodies can cause mild fetal anaemia and postnatal jaundice.

Manifestations of rhesus disease

As antibody levels rise in a sensitized woman, the antibodies will cross the placenta and cause haemolysis, but only if the fetus is rhesus positive. In mild disease, this may lead to *neonatal jaundice* only. Or there may be sufficient haemolysis to cause neonatal anaemia (haemolytic disease of the newborn). More severe disease causes *in utero* anaemia and, as this worsens, cardiac failure, ascites and oedema (hydrops) and fetal death follow. Rhesus disease usually worsens with successive pregnancies as maternal antibody production increases.

Management of isoimmunization

The management of rhesus isoimmunization varies widely but comprises:
1 Identification of women at risk of fetal haemolysis and anaemia;
2 Assessing if/how severely the fetus is anaemic; and
3 Blood transfusion *in utero* or delivery for affected fetuses.

Identification

Unsensitized women are screened for antibodies at booking and at 28 and 34 weeks' gestation. If anti-D levels are <10 IU/mL, a significant fetal problem is very unlikely and levels are subsequently checked every 2–4 weeks. Higher levels warrant further investigation.

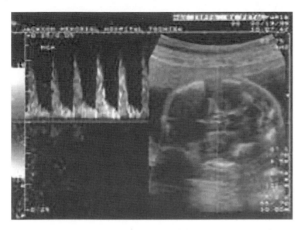

Fig. 22.3 Middle cerebral artery (MCA).

Amniocentesis, and more recently, maternal blood sampling for fetal cells (*Prenat Diagn* 2001; **21**: 321), is sometimes used to test for fetal rhesus status where the father is a heterozygote. Anti-Kell antibody levels are less predictive of disease severity and ultrasound is used earlier.

Assessing severity of fetal anaemia

Pregnancies at risk of fetal anaemia are assessed using ultrasound. Only severe anemia (e.g. <5 g/dL) is detectable as fetal hydrops or excessive fetal fluid. Doppler ultrasound of the peak velocity in systole (PSV) of the fetal middle cerebral artery (MCA) (Fig. 22.3) has a high sensitivity for significant anaemia (*NEJM* 2000; **342**: 9), at least before 36 weeks. It is therefore used at least fortnightly in at-risk pregnancies.

If anaemia is suspected from this, fetal blood sampling is performed under ultrasound guidance, using a needle in the umbilical vein at the cord insertion in the placenta, or in the intrahepatic vein. The risk of fetal loss is 1%, and after 28 weeks it should be performed with facilities for immediate delivery if complications arise.

Treatment of fetal anemia: *in utero* transfusion

Fetal blood sampling is performed with rhesus negative, high haematocrit, cytomegalovirus-negative blood ready, which can be injected down the needle into the umbilical vein if anaemia is confirmed. This process of quantification of anaemia and transfusion will need to be repeated at increasing intervals until about 36 weeks, after which time delivery is undertaken. Blood is more easily administered to the neonate: both top-up (for anaemia) and exchange (for hyperbilirubinaemia) transfusions may be required.

All neonates born to rhesus negative women should have a full blood count (FBC), blood film, bilirubin and indirect Coombs' test: these detect lesser degrees of isoimmunization.

Further reading

Crowther CA, Keirse MJ. Anti-D administration in pregnancy for preventing rhesus alloimmunization. *Cochrane Database of Systematic Reviews (Online: Update Software)* 2000; **2**: CD000020.

Moise KJ. Red blood cell alloimmunization in pregnancy. *Seminars in Hematology* 2005; **42**: 169–78.

Rhesus Isoimmunization at a Glance

Definition	Maternal antibody response against fetal red cell antigen entering her circulation; passage of antibodies into fetus leads to haemolysis
Aetiology	Anti-D still prevalent because of inadequate/failed prophylaxis Other major antibodies: anti-c and anti-Kell
Epidemiology	15% of Caucasian women are rhesus negative; anti-D responses in 1.7%
Pathology	Haemolysis causes anaemia. Neonatal jaundice ± anaemia if less severe; hydrops and fetal death if severe
Prevention	Administer anti-D to rhesus-negative women at 28 and 34 weeks, and after potentially sensitizing events
Management	Identification: Antibody testing and past obstetric history Assess severity: Doppler of fetal middle cerebral artery (MCA); fetal blood sampling to confirm Treat: Transfuse if fetus anaemic, deliver if >36 weeks Postnatally: Check full blood count (FBC), bilirubin, rhesus group, Coombs' test

Preterm delivery

Definitions and epidemiology

Delivery is preterm if it occurs between 24 and 37 weeks' gestation. However, it is most important before 34 weeks because that is when the neonatal risks are greater. Before 24 weeks, labour is tantamount to a miscarriage, although exceptionally fetal survival occurs at 23 weeks. Some 5–8% of deliveries are preterm. A further 6% of deliveries present preterm with contractions but deliver at term. Preterm delivery can be the result of spontaneous labour or, usually at later gestations, can be iatrogenic. This is where delivery is expedited by the obstetrician because the fetal or maternal risks of continuation justify exposing the fetus to the risks of preterm delivery. As these risks lessen with increasing gestation, the threshold for such intervention changes. The most common example is pre-eclampsia [→ p.165], where delivery is the only cure, and a pregnancy affected at, say, 28 weeks would have a high risk of both maternal and fetal death if it continued to term.

Complications

Neonatal: Prematurity accounts for 80% of neonatal intensive care occupancy, 20% of perinatal mortality and up to 50% of cerebral palsy. Other long-term morbidity, including chronic lung disease, blindness and minor disability is common (Fig. 23.1). It is possibly the most important and least understood area of pregnancy.

Maternal: Infection is frequently associated with preterm labour and can cause occasionally severe maternal illness and postnatally, endometritis is common. Caesarean section is more commonly used.

Obstetrics and Gynaecology, 3rd edition. By Lawrence Impey and Tim Child. Published 2008 by Blackwell Publishing, ISBN: 978-1-4051-6095-7.

Aetiology of spontaneous preterm labour (Fig. 23.2)

Risk factors: These are multiple and include a previous history, lower socioeconomic class, extremes of maternal age, a short inter-pregnancy interval, maternal medical disease such as renal failure or diabetes, pregnancy complications such as pre-eclampsia or intrauterine growth restriction (IUGR), male fetal gender, a high haemoglobin, sexually transmitted disease (STDs) and vaginal infection (such as bacterial vaginosis), previous cervical surgery, multiple pregnancy, uterine abnormalities and fibroids, urinary infection, polyhydramnios, congenital fetal abnormalities and antepartum haemorrhage.

Mechanisms: To rationalize these disparate risks, the uterus can be thought of as a castle, with the cervix as the castle wall holding the 'defenders' in (Fig. 23.2). Three groups of mechanisms, affecting the defenders, the castle walls, or the enemy, lead to the wall being breached.

Too many defenders: Multiple pregnancy is an increasing contributor because of assisted conception. Delivery before 34 weeks occurs in 20% of twins and is the mean time for delivery of triplets. Excess liquor, polyhydramnios [→ p.157] has the same effect, probably largely mediated by increased stretch.

The defenders jump out: The fetal survival response. Spontaneous preterm labour is more common where the fetus is at risk, e.g. pre-eclampsia and IUGR, or if there is infection. Likewise, a placental abruption will often be followed by labour. Iatrogenic preterm delivery attempts to improve upon this mechanism.

The castle design is poor: Uterine abnormalities such as fibroids or congenital (müllerian duct) abnormalities.

The wall is weak: The phrase '*cervical incompetence*' describes the painless cervical dilatation that precedes some preterm deliveries. Some follow cervical surgery including treatments for cervical intraepithelial neoplasia (CIN) [→ p.32] or cervical cancer, or multiple termi-

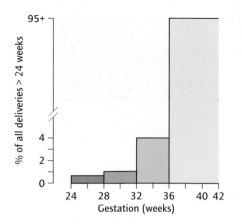

Fig. 23.1 Incidence of preterm delivery. Source: Oxford data.

nations of pregnancy, but in many no risk factors are known.

The enemy knock down the walls: Infection is implicated in about 60% of preterm deliveries, and is often subclinical. Choriomanionitis, offensive liquor, neonatal sepsis and endometritis after delivery are all manifestations. Bacterial vaginosis is a well-known risk factor, but many bacteria including group B streptococcus (GBS) [→ p.160], *Trichomonas*, *Chlamydia* and even commensals have been implicated. The effects of infection are partly dependent on the cervix: whether a castle wall falls down depends on both its strength and that of the enemy. In practice, therefore, a cervical problem and infection often coexist.

The enemy get around the walls: Urinary tract infection and poor dental health (*J Periodontol* 2005; **76**: 2144) are risk factors.

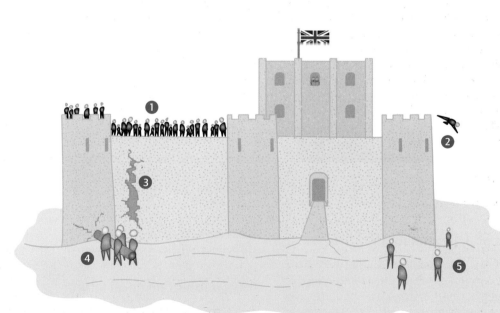

❶ 'Too much inside':	Multiple pregnancy polyhydramnios
❷ 'Defenders escape' (fetal survival response)	IUGR, pre eclampsia
❸ Weak wall:	Cervix
❹ Enemy:	Bateria in vagina
❺ Enemy:	Bateria elsewhere

Fig. 23.2 Risk factors for preterm delivery.

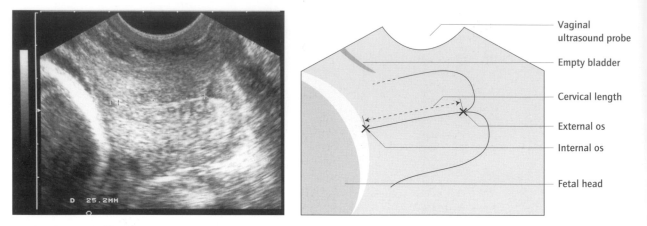

Fig. 23.3 Cervical length.

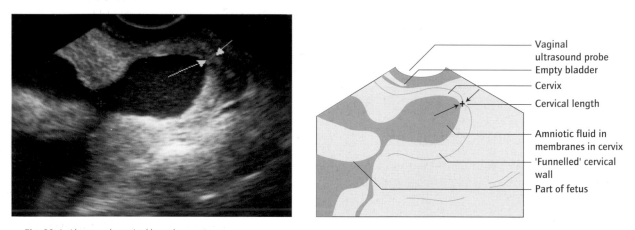

Fig. 23.4 Abnormal cervical length.

Prediction of preterm labour

History: Those at increased risk (see above), particularly those with a previous history of late miscarriage or preterm labour, may undergo investigations and attempts to prevent preterm delivery. Nevertheless, most women who deliver preterm are not identified as high risk on history alone.

Investigations: Even in women apparently at low risk for preterm delivery the *cervical length* on transvaginal sonography (TVS) (Figs 23.3 & 23.4) is sensitive and specific: at 23 weeks, a cervical length of <15 mm on TVS predicts 85% of spontaneous deliveries before 28 weeks (*Ultrasound Obstet Gynecol* 1998; **12**: 312), with a false positive rate of 1.5%. Prediction of preterm delivery is therefore relatively effective, although prediction is not the same as prevention.

Prevention of preterm labour

Preventative strategies are usually limited to women at high risk. It is unclear if universal screening of all women with a cervical scan could lead to an overall reduction in the incidence of preterm labour. In women at high risk, because preterm labour is usually the culmination of events initiated many weeks earlier, strategies should begin at 12 weeks.

The cervix. Cervical cerclage is the insertion of one or more sutures in the cervix to strengthen it and keep it closed (Fig. 23.5). It is commonly used although its

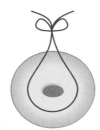

Fig. 23.5 Cervical suture. Transverse section of the cervix.

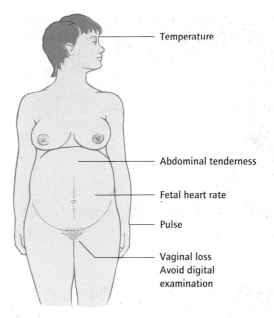

Fig. 23.6 Monitoring the patient with preterm prelabour rupture of the membranes.

effectiveness in isolation is disputed (*Cochrane* 2003: CD003253). The vaginal route is usual, but it can be placed abdominally if the cervix is very short or scarred. It is inserted in one of three situations. It can be elective, at 12–14 weeks, particularly in women who presented previously with a history or risk factors suggestive of cervical weakness or in whom the cervix is very short. Or, the cervix can be scanned regularly and only sutured if there is significant shortening (*Obstet Gynecol* 2005; **106**: 181). Finally, it can be used as a 'rescue suture' that will, in expert hands, occasionally prevent delivery even when the 'incompetent' cervix is dilated.

Infection. Although infection is common, it is likely that some bacteria are beneficial. For example, metronidazole actually increases the risk of preterm labour. In practice, screening and treatment of sexually transmitted disease, urinary tract infections (UTIs) and *bacterial vaginosis* (*Lancet* 2003; **361**: 983) is beneficial, although the role of antibiotics for other bacteria is disputed. Evidence that treatment of periodontal disease is effective is also disputed (*NEJM* 2006; **355**: 1885).

Fetal reduction. Reduction of higher order multiples [→ p.221] is offered at 10–14 weeks.

Treatment of polyhydramnios. Very high amniotic fluid volumes, usually as a result of a fetal abnormality, can be treated by needle aspiration (amnioreduction) or, providing fetal surveillance is intensive, non-steroidal anti-inflammatory drugs (NSAIDs). These reduce fetal urine output, but may also cause premature closure of the fetal ductus arteriosus.

Progesterone supplementation. Suppositories from early pregnancy reduce the risk of preterm labour in women at high risk (*AmJOG* 2006; **194**: 1234).

Ineffective treatments. These include bedrest and prolonged oral tocolysis.

Clinical features

History. Typically, women present with painful contractions. In over half of such women, however, the contractions will stop spontaneously and labour will not ensue until term. With 'cervical incompetence', painless cervical dilatation may occur or the woman may experience only a dull suprapubic ache. Antepartum haemorrhage and fluid loss are common: the latter suggests ruptured membranes.

Examination. Fever may occur. The lie and presentation of the fetus are checked with abdominal palpation (Fig. 23.6). Digital vaginal examination is performed unless the membranes have ruptured. An effaced or dilating cervix confirms the diagnosis, but the course of preterm labour is unpredictable and may be extremely rapid or very slow.

Investigations

To assess fetal state, cardiotocography (CTG) and ultrasound are used.

To assess the likelihood of delivery if the cervix is uneffaced, fetal fibronectin assay is helpful (*BMJ* 2002; **325**: 301): a negative result means preterm delivery is unlikely. Transvaginal scanning (TVS) of cervical length is also predictive: delivery is extremely unlikely if the cervix is >15 mm long.

To look for infection, vaginal swabs should be taken, using a sterile speculum if the membranes have ruptured. The maternal C-reactive protein (CRP) usually rises with chorioamnionitis; white cell count estimation is often unhelpful because steroids may cause it to rise.

Management

Promoting pulmonary maturity

Steroids are given between 24 and 34 weeks. These reduce perinatal morbidity and mortality by promoting pulmonary maturity (*Cochrane* 2000: CD000065). They do not increase the risk of infection, but careful glucose control is needed in diabetic patients. As they take 24 h to act, delivery is often artificially delayed using tocolysis. Long-term follow-up has confirmed the safety of one course (*BMJ* 2005; **331**: 665), but repeated doses are not advised.

Tocolysis: Nifedipine or atosiban, an oxytocin-receptor antagonist, can be given to allow steroids time to act or to allow *in utero* transfer to a unit with neonatal intensive care facilities. These delay rather than stop preterm labour and should not be used for more than 24 h. Ritodrine or salbutamol and NSAIDs also delay delivery but are seldom used because of side effects.

Detection and prevention of infection

The presence of infection within the uterus risks maternal health and considerably worsens the outlook for the neonate (*Lancet* 1995; **346**: 1449). This may occur even where the membranes have not ruptured: chorioamnionitis warrants intravenous antibiotics and immediate delivery, whatever the gestation.

Delivery

Mode of delivery: Vaginal delivery reduces the incidence of respiratory distress syndrome in the neonate and Caesarean section is undertaken only for the usual obstetric indications. Breech presentation [→ p.212] is more common in preterm labour: at term, elective Caesarean section is safer for breech babies. This has meant a loss of operator skills, and although the evidence in preterm

labour is lacking, most preterm breeches now undergo Caesarean section.

Conduct of delivery: Paediatric facilities are mobilized. The membranes are not ruptured in labour, at least up to 32 weeks: labour may be slow, allowing steroids more time to act, and the membranes might cushion the delicate preterm fetus against trauma. Forceps are used only for the usual obstetric indications, and the ventouse is contraindicated.

Antibiotics for delivery are recommended, because of the increased risk and morbidity of GBS [→ p.241].

Preterm prelabour rupture of the membranes

Definition

The membranes rupture before labour at <37 weeks. Often the cause is unknown, but all the causes of preterm labour may be implicated. It occurs before one-third of preterm deliveries.

Complications

Preterm delivery is the principal complication and follows within 48 h in >50% of cases. *Infection* of the fetus or placenta (chorioamnionitis) or cord (funisitis) is common. This may occur before, and therefore be the cause of the membranes rupture, or it may follow membrane rupture. *Prolapse of the umbilical cord* may occur rarely. Absence of liquor (usually before 24 weeks) can result in *pulmonary hypoplasia* and postural deformities.

Clinical features

History: A gush of clear fluid is normal, followed by further leaking.

Examination: The lie and presentation are checked. A pool of fluid is visible in the posterior fornix on speculum examination. Digital examination is best avoided, although it is performed to exclude cord prolapse if the presentation is not cephalic. Chorioamnionitis is characterized by contractions or abdominal pain, fever, tachycardia, uterine tenderness and coloured or offensive liquor, although clinical signs often appear late.

Investigations

To confirm the diagnosis in doubtful cases, commercially available tests are available but not entirely reliable. Ultrasound may reveal reduced liquor, but the volume can also be normal as fetal urine production continues.
To look for infection, a high vaginal swab (HVS), full blood count (FBC) and CRP are taken. In doubtful cases, amniocentesis [→ p.151] with Gram staining and culture is occasionally used.
Fetal well-being is assessed by CTG. A persistent fetal tachycardia is suggestive of infection.

Management

The risk of preterm delivery must be balanced against the risk of infection, which, if present, greatly increases neonatal mortality and long-term morbidity. Prevention and identification are therefore essential. The woman is admitted and given steroids. Close maternal (signs of infection) and fetal surveillance is performed, and if the gestation reaches 36 weeks, induction is normally performed.

Identification and management of infection

Early chorioamnionitis produces few signs. If signs of infection appear, intravenous antibiotics are given immediately and the fetus is delivered whatever the gestation: antibiotics alone will not eliminate chorioamnionitis.

Prevention of infection

The prophylactic use of erythromycin in women even without clinical evidence of infection is recommended (*Cochrane* 2003: CD001058). Co-amoxiclav is contraindicated, as the neonate is more prone to necrotizing enterocolitis (NEC).

Further reading

Berghella V, Odibo A, To M, Rust O, Althuisius S. Cerclage for short cervix on ultrasonography: a meta-analysis of trials using individual-level patient data. *Obstetrics and Gynecology* 2005; **106**: 181–9.
Chandiramani M, Shennan A. Preterm labour: update on prediction and prevention strategies. *Current Opinions in Obstetrics and Gynecology* 2006; **18**: 618–24.
Slattery MM, Morrison JJ. Preterm delivery. *Lancet* 2002; **360**. 1409–97.
Welsh A, Nicolaides K. Cervical screening for preterm delivery. *Current Opinions in Obstetrics and Gynecology* 2002; **14**: 195–202.

Preterm Delivery at a Glance	
Epidemiology	8% of deliveries, 20% of perinatal mortality
Aetiology	Subclinical infection, cervical incompetence, iatrogenic, multiple pregnancy, antepartum haemorrhage, diabetes, polyhydramnios, fetal compromise, uterine abnormalities, idiopathic
Prediction	History; ultrasound (transvaginal) of cervical length at 23 weeks
Prevention	Antibiotics if bacterial vaginosis, urinary tract infection (UTI), sexually transmitted disease (STD) or history of infection in previous preterm labour Cervical suture if cervical incompetence likely: either at 12 weeks or if cervix shortens Progesterone pessaries Specific strategies, e.g. fetal reduction, amnioreduction
Features	Abdominal pain, antepartum haemorrhage, ruptured membranes. Cervical incompetence silent
Investigations	Fibronectin assay or cervical scan if cervix uneffaced to rule out false diagnosis. High vaginal swab (HVS), cardiotocography (CTG), ultrasound
Management	Steroids if <34 weeks, tocolysis for max. 24 h Antibiotics in labour Caesarean for normal indications Inform neonatologists

24 Antepartum haemorrhage

Definition

Antepartum haemorrhage (APH) is bleeding from the genital tract after 24 weeks' gestation. This is the time at which neonatal survival is better than anecdotal.

Causes of antepartum haemorrhage (APH)	
Common:	Undetermined origin
	Placental abruption
	Placenta praevia
Rarer:	Incidental genital tract pathology
	Uterine rupture
	Vasa praevia
	Placenta praevia

Placenta praevia

Definitions and epidemiology

Placenta praevia occurs when the placenta is implanted in the lower segment of the uterus. It complicates 0.4% of pregnancies at term. At 20 weeks the placenta is 'low-lying' in many more pregnancies, but appears to 'move' upwards as the pregnancy continues. This is because of the formation of the lower segment of the uterus in the third trimester: it is the myometrium where the placenta implants that moves away from the internal cervical os. Therefore, only 1 in 10 apparently low-lying placentas will be praevia at term.

Classification of placenta praevia	
Marginal (previously types I–II):	Placenta in lower segment, not over os (Fig. 24.1a)
Major (previously types III–IV):	Placenta completely or partially covering os (Fig. 24.1b)

Obstetrics and Gynaecology, 3rd edition. By Lawrence Impey and Tim Child. Published 2008 by Blackwell Publishing, ISBN: 978-1-4051-6095-7.

Classification

Placenta praevia is classified according to the proximity of the placenta to the internal os of the cervix. It may be predominantly on the anterior or posterior uterine wall.

Aetiology

This is unknown, but placenta praevia is slightly more common with twins, in women of high parity and age, and if the uterus is scarred (e.g. previous Caesarean) (*J Matern Fetal Neonatal Med* 2003; **13**: 175).

Complications

The placenta in the lower segment obstructs engagement of the head: except for some marginal praevias, this necessitates *Caesarean section* and may also cause the lie to be *transverse*. *Haemorrhage* can be severe and may continue during and after delivery as the lower segment is less able to contract and constrict the maternal blood supply. If a placenta implants in a previous Caesarean section scar, it may be so deep as to prevent placental separation (placenta accreta) or even penetrate through the uterine wall into surrounding structures such as the bladder (placenta percreta). These may provoke massive haemorrhage at delivery, which is conducted only by experienced personnel. Haemorrhage may require *hysterectomy*.

Clinical features

History: Typically, there are intermittent painless bleeds, which increase in frequency and intensity over several weeks. Such bleeding may be catastrophic. One-third of women, however, have not experienced bleeding before the diagnosis is made.

Examination: Breech presentation and transverse lie are common. The fetal head is not engaged and high.

Vaginal examination can provoke massive bleeding and is *never* performed in a woman who is bleeding vaginally unless placenta praevia has been excluded.

Presentation of placenta praevia
Incidental finding on ultrasound scan
Vaginal bleeding
Abnormal lie, breech presentation

Investigations

To make the diagnosis, ultrasound is used (Fig. 24.2). If a low-lying placenta has been diagnosed at a second trimester ultrasound, this is repeated at 34 weeks to exclude placenta praevia.

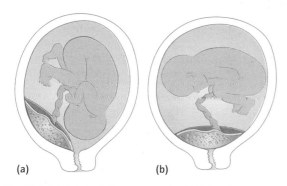

(a)   (b)

Fig. 24.1 (a) Marginal placenta praevia. (b) Major placenta praevia (abnormal lie and malpresentation are common).

To assess fetal and maternal well-being, cardiotocography (CTG), a full blood count (FBC), clotting studies and cross-match are needed. Fetal distress [→ p.203] is uncommon.

Management

Admission

This is necessary for all women with bleeding. If placenta praevia is then found on ultrasound, such women normally stay in hospital until delivery because of the risk of massive haemorrhage. Blood is kept available; anti-D is administered to rhesus negative women; intravenous access is maintained; steroids [→ p.194] are administered if the gestation is <34 weeks. In women with asymptomatic placenta praevia, admission can be delayed until 37 weeks, provided they can get to hospital easily.

Delivery

This is by elective Caesarean section at 39 weeks by the most senior person available. Blood loss may be great during delivery; postpartum haemorrhage is also common because the lower segment does not contract well after delivery. Earlier, emergency delivery is needed if bleeding is severe before this time. However, pregnancy can often be prolonged with observation and, if necessary, blood transfusion. Only if the degree of praevia is marginal and the fetal head is past the lower

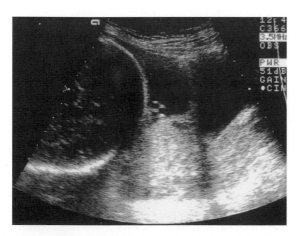

Fig. 24.2 Ultrasound of placenta praevia and labelled drawing.

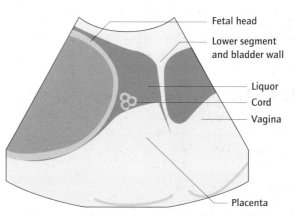

Fetal head

Lower segment and bladder wall

Liquor

Cord

Vagina

Placenta

edge (on ultrasound) can vaginal delivery be contemplated. In exceptional, doubtful cases, vaginal examination is performed in theatre with full facilities for an immediate Caesarean.

Placenta accreta [→ p.260] can be diagnosed using ultrasound and should be anticipated, although the placenta may also occasionally invade the myometroium even if it is not praevia or over a scar. At the time of delivery, the placenta will not separate and massive haemorrhage may follow its partial separation. Treatment involves either compression of the inside of the scar after removal of the placenta with an inflatable (e.g. Rusch) balloon or, frequently, hysterectomy.

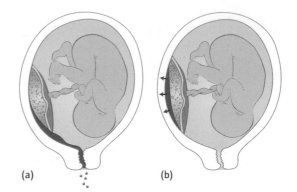

Fig. 24.3 (a) Revealed abruption. (b) Concealed abruption.

Differentiation between placental abruption and placenta praevia		
	Abruption	*Placenta praevia*
Shock:	Inconsistent with external loss	Consistent with external loss
Pain:	Common, often severe Constant with exacerbations	No. Contractions occasionally
Bleeding:	May be absent Often dark	Red and often profuse Often smaller previous antepartum haemorrhage (APHs)
Tenderness:	Usual, often severe Uterus may be hard	Rare
Fetus:	Lie normal, often engaged May be dead or distressed	Lie often abnormal/ head high Heart rate usually normal
Ultrasound:	Often normal, placenta not low	Placenta low

Placental abruption

Definition

Placenta abruption is when part (or all) of the placenta separates before delivery of the fetus. It occurs in 1% of pregnancies. However, it is likely that many antepartum haemorrhages of 'undetermined origin' are in fact small placental abruptions and that this figure is therefore higher.

Pathology

When part of the placenta separates, considerable maternal bleeding may occur behind it. This can have several consequences. Further placental separation and acute fetal distress may follow. Blood usually also tracks down between the membranes and the myometrium to be revealed as APH. It may also enter the liquor. Or it may simply enter the myometrium: visible haemorrhage is absent in 20% (Fig. 24.3).

Complications

Fetal death is common (30% of proven abruptions). Haemorrhage often necessitates blood transfusion; this, disseminated intravascular coagulation (DIC) and renal failure may rarely lead to maternal death.

Aetiology

Many affected women have no risk factors. However, intrauterine growth restriction (IUGR), pre-eclampsia, autoimmune disease, maternal smoking, cocaine usage, a previous history of placental abruption (risk 6%), multiple pregnancy and high maternal parity all predispose to abruption. It has also been occasionally associated with trauma, external cephalic version (ECV) [→ p.213] or a sudden reduction in uterine volume (e.g. rupture of the membranes in a woman with polyhydramnios).

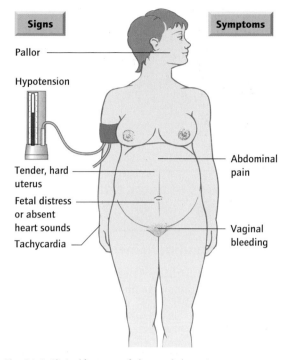

Signs | Symptoms

Pallor

Hypotension

Tender, hard uterus

Fetal distress or absent heart sounds

Tachycardia

Abdominal pain

Vaginal bleeding

Fig. 24.4 Clinical features of placental abruption

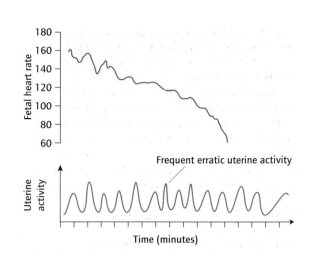

Fig. 24.5 Terminal fetal heart bradycardia with placental abruption.

Major risk factors for placental abruption
Intrauterine growth restriction (IUGR)
Pre-eclampsia
Pre-existing hypertension
Maternal smoking
Previous abruption

Clinical features (Fig. 24.4)

History: Classically, there is painful bleeding. The pain is due to blood behind the placenta and in the myometrium, and is usually constant with exacerbations; the blood is often dark. The degree of vaginal bleeding does not reflect the severity of the abruption because some may not escape from the uterus. Indeed, pain or bleeding may occur alone. If pain occurs alone, the abruption is 'concealed'. If vaginal bleeding is evident, it is 'revealed'.

Examination: Tachycardia suggests profound blood loss, which may be out of proportion to the vaginal loss because of 'concealed' loss. Hypotension only occurs after massive blood loss. The uterus is tender and often contracting: labour usually ensues. In severe cases, the uterus is 'woody' hard and the fetus is very difficult to feel. Fetal heart tones are often abnormal or even absent. If coagulation failure has occurred, widespread bleeding is evident.

Investigations

The diagnosis is usually made on clinical grounds. Investigations help to establish the severity of the abruption, to plan appropriate resuscitation, and whether and how to deliver the fetus.

To establish fetal well-being, CTG [→p.207] is performed. In addition to fetal distress, frequent uterine activity may be evident on the tocograph (Fig. 24.5).

To establish maternal well-being, FBC, coagulation screen and cross-match are performed. Catheterization with hourly urine output, central venous pressure (CVP) monitoring, regular FBC, coagulation, and urea and creatinine (U&E) estimations are required in severe cases. Ultrasound has little place in the diagnosis of placental abruption, except to exclude placenta praevia.

Features of major placental abruption
Maternal collapse
Coagulopathy
Fetal distress or demise
'Woody' hard uterus
Poor urine output or renal failure
N.B. Degree of vaginal loss is often unhelpful

Principles of management of major placental abruption
Fetal condition: cardiotocography (CTG)
Maternal condition: fluid balance, renal function, full blood count (FBC) and clotting. Central venous pressure (CVP) if appropriate
Early delivery
Blood ± blood products transfusion

Management

Assessment and resuscitation

Admission is required, even without vaginal bleeding if there is pain and uterine tenderness. Intravenous fluid is given, with steroids if the gestation is <34 weeks. Blood transfusion must be considered. Opiate analgesia is used; anti-D is given to rhesus negative women.

Delivery

This depends on the fetal state and gestation. The mother must be stabilized first.

If there is fetal distress, urgent delivery by Caesarean section is required.

If there is no fetal distress, but the gestation is 37 weeks or more, induction of labour with amniotomy is performed. The fetal heart is monitored continuously, maternal condition is closely observed and Caesarean section is performed if fetal distress ensues.

If the fetus is dead, coagulopathy is also likely. Blood products are given and labour is induced.

Conservative management

If there is no fetal distress, the pregnancy is preterm and the degree of abruption appears to be minor, steroids are given (if <34 weeks) and the patient is closely monitored on the antenatal ward. If all symptoms settle, she may be discharged, but the pregnancy is now 'high risk': ultrasound scans for fetal growth are performed.

Postpartum management

Whatever the mode of delivery, postpartum haemorrhage [→ p.267] is a major risk.

Other causes of antepartum haemorrhage

Bleeding of undetermined origin

When APH is small and painless but the placenta is not praevia, it may be difficult to find a cause. Ultrasound is of little diagnostic use. Many episodes are likely to be minor degrees of placental abruption: there is no such thing as a 'heavy show' (a show is the occasionally slightly blood-stained mucus plug that usually drops from the cervix around the time that labour begins). This, and indeed the 'recurrent show', are likely to be minor abruptions, and patients should be managed as such.

Ruptured vasa praevia

Vasa praevia occurs when a fetal blood vessel runs in the membranes in front of the presenting part (Fig. 24.6a). Such vessels are rare, but typically occur when the umbilical cord is attached to the membranes rather than the placenta (velamentous insertion). They can be detected on ultrasound but seldom are. When the membranes rupture, the vessel may rupture too, with massive fetal bleeding. This occurs in about 1 in 5000 pregnancies. The typical presentation is painless, moderate vaginal bleeding at amniotomy or spontaneous rupture of the membranes, which is accompanied by severe fetal distress. Caesarean section is often not fast enough to save the fetus.

Uterine rupture [→ p.264]

This condition (Fig. 24.6b) very occasionally occurs before labour in women with a scarred or congenitally abnormal uterus.

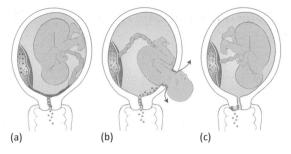

(a)   (b)   (c)

Fig. 24.6 Other causes of antepartum haemorrhage (APH). (a) Vasa praevia. (b) Ruptured uterus (intra-abdominal loss usually predominates). (c) Cervical carcinoma.

Bleeding of gynaecological origin

Cervical carcinoma can present in pregnancy (Fig. 24.6c). If a cervical smear is overdue, the woman with small recurrent or postcoital haemorrhage should undergo speculum examination and colposcopy. Cervical polyps, ectropions and vaginal lacerations may also

be evident but bleeding should not usually be attributed to them.

Further reading

Ananth CV, Smulian JC, Vintzileos AM. The effect of placenta previa on neonatal mortality: a population-based study in the United States, 1989 through 1997. *American Journal of Obstetrics and Gynecology* 2003; **188**: 1299–304.

Ananth CV, Wilcox AJ. Placental abruption and perinatal mortality in the United States. *American Journal of Epidemiology* 2001; **153**: 332–7.

Kayani SI, Walkinshaw SA, Preston C. Pregnancy outcome in severe placental abruption. *BJOG: an International Journal of Obstetrics and Gynaecology* 2003; **110**: 679–83.

Neilson JP. Interventions for suspected placenta praevia. *Cochrane Database of Systematic Reviews (Online: Update Software)* 2003; **2**: CD001998.

Oyelese Y, Ananth CV. Placental abruption. *Obstetrics and Gynecology* 2006; **108**: 1005–16.

Placenta Praevia at a Glance	
Definition	Placenta implanted in uterine lower segment. 'Low-lying' refers to placental site before lower segment formation
Types	Marginal praevia: Near/adjacent to cervical os Major praevia: Over/partly covering cervical os
Epidemiology	0.4% of pregnancies. Low-lying placenta in early pregnancy 5%
Aetiology	Usually idiopathic. Large placenta, scarred uterus, high parity/age
Complications	Haemorrhage. Need for preterm or Caesarean delivery
Features	Painless antepartum haemorrhage (APH), often multiple and increasing in frequency and severity Also abnormal lie, incidental ultrasound finding
Investigations	Ultrasound to locate the placenta. Full blood count (FBC) and cross-match if bleeding
Management	If low-lying placenta on early ultrasound, repeat at 36 weeks Asymptomatic: Admission at 37 weeks Bleeding: Admit whatever gestation. Have blood ready. Steroids if <34 weeks. Blood transfusion if necessary Delivery: Caesarean at 39 weeks; before if bleeding heavy

Placental Abruption at a Glance

Definition	Separation of part/all of placenta before delivery; after 24 weeks
Epidemiology	1% of pregnancies
Aetiology	Idiopathic; common associations: intrauterine growth restriction (IUGR), pre-eclampsia, autoimmune disease, smoking, previous abruption
Complications	Fetal death, massive haemorrhage causing disseminated intravascular coagulation (DIC), renal failure, maternal death
Features	Painful antepartum haemorrhage (APH), but pain or bleeding can be in isolation. Uterine tenderness and contractions: if major, absent fetal heart, 'woody' uterus, maternal collapse, coagulopathy
Investigations	Cardiotocography (CTG) to assess fetus. Full blood count (FBC), clotting to assess maternal state. Ultrasound scan excludes placenta praevia if diagnosis in doubt. If severe, intensive maternal monitoring (renal and liver function, central venous pressure [CVP], urine output)
Management	Admit: If severe, resuscitate with blood Fetal distress present: Deliver by Caesarean section Fetal distress absent: >37 weeks, induce labour Fetus dead: Induce labour. Coagulopathy likely Minor preterm abruption: Wait. Serial ultrasound scans

25 Fetal growth, compromise and surveillance

The aim of pregnancy care of the fetus is to prevent bad outcomes: particularly death or morbidity. Pursuit of this aim must take account of maternal health, resources and the fact that most pregnancies are normal. Morbidity encompasses cerebral palsy particularly, but also the need for neonatal care or resuscitation. Furthermore, there is growing evidence that *in utero* health and growth influences health, particularly cardiac disease, in later life (*Lancet* 1993; **341**: 938). The principal causes of perinatal mortality and cerebral palsy are outlined in the boxes below.

Principal causes of perinatal mortality

Unexplained
Preterm delivery
Intrauterine growth restriction (IUGR)
Congenital abnormalities
Intrapartum fetal distress
Placental abruption

Principal associations of cerebral palsy

Major: Prematurity (see Chapter 23)
          Intrauterine growth restriction (IUGR)
          Infection
          Pre-eclampsia (see Chapter 20)
          Congenital abnormalities (see Chapter 18)
          Intrapartum 'fetal distress' (see Chapter 29)
          Postnatal events

Other: Autoimmune disease (see Chapter 21)
          Multiple pregnancy (see Chapter 27)
          Placental abruption (see Chapter 24)

Fetal growth and terminology

Because there are so many associations of adverse neo-

Obstetrics and Gynaecology, 3rd edition. By Lawrence Impey and Tim Child. Published 2008 by Blackwell Publishing, ISBN: 978-1-4051-6095-7.

natal outcomes, and because their mechanisms of action are poorly understood, our use of terms such as compromise and fetal distress is simplistic.

Fetal compromise is a chronic situation and should be defined as when conditions for the normal growth and neurological development are not optimal. Most identifiable causes involve poor nutrient transfer through the placenta, often called 'placental dysfunction'. Commonly there is intrauterine growth restriction (IUGR), but this may also be absent (e.g. maternal diabetes or prolonged pregnancy).

Small for dates (gestational age) means that the weight of the fetus is less than the tenth centile for its gestation (if at term: 2.7 kg). Other cut-off points (e.g. third centile) can also be used. Traditionally, small size was felt to reflect chronic compromise due to placental dysfunction. However, most fetuses are simply constitutionally small, have grown consistently (Fig. 25.1) and are not compromised. Assessment of fetal weight is better at identifying IUGR if customized (www.preg.info) according to what would be expected for the individual [→ p.206] rather than the overall population.

Intrauterine growth restriction (IUGR) describes fetuses that have failed to reach their own 'growth potential'. Their growth *in utero* is slowed: many end up 'small for dates' (SFD), but some do not: many stillbirths or fetuses distressed in labour are of apparently 'normal' weight. If a fetus was genetically determined to be 4 kg at term and delivers at term weighing 3 kg, its growth has been restricted, and it may have placental dysfunction (Fig. 25.2) (www.gestation.net). Similarly, an ill, malnourished, tall adult may weigh more than a healthy shorter one. This means that whilst most IUGR babies are SFD, a proportion do not appear to be.

Fetal distress refers to an acute situation, such as hypoxia, that may result in fetal damage or death if it is not reversed, or if the fetus delivered urgently. As such it is usually used in labour (see Chapter 29). Nevertheless, most babies that subsequently develop cerebral palsy were not born hypoxic.

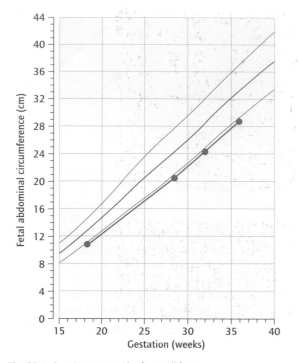

Fig. 25.1 Consistent growth of a small fetus.

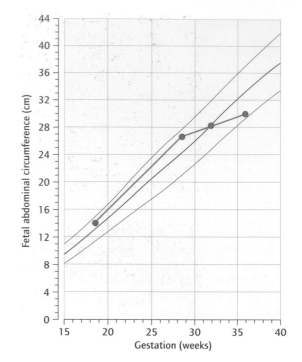

Fig. 25.2 Slowed growth suggestive of fetal compromise.

Fetal surveillance

Aims of fetal surveillance

1 Identify the 'high-risk' pregnancy using history or events during pregnancy, or using specific investigations.
2 Monitor the fetus for growth and well-being. The methods used will vary according to pregnancy risk and events during the pregnancy.
3 Intervene (usually expedite delivery) at an appropriate time, balancing the risks of *in utero* compromise against those of intervention and prematurity. The latter is itself a major cause of mortality and morbidity.

Problems with fetal surveillance

All methods of surveillance have a false positive rate (i.e. they can be overinterpreted). Whilst they may identify problems, they do not necessarily solve them and prevent adverse outcomes. In addition, they 'medicalize' pregnancy by concentrating on the abnormal, and they are expensive. For these reasons, identification of pregnancy risk is important to try to target the pregnancy at higher risk with more intensive surveillance (Fig. 25.3).

Identification of the high-risk pregnancy	
Pre-pregnancy:	Poor past obstetric history or very small baby Maternal disease Assisted conception Extremes of reproductive age Heavy smoking or drug abuse
During pregnancy:	Hypertension/proteinuria Vaginal bleeding Small for dates (SFD) baby Prolonged pregnancy Multiple pregnancy Recurrent urinary tract infections (UTIs)
Available investigations:	Cervical scan at 23 weeks [→ p.192] Uterine artery Doppler at 23 weeks Maternal blood tests, e.g. PAPP-A [→ p.205]

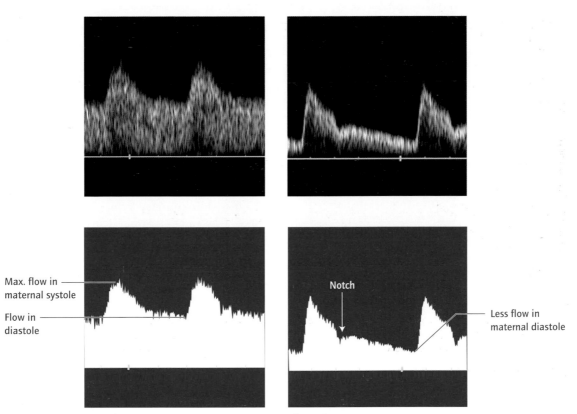

Fig. 25.3 Normal and abnormal uterine artery Doppler.

Identification of pregnancy risk

Prepregnancy risks

History: The traditional methods have centred on history: the mother's age, her previous medical history and obstetric history (see box above). Unfortunately, most women who develop pregnancy complications such as IUGR do not have any such risk factors: i.e. the use of history as a screening tests is not very sensitive. Further, taking all minor risk factors such as age >35 years will mean that many women who would have had normal pregnancy outcomes are considered high risk, i.e. the use of history as a screening test is not specific.

Early pregnancy

Blood tests: Pregnancy-associated plasma protein A (PAPP-A) is a placental hormone, the maternal level of which is reduced in the first trimester with chromosomal abnormalities. It is therefore used in screening for Down's syndrome [→ p.149]. It is now known that a low level constitutes a high risk of IUGR, placental abruption and consequent stillbirth (*JAMA* 2004; **292**: 2249). Levels of human chorionic gonadotrophin (hCG) and alpha fetoprotein (AFP), also used for screening for chromosomal abnormalities, also predict other pregnancy problems, albeit less consistently.

Maternal uterine artery Doppler at 23 weeks: The uterine circulation normally develops a very low resistance in normal pregnancy. Abnormal waveforms, indicating failure of development of a low resistance circulation, identify 75% of pregnancies at risk of adverse neonatal outcomes in the early third trimester, particularly early pre-eclampsia, IUGR or placental abruption (*Ultrasound Obstet Gynecol* 2001; **18**: 441). This test is less predictive of later problems.

Integrated screening for pregnancy risk: Using integration of (the above) multiple independent risk factors as in screening for chromosomal abnormalities [→ p.149] will increase the accuracy of screening (*AmJOG* 2006; **195**: 330). In this way, factors in the history and investigations can be used to identify more high risk women (with a lower false positive rate). This is currently under evaluation but is likely to enable more appropriate targeting of hospital-based and high risk antenatal care.

Later pregnancy

Pregnancy events: The occurrence of pre-eclampsia or vaginal bleeding, or if routine abdominal palpation suggests an SFD fetus, more close examination is required and the risk level will change.

Methods of fetal surveillance

Routine pregnancy care

The tests outlined below are not routine in low risk pregnancy. Here, the cornerstone of the identification of the small or compromised fetus is serial measurement of the symphisis fundal height and other aspects of antenatal visits [→ p.146].

Kick chart

What it is: The mother records the number of individual movements that she experiences every day. Ten is considered normal, but it is a change in number rather than the actual number of movements that is important.
Benefits: Most compromised fetuses have reduced movements in the days or hours before demise. A reduction in fetal movements is an indication for more sophisticated testing. Kick charts are simple and cheap.
Limitations: Compromised fetuses stop moving only shortly before death. Routine counting is of very limited benefit in reducing perinatal mortality. The high false positive rate can lead to unnecessary intervention, and maternal anxiety is common. As a result of these limitations, kick charts should not be used routinely.

Ultrasound assessment of fetal growth

What it is: Ultrasound scan is used to measure fetal size after the first trimester, using the abdominal and head circumferences. These changes are recorded on centile charts (Fig. 25.4). Three factors help to differentiate between the healthy small fetus and the 'growth-restricted' fetus:
1 The rate of growth can be determined by previous scans, or a later examination, at least 2 weeks apart.
2 The pattern of 'smallness' may help: the fetal abdomen will often stop enlarging before the head, which is 'spared'. The result is a 'thin' fetus or 'asymmetrical' growth restriction.
3 Allowance for constitutional non-pathological determinants of fetal growth enables 'customization' of individual fetal growth (*BJOG* 2001; **108**: 830), assessing actual growth according to expected growth.
Benefits: Serial ultrasound is safe and useful in confirming consistent growth in high risk and multiple pregnancies, and is essential to the management of such pregnancies. The use of ultrasound in dating and identification of abnormalities is discussed elsewhere [→ p.149].
Limitations: 'One-off' ultrasound scans in later pregnancy are of limited benefit in 'low risk' pregnancies (*Cochrane* 2000: CD001451). Inaccurate measurements are common, misleading and potentially harmful.

Doppler umbilical artery waveforms

What it is: Doppler is used to measure velocity waveforms in the umbilical arteries (Fig. 25.5). Evidence of a high resistance circulation, i.e. reduced flow in fetal diastole compared to systole, suggests placental dysfunction.
Benefits: Umbilical artery waveforms help identify which small fetuses are actually growth restricted and therefore compromised (*Cochrane* 2000: CD000073). Its usage improves perinatal outcome in high risk pregnancy whilst reducing intervention in those not compromised. In addition, the absence of flow in diastole usually predates cardiotocograph (CTG) abnormalities and correlates well with severe compromise.
Limitations: Doppler is not a useful screening tool in low risk pregnancies (*Cochrane* 2000: CD001450) and is less effective at identifying the normal-weight but compromised fetus.

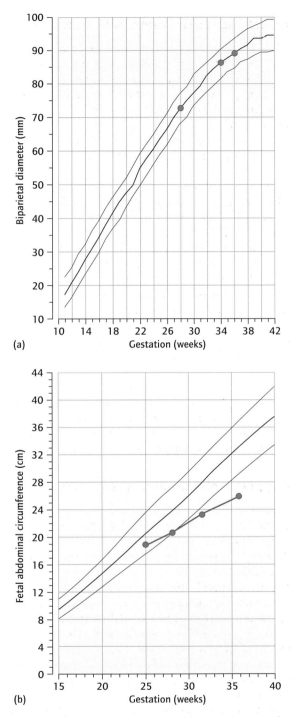

(a)

(b)

Fig. 25.4 (a) Normal growth of the head; (b) slowed growth of the abdomen.

Doppler waveforms of the fetal circulation

What it is: All major fetal vessels can be seen, but the most commonly measured are the middle cerebral arteries and the ductus venosus. With fetal compromise, the middle cerebral artery often develops a low resistance pattern in comparison to the thoracic aorta or renal vessels. This reflects a head-sparing effect. The velocity of flow also increases with fetal anaemia [→ p.189]. The ductus venosus waveform has been used as an alternative to antepartum CTG.

Benefits: The use of these is restricted to high risk pregnancy and generally contributes to, rather than dictates, decisions regarding intervention.

Limitations: There is currently little evidence that their use reduces perinatal mortality or morbidity.

Ultrasound assessment of biophysical profile/amniotic fluid volume

What it is: Four variables (limb movements, tone, breathing movements and liquor volume) are 'scored' zero or two each, to a total out of eight. In the traditional biophysical profile, CTG is also included and the total score is out of 10. It takes up to 30 minutes. A low score suggests severe compromise. Reduced liquor (oligohydramnios) is a non-specific finding that is more common in compromised fetuses.

Benefits: It is useful in high-risk pregnancy where CTG or Doppler give equivocal results.

Limitations: It is time consuming and is of little use in the low risk pregnancy.

Cardiotocography or non-stress test

What it is: The fetal heart is recorded electronically for up to an hour (this can be combined with ultrasound as a biophysical profile). Accelerations and variability >5 beats/minute should be present, decelerations absent and the rate in the range of 110–160 (Fig. 25.6).

Benefits: Antenatal abnormalities represent a late stage in fetal compromise and delivery is indicated. Computerized interpretation of variability is of benefit in 'buying time': delaying delivery of chronically compromised premature fetuses.

Limitations: CTGs alone are of no use as an antenatal screening test. Indeed, reliance on occasional CTGs as tests of well-being leads to increased perinatal mortality.

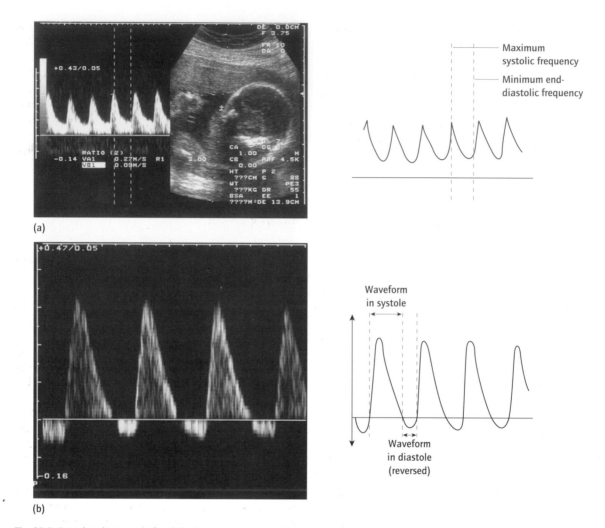

Fig. 25.5 Doppler ultrasound of umbilical artery: (a) normal; (b) reversed end-diastolic flow.

The best a normal antenatal CTG means is that, barring an acute event, the fetus will not die in the next 24 h. Therefore, to be useful in high-risk pregnancy it needs to be performed daily. CTG analysis is discussed on p. 239.

The small for dates fetus

Epidemiology

Small for dates (SFD) means small for the gestation. By definition, 10% of babies are below the tenth centile, 3% below the third, for that gestation. These centiles are used for the whole population, and therefore do not take account of genetic and ethnic differences. Because of the difficulties quantifying IUGR [→ p.203], its frequency is uncertain.

Aetiology

Fetal size and health is determined by a combination of factors that are genetic or acquired.

Constitutional determinants affect growth and birth weight without causing IUGR. Low maternal height and weight, nulliparity, Asian (as opposed to Caucasian or Afro-Carribean) ethnic group and female fetal gender are all associated with smaller babies.

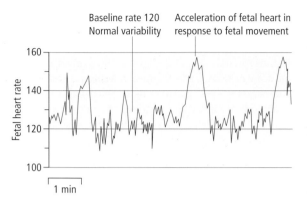

Baseline rate 120
Normal variability

Acceleration of fetal heart in
response to fetal movement

Fig. 25.6 Normal antenatal cardiotocograph (CTG).

Pathological determinants of fetal growth include preexisting maternal disease (e.g. renal disease and autoimmune disease), maternal pregnancy complications (e.g. pre-eclampsia) [→p. 165], multiple pregnancy, smoking, drug usage, infection such as cytomegaolovirus (CMV) [→ p. 158], extreme malnutrition and congenital (including chromosomal) abnormalities. These may cause IUGR. In addition, maternal obesity and male gender are associated with an increased risk of adverse outcomes.

Complications

If adjustment is made for constitutional determinants, about half of all so-called 'unclassified' stillbirths weigh less than tenth centile (www.gestation.net); the risk of cerebral palsy is also increased. Preterm delivery, both iatrogenic and spontaneous is more common. Maternal risks are greater because pre-eclampsia may coexist and because Caesarean delivery is often used.

Diagnosis

History: The SFD fetus may move less. This is not a reliable feature of IUGR because a compromised fetus stops moving only when it is very unwell, and because most events of reduced movements are transient, insignificant and in well babies.

Examination: Serial measurement of the symphisis fundal height [→ p. 136] may be reduced or slow down. The blood pressure and urine must be checked as pre-eclampsia commonly coexists with IUGR.

Investigations: The diagnosis of SFD is made using *ultrasound*. Occasionally, congenital malformations will be apparent. To tell which SFD fetuses are actually IUGR, serial ultrasound and particularly *umbilical artery Doppler* are used. The amniotic fluid volume is often reduced (oligohydramnios), with fetal redistribution of blood flow apparent in the middle cerebral artery, as 'head sparing'. In occasional cases, testing for infection (e.g. CMV), or for chromosomal abnormalities with fetal blood sampling or *amniocentesis*, is used. *Cardiotocography* is also used but will become abnormal usually only when severe compromise or 'fetal distress' is present.

Management

SFD only: Growth is rechecked at fortnightly intervals. The small but consistently growing fetus with normal umbilical artery Doppler values does not need intervention.

Fetal compromise at term: Small for dates with abnormal Doppler values is delivered if beyond 36 weeks. Labour induction or Caesarean section are required.

Fetal compromise preterm: The aim is to prevent *in utero* demise or neurological damage associated with ongoing placental dysfunction, whilst maximizing the gestation to avoid complications of prematurity. The threshold for intervention therefore varies with gestation; further, criteria for intervention are debated. In general, the IUGR fetus with abnormal Doppler values is reviewed at least twice a week; if absent end-diastolic flow is seen the mother is admitted for steroids (if pre-34 weeks) and daily CTG. At severely preterm gestations, delivery is delayed until this, or the CTG becomes abnormal; beyond 34 weeks, delivery is often undertaken anyway. Bedrest does not increase fetal growth, but admission or even delivery may be needed for other indications, particularly severe pre-eclampsia. The severely IUGR fetus is usually delivered by Caesarean.

Small for dates (SFD) and intrauterine growth restriction (IUGR)

'*Small for dates*' means the fetus's weight or estimated weight is below the tenth/fifth/third centile

Intrauterine growth restriction implies compromise: growth has slowed or is less than is expected taking account of constitutional factors

The prolonged pregnancy

Epidemiology and aetiology

A pregnancy is prolonged if ≥42 weeks' gestation are completed. However, the risk of perinatal mortality and morbidity starts increasing between 41 and 42 weeks. Approximately 10% of pregnancies reach 42 weeks, although with accurate early pregnancy dating with ultrasound the figure is nearer 6%. The aetiology of prolonged pregnancy is not understood, but it is more common if previous pregnancies have been prolonged and in nulliparous women, and is rarer in South Asian and black women.

Risks

The rate of stillbirth per 1000 continuing pregnancies rises from 0.35 at 37 weeks to 2.12 at 43 weeks (*BJOG* 1999; **105**: 169). Neonatal illness and encephalopathy, meconium passage and a clinical diagnosis of fetal distress are more common. The risks are greater in women of South Asian origin (*BMJ* 2007; **334**: 833). The absolute risk of a problem nevertheless remains small.

Management

The problem is that induction of labour, particularly in nulliparous patients, may fail to establish labour and lead to Caesarean section. However, prolonged pregnancy increases the chances of fetal distress when labour does start: this also leads to an increased chance of a Caesarean section. The aim is to balance the risks of obstetric intervention against those of prolonged pregnancy.

By 41–42 weeks, this balance is in favour of induction of labour. This prevents one fetal death for every 500 women induced, and is associated with a *lower* Caesarean rate than waiting (*Cochrane* 2006: CD004945).

Induction before 41 weeks does not have this effect, and is probably associated with increased intervention. It is therefore usual to induce labour at or after 41 weeks, but in appropriately counselled women who prefer not to be induced, or in nulliparous women with a very unfavourable cervix [→ p.251], surveillance with daily CTG is an acceptable alternative. 'Sweeping' the cervix (usually at 40–41 weeks) helps spontaneous labour start earlier (*Cochrane* 2001: CD000451).

Management of the prolonged pregnancy	
Check the gestation carefully; counsel patient appropriately If correct, induction before 41 weeks is inappropriate unless complications are present	
At 41 weeks:	Examine the patient vaginally and induce *unless* cervix very unfavourable (not ripe), *or* patient prefers to wait
If no induction:	Sweep cervix and arrange daily cardiotocography (CTG)
If CTG abnormal:	Deliver whatever the condition of the cervix, consider Caesarean

Further reading

Alberry M, Soothill P. Management of fetal growth restriction. *Archives of Disease in Childhood. Fetal and Neonatal Edition* 2007; **92**: F62–7.

Baschat AA. Pathophysiology of fetal growth restriction: implications for diagnosis and surveillance. *Obstetrical and Gynecological Survey* 2004; **59**: 617–27.

Gulmezoglu AM, Crowther CA, Middleton P. Induction of labour for improving birth outcomes for women at or beyond term. *Cochrane Database of Systematic Reviews* 2006; **4**: CD004945.

http://www.gestation.net

Stanley F, Blair E, Alberman E. *Cerebral Palsies: Epidemiology and Causal Pathways*. Cambridge: Cambridge University Press, 2000.

Fetal Surveillance at a Glance

Screening for the high-risk pregnancy	Maternal, past obstetric and pregnancy history for risk factors
	Uterine artery Doppler at 23 weeks to identify some high-risk pregnancies
	Maternal blood tests abnormal (e.g. pregnancy-associated plasma protein A [PAPP-A], alpha fetoprotein [AFP], human chorionic gonadotrophin [hCG]): high risk if in absence of an anomaly
	Integration of above 3 likely to prove best in future
	Antenatal care including symphysis–fundal height measurements: refer for ultrasound if less than expected, and repeat at 2-week intervals if fetus small for dates (SFD)
	'One-off' ultrasound, umbilical artery Doppler or cardiotocography (CTG) poor as screening
Methods of surveillance in the high-risk pregnancy	Fortnightly (max.) ultrasound to establish consistent growth
	Umbilical artery Doppler to identify the compromised fetus, if SFD
	CTG on a daily basis in preterm compromised fetus, or to establish that fetus healthy at time of test
	Methods specific to disorder, e.g. blood pressure in pre-eclampsia

Small for Dates and Intrauterine Growth Restriction at a Glance

Definition	Small for dates:	Smaller than the tenth centile for the gestation
	IUGR:	Small compared to genetic determination, and compromised
Aetiology		Predominantly physiological determinants of size are race, parity, fetal gender, maternal size
		Pathological determinants of fetal growth are maternal illness, e.g. renal disease, pre-eclampsia; also multiple pregnancy, chromosomal abnormalities, infections, smoking
Clinical features		Low symphisis–fundal height, reduced fetal movements
Investigations		Ultrasound of fetal size, liquor volume
		Doppler ultrasound of umbilical artery ± fetal Doppler
		Cardiotocography (CTG)
		Occasionally, amniocentesis for karyotype or fetal infection
Management	Small for dates:	Monitor growth. No intervention if consistent and umbilical artery Doppler normal
	IUGR:	At term, deliver
	34–37 weeks:	Regular umbilical Doppler; daily CTG; consider delivery
	<34 weeks:	Give steroids. As for 34–37 weeks but deliver usually only if abnormal CTG

Abnormal lie and breech presentation

Abnormal (transverse and oblique) lie

Definitions and epidemiology

The lie of the fetus describes the relationship of the fetus to the long axis of the uterus: if it is lying longitudinally within the uterus, the lie is longitudinal (Fig. 26.1a) and the *presentation* will be cephalic (head) or breech: either will be palpable at the pelvic inlet. If neither is present, the fetus must be lying across the uterus, with the head in one iliac fossa (oblique lie) or in the flank (transverse lie; Fig. 26.1b). Abnormal lie occurs at 1 in 200 births, but is more common earlier in the pregnancy: before term, it is normal.

Aetiology

Preterm labour is more commonly complicated by an abnormal lie than labour at full term. *Circumstances that allow more room to turn*, e.g. polyhydramnios [→ p.157] or high parity (more lax uterus), are the most common causes, frequently resulting in an 'unstable' or continually changing lie. *Conditions that prevent turning*, e.g. fetal and uterine abnormalities and twin pregnancies, may also cause persistent transverse lie, as may *conditions that prevent engagement*, e.g. placenta praevia and pelvic tumours or uterine deformities (Fig. 26.2).Unstable lie in nulliparous women is rare.

Complications

If the head or breech cannot enter the pelvis, labour cannot deliver the fetus. An arm or the umbilical cord

Obstetrics and Gynaecology, 3rd edition. By Lawrence Impey and Tim Child. Published 2008 by Blackwell Publishing, ISBN: 978-1-4051-6095-7.

(Fig. 26.3) may prolapse when the membranes rupture, and if neglected the obstruction eventually causes uterine rupture. Both fetus and mother are therefore at risk.

Management

No action is required for transverse or unstable lie before 37 weeks unless the woman is in labour. After 37 weeks, the woman is usually admitted to hospital in case the membranes rupture and an ultrasound scan performed to exclude particular identifiable causes, notably polyhydramnios and placenta praevia. External cephalic version (ECV [→ p.213]) is unjustified because the fetus usually turns back. Only if spontaneous version occurs and persists for more than 48 h is the mother discharged. In the absence of pelvic obstruction, an abnormal lie will usually stabilize before 41 weeks. At this stage, or if the woman is in labour, the persistently abnormal lie is delivered by Caesarean, but in expert hands ECV and then amniotomy (stabilizing induction) is an alternative.

Breech presentation

Definitions and epidemiology

The presentation refers to the part of the fetus that occupies the lower segment of the uterus or the pelvis. Presentation of the buttocks is breech presentation (Fig. 26.4). It occurs in 3% of term pregnancies, but, like the abnormal lie, is common earlier in the pregnancy and is therefore more common (25%) if labour occurs prematurely. The extended breech (70%) has both legs extended at the knee. The flexed breech (15%) has both legs flexed at the knee. In the footling breech (15%, more common if preterm) one or both feet present below the buttocks.

Aetiology

No cause is found with most. A previous breech presentation has occurred in 8%. *Prematurity* is commonly associated with breech presentation. Conditions that prevent movement, such as *fetal* and *uterine abnormalities* or *twin pregnancies*, or that prevent engagement of the head, such as *placenta praevia*, *pelvic tumours* and *pelvic deformities* are more common (Fig. 26.2).

Diagnosis

Breech presentation is commonly (30%) missed, but diagnosis is only important from 37 weeks or if the patient is in labour. Upper abdominal discomfort is common: the hard head is normally palpable and ballottable at the fundus. Ultrasound confirms the diagnosis, helps detection of a fetal abnormality, pelvic tumour or a placenta praevia and ensures the prerequisites for ECV are met.

Complications

Perinatal and long-term morbidity and mortality are increased. Fetal abnormalities are more common, but even 'normal' breech babies have higher rates of long-term neurological handicap (*BMJ* 1996; **312**: 1451), which is independent of the mode of delivery. In addition, labour has potential hazards. The relatively poor 'fit' of the breech or feet leads to an increased rate of cord prolapse [→ p.262]. The after-coming head may get trapped: in cephalic presentations a head that is too big or extended [→ p.226] will cause a cessation of progress in labour that is easily managed by Caesarean section, but with a breech only after the body has been delivered will the problem be evident. At this stage, a baby with a trapped head will rapidly die.

Management

External cephalic version

After 37 weeks, an attempt is made to turn the baby to a cephalic presentation (Fig. 26.5). The advantage is a reduction in breech presentation at term and therefore

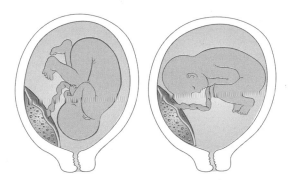

Fig. 26.1 (a) Longitudinal lie. (b) Transverse lie.

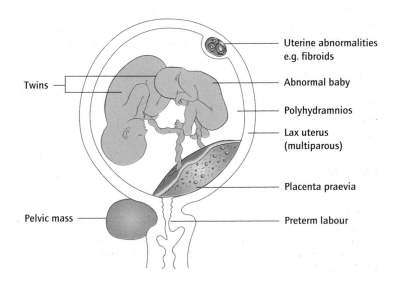

Twins

Pelvic mass

Uterine abnormalities e.g. fibroids

Abnormal baby

Polyhydramnios

Lax uterus (multiparous)

Placenta praevia

Preterm labour

Fig. 26.2 Causes of transverse lie and breech presentation.

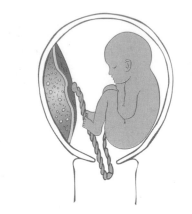

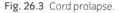

Fig. 26.3 Cord prolapse.

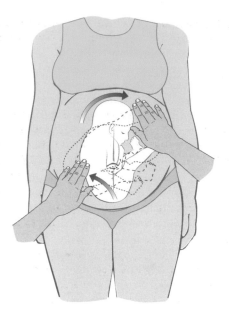

Fig. 26.5 External cephalic version (ECV).

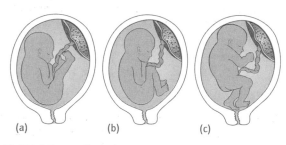

(a)   (b)   (c)

Fig. 26.4 Types of breech presentation. (a) Extended. (b) Flexed. (c) Footling.

attempted. This is performed under ultrasound guidance and in hospital to allow immediate delivery if complications occur. Cardiotocography (CTG) is performed straight after and anti-D is given to rhesus negative women [→ p.187]. The usage of moxabustion as an alternative to ECV is probably ineffective (*Cochrane* 2005: CD003928).

Safety of ECV: The risk of fetal damage is minimal, provided care is taken, although placental abruption and uterine rupture have been reported; the risk of an emergency Caesarean section being required after the procedure is 0.5% (*BJOG* 2007; **114**: 636).

Factors affecting success of ECV: lower success rates are seen in nulliparous women, in Caucasians, where the breech is engaged, where the head not easily palpable or uterine tone is high (*BJOG* 1997; **104**: 798), with obese women and if the liquor volume is reduced. Fetal size makes little difference.

Contraindications to ECV: ECV is not performed if the fetus is compromised [→ p.203], if vaginal delivery would be contraindicated anyway (e.g. placenta praevia), if there are twins, if the membranes are ruptured or if

Caesarean or vaginal breech delivery (*Cochrane* 2000: CD000184). External cephalic version before 37 weeks does not have this effect and is not currently advised, although ECV at 34 weeks in more difficult cases is undergoing evaluation. The success rate is about 50%; approximately 3% of successfully turned breeches will turn back.

Technique: ECV is done without anaesthetic, but is made easier and more successful by administering a uterine relaxant (tocolytic) to the mother (*Cochrane* 2002: CD000184) if uterine tone is high or if an initial attempt has failed. With both hands on the abdomen, the breech is disengaged from the pelvis, pushed upwards and to the side, and rotation in the form of a forward somersault is

there has been recent antepartum haemorrhage. One previous Caesarean section is not a contraindication.

Caesarean section

If ECV has failed or is contraindicated, or the breech presentation was missed, the safest method of delivery for the singleton term breech is by Caesarean section (*Cochrane* 2003: CD000166). This reduces neonatal mortality and short-term morbidity, although does not affect long-term outcomes (*AmJOG* 2004; **191**: 864). The beneficial effect of Caesarean section remains even with experienced operators and is greater in 'developed' countries. Maternal morbidity is not increased by this policy: indeed, more than one-third of attempts at vaginal breech delivery end in emergency Caesarean section, which carries even greater maternal risks than an elective procedure. Parents should be counselled as to these findings, although the final decision rests with them. Most in the West undergo Caesarean section.

Some women, however, still wish to deliver vaginally; further, breech presentation is often diagnosed only in late labour and second twins often present as breech. Under such circumstances, vaginal breech delivery may still be appropriate, yet skills are being lost due to lack of experience. Knowledge of the technique of vaginal breech delivery remains essential for any obstetrician and is therefore described.

Vaginal breech birth

Patient selection: Vaginal breech birth is probably yet more risky with a fetus >4.0 kg, with evidence of fetal compromise, an extended head or footling legs.

Intrapartum care: In about 30%, there is slow cervical dilatation in the first stage or, particularly, poor descent in the second. Under these circumstances augmentation with oxytocin is unwise and Caesarean section is performed. Pushing is not encouraged until the buttocks are visible. Cardiotocography is advised. Epidural analgesia is common but not mandatory.

Breech delivery (Fig. 26.6): Most breech babies deliver easily: it is the perhaps in 10% where real skill is required. A difficult delivery is often the result of injudicious traction causing extension of the head. Once the buttocks distend the perineum, an episiotomy [→ p.245] is made. The fetus delivers with maternal effort as far as the umbilicus, and should not be touched. The legs can be flexed out of the vagina, whilst the back is kept anterior. Once

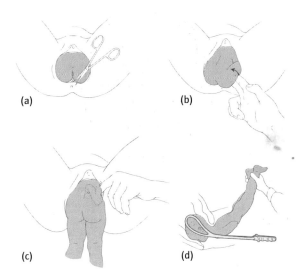

Fig. 26.6 Breech delivery. (a) As buttocks distend the perineum, perform the episiotomy. (b) A finger behind the knee delivers the legs. (c) A finger hooks each arm down. (d) Forceps deliver the head once the arms are delivered.

the scapula is visible, the anterior and then the posterior arms are 'hooked' down by a finger over the shoulder sweeping it across the chest. If the arms cannot be reached because they are extended above the neck, then *Lovset's procedure* is required. This involves placing the hands around the body with the thumbs on the sacrum and rotating the baby 180° clockwise and then counter-clockwise with gentle downward traction. This allows the anterior shoulder and then the posterior shoulder to enter the pelvis. Once the back of the neck is visible, the operator supports the entire weight of the fetus on one palm and forearm, with his or her finger in its mouth to guide the head over the perineum and maintain flexion. With the same intent, his or her other hand presses against the occiput. This is the *Mauriceau–Smellie–Veit manoeuvre*. If this fails to deliver the head, an assistant holds the legs up whilst forceps are applied, and with the next contraction the head is lifted slowly out of the vagina.

It is maintained by advocates of vaginal breech birth that an upright position for birth is most effective. Whilst this may be so, it has not yet been subjected to scientific scrutiny.

Further reading

Hannah ME, Hannah WJ, Hewson SA, *et al.* for the Term Breech Trial Collaborative Group. Planned Caesarean section versus planned vaginal birth for breech presentation at term: a randomised multicentre trial. *Lancet* 2000; **356**: 1375–83.

Royal College of Obstetricians and Gynaecologists. External cephalic version and reducing the incidence of breech presentation. Green Top Guideline 2006. http://www.rcog.org.uk/index.asp?PageID=1811

Royal College of Obstetricians and Gynaecologists. The management of breech presentation. Green Top Guideline 2006. http://www.rcog.org.uk/index.asp?PageID=1812

Transverse/Oblique Lie at a Glance

Definition	Lie of fetus not parallel to long axis of uterus
Epidemiology	1 in 200 births
Aetiology	Preterm labour, polyhydramnios, multiparity, placenta praevia, pelvic mass, fetal or uterine abnormality, twins
Management	Admit if >37 weeks. Ultrasound to find cause If not stabilized by 41 weeks, or if pelvis obstructed, elective Caesarean

Breech Presentation at a Glance

Types	Extended (70%), flexed (15%), footling (15%)
Epidemiology	3% at term, more if preterm labour or previous breech presentation
Aetiology	Idiopathic, uterine/fetal anomalies, placenta praevia, pelvic mass, twins More common preterm

Complications	Increased perinatal mortality and morbidity due to:
	    Unknown but unrelated to vaginal delivery
	    Congenital anomalies
	    Intrapartum problems

Management	External cephalic version (ECV) after 37 weeks, 50% success. Not if antepartum haemorrhage, ruptured membranes, fetal compromise, twins Elective Caesarean section safest

27 Multiple pregnancy

Epidemiology

Twins occur in 1 in 80 pregnancies, triplets in 1 in 1000. There is considerable geographic variation. The incidence of twins is increasing because of subfertility treatment [→ p.85] and the increasing number of older mothers, although in the UK triplets and higher order multiples have become fewer again with better fertility treatment regulation.

Types of multiple pregnancy

Dizygotic (DZ) twins (two-thirds of all multiple pregnancies) or triplets result from fertilization of different oocytes by different sperm (Fig. 27.1). Such fetuses may be of different sex and are no more genetically similar than siblings from different pregnancies.

Monozygotic (MZ) twins result from mitotic division of a single zygote into 'identical' twins. Whether they share the same amnion or placenta depends on the time at which division into separate zygotes occurred (Fig. 27.1). Division before day 3 (approx. 30%) leads to twins with separate placentas and amnions (dichorionic diamniotic [DCDA]). Division between days 4 and 8 (approx. 70%) leads to twins with a shared placenta but separate amnions (monochorionic diamniotic [MCDA]). Later division (9–13 days) is very rare and causes twins with a shared placenta and a single amniotic sac (monochorionic monoamniotic [MCMA]). Incomplete division leads to conjoined twins. Monochorionic (MC) twins have a higher fetal loss rate, particularly before 24 weeks.

Aetiology

Assisted conception, genetic factors and increasing

maternal age and parity are the most important factors, largely affecting DZ twinning. About 20% of all *in vitro* fertilization (IVF) [→ p.90] conceptions and 5–10% of clomiphene-assisted conceptions are multiple. Embryo transfer of more than two fertilized ova at IVF is now performed in the UK only under exceptional circumstances.

Diagnosis

Vomiting may be more marked in early pregnancy. The uterus is larger than expected from the dates and palpable before 12 weeks. Later in pregnancy, three or more fetal poles may be felt. Many are diagnosed only at ultrasound (Fig. 27.2): as this is now performed in most pregnancies, the diagnosis is seldom missed.

Antepartum complications

The perinatal mortality and long-term handicap rate of multiple pregnancies is greatly increased. Triplets fare even worse. The major risk factors are preterm delivery, intrauterine growth restriction (IUGR) and monochorionicity (see below).

Maternal: *Gestational diabetes* and *pre-eclampsia* particularly are more frequent. *Anaemia* is common, partly because of a greater increase in blood volume causing a dilutional effect and partly because more iron and folic acid are needed.

All multiples: Virtually all obstetric risks are exaggerated in multiple pregnancies (Fig. 27.3).

Congenital abnormalities, particularly cardiac ones, are more common in MC twins.

Miscarriage: One of a twin or more of a higher multiple pregnancy can 'vanish', where there is first trimester death. Late miscarriage is also more common.

Preterm labour is the main cause of perinatal mortality: 40% of twin and 80% of triplet pregnancies deliver before 37 weeks; 10% of twins deliver before 32 weeks. Multiples usually but not invariably grow at the same

Obstetrics and Gynaecology, 3rd edition. By Lawrence Impey and Tim Child. Published 2008 by Blackwell Publishing, ISBN: 978-1-4051-6095-7.

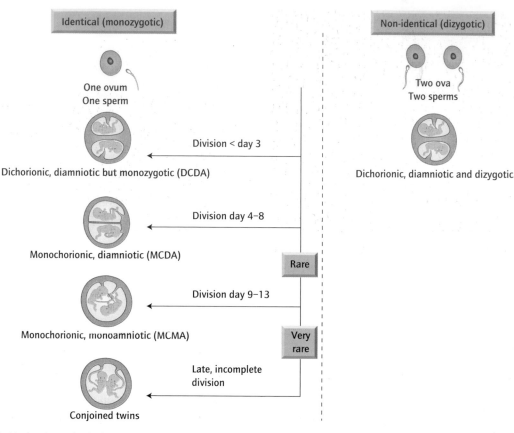

Fig. 27.1 Mechanisms of twinning.

rate as singletons until about 28 weeks, but thereafter slower growth is common (Fig. 27.4) and may be discordant, usually as a result of placental insufficiency. *IUGR* is therefore common.

Monochorionic twin complications including twin–twin transfusion syndrome (TTTS) (Fig. 27.5): In MCDA twins, the most common form of identical twins, the circulation is shared via a single placenta. TTTS occurs in about 15% of these and results from unequal blood distribution through vascular anastomoses of the shared placenta. One twin, the 'donor', is volume depleted and develops anaemia, IUGR and oligohydramnios. The other or 'recipient' twin gets volume overloaded and may develop polycythaemia, cardiac failure and polyhydramnios. This causes massive distension of the uterus. Disease is staged according to Quintero in stages 1–5

(*J Perinatal* 1999; **19**: 550). Both twins are at very high risk of *in utero* death, late miscarriage or severely preterm delivery. Even with optimal treatment, survival of both twins occurs in only 60%, with one twin in 85% and up to 20% of survivors having neurological disability (*NEJM* 2004; **35**: 136).

If one of an MC twin pair dies, either due to TTTS or any other cause, the drop in its blood pressure allows acute transfusion of blood from the other one: this rapidly leads to hypovolaemia and, in about 30% of cases, death or neurological damage.

Intrapartum complications

Malpresentation of the first twin occurs in 20% (Fig. 27.6): this is an indication for Caesarean section.

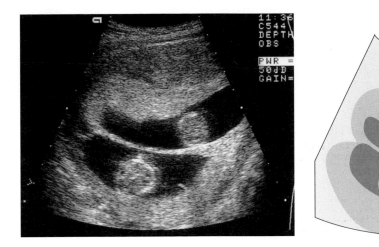

Fig. 27.2 Ultrasound showing dichorionic twins in early pregnancy.

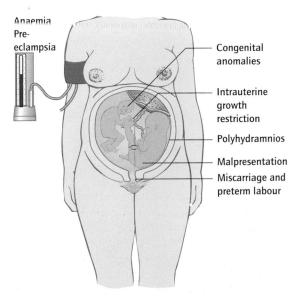

Fig. 27.3 Complications of twin pregnancies.

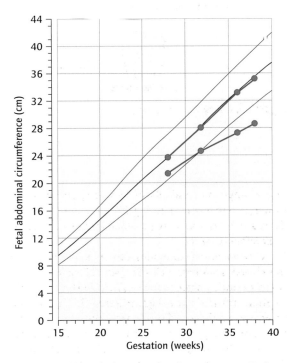

Fig. 27.4 Fetal growth chart showing discordant growth of twins.

Fetal distress [→ p.203] in labour is more common. The *second twin* is particularly vulnerable after the first has been delivered because of an increased risk of hypoxia, cord prolapse, tetanic uterine contraction or placental abruption, and may present as a breech. *Postpartum haemorrhage* is more common (10%).

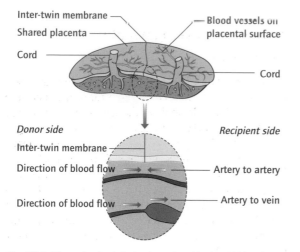

Fig. 27.5 Monochorionic twin placenta with shared blood vessels.

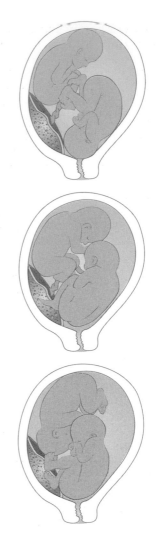

Fig. 27.6 Presentation of twins.

Complications of twin pregnancies

Perinatal mortality increased fourfold
Preterm labour and miscarriage
Congenital abnormalities
Placental insufficiency/intrauterine growth restriction (IUGR)
Twin–twin transfusion syndrome (monochorionic [MC] twins only)
Antepartum and postpartum haemorrhage
Pre-eclampsia, diabetes, anaemia
Malpresentation

Outcomes of multiple pregnancies

Type	8–24 week loss 1+ baby*	Perinatal mortality (per baby)*	Cerebral palsy (per baby)*
DC twins	2.5%	3–5%	1%
MCDA twins	15%	5–12%	2–5%
Triplets	5–15%	10%	2–3%

DC, dichorionic; MCDA, monochorionic diamniotic.
* Approximate figures.

Antepartum management

All multiples

General: The pregnancy should be considered 'high risk': care should be consultant-led, although not every visit need be in the hospital. Iron and folic acid supplements are prescribed. Multiple pregnancies increase maternal tiredness and anxiety, and may result in financial problems. Postnatal home help should be discussed.

Early ultrasound: Screening for chromosomal abnormalities is offered using nuchal translucency scanning [→ p.149]; anomalies are sought at the 20-week scan as normal. Chorionicity is most accurately ascertained in the first trimester: the dividing membrane is thin and forms a 'T' as it meets the single placenta in perpendicular fashion. If the uterus is palpable abdominally before 12 weeks, early ultrasound scan is advised. Twins of opposite gender are always DZ.

Selective reduction to a twin pregnancy at 12 weeks should be discussed with women with triplets or higher order pregnancies. Whilst this slightly increases early miscarriage rates, it reduces the chances of preterm birth and therefore cerebral palsy (*Hum Reprod* 2006; **21**: 1912). Reduction of a twin to a singleton is not advised.

Identification of risk of preterm delivery: Transvaginal ultrasound of cervical length may identify those at most risk [→ p.192]. A policy of inserting cervical sutures in all women with a short cervix is not currently advised but is probably appropriate if the cervix is very short, very early.

Identification of IUGR: As this is both more common and more difficult to detect in multiple pregnancies compared with singleton pregnancies, serial ultrasound examinations for growth are usually routinely performed at 28, 32 and 36 weeks.

Monochorionic twins

Ultrasound surveillance of MC twin pregnancies starts by 12 weeks. TTTS is most commonly diagnosed between 18 and 22 weeks, either by careful ultrasound surveillance or because polyhydramnios around the recipient causes massive abdominal distension. Except where disease is very mild, laser photocoagulation of the placental anastomoses in a fetal medicine centre is the preferred treatment, resulting in a lower rate of neonatal handicap (*AmJOG* 1999; **180**: 717) than the traditional treatment of amnioreduction. Monochorionic twins are also at higher risk of IUGR and *in utero* death, and usually are scanned every 2 weeks.

Fetal abnormality

Where one twin has an abnormality selective termination should be discussed. In DC twins this can be by intracardiac injection of KCl; in monochorionic the cord must be occluded (*BJOG* 2005; **112**: 1344) because the circulation is shared and death or damage to the remaining twin may follow. Both, particularly cord occlusion, risk miscarriage: the risk of this is lowest early in the pregnancy. Where late (>24 weeks' gestation) termination of pregnancy is legal, as in the UK, it can be performed at about 34 weeks so that if delivery ensues the remaining twin will survive.

Intrapartum management

Mode of delivery

Caesarean section is increasingly used for all, even uncomplicated twins. This is because of the increased risk of death and hypoxia in the second twin compared to the first (*BMJ* 2007; **334**: 576), and a trial is ongoing to determine if elective Caesarean section is safer. Caesarean section is certainly indicated if the first fetus is a breech or a transverse lie, with triplets, if there have been antepartum complications and, in some hospitals, with all monochorionic twins. Vaginal delivery when the first fetus is cephalic, whatever the lie or presentation of the second (Fig. 27.6), remains commonplace and is therefore discussed.

Method of delivery

Induction, or Caesarean, is usual at 38 weeks (DC twins) or 36–37 weeks (MC twins), after which time perinatal mortality is increased. Cardiotocography (CTG) [→ p.239] is advised as the risk of intrapartum hypoxia is increased, particularly for the second twin. Epidural analgesia is helpful as difficulty is occasionally encountered with delivery of the second twin. The first twin is delivered in the normal manner.

Good communication with, and a comfortable position for the mother are essential. CTG must continue. Contractions often diminish after the first twin. Usually contractions return within a few minutes; oxytocin can be started if not. The lie of the second twin is checked and external cephalic version (ECV) is performed if it is not longitudinal. Once the head or breech enters the pelvis, the membranes are ruptured and pushing again begins. Delivery is usually easy whether cephalic or breech [→ p.215] and achieved within 20 minutes of the first fetus. Excessive delay is associated with increased morbidity for the second twin, but excessive haste is equally dangerous. If the head does not descend, a malpresentation (particularly a brow) is likely and Caesarean section is very occasionally required. If fetal distress or cord prolapse occur, vaginal delivery can be expedited with a ventouse [→ p.256] or breech extraction. The latter must be performed under general, epidural or spinal anaesthesia, and only by experienced personnel. It involves inserting a hand into the uterus, grasping the feet and guiding them down. After delivery, a prophylactic oxytocin infusion is used to prevent postpartum haemorrhage.

Further reading

Gerris JM. Single embryo transfer and IVF/ICSI outcome: a balanced appraisal. *Human Reproduction Update* 2005; **11**: 105–21.

Harkness UF, Crombleholme TM. Twin twin transfusion syndrome: where do we go from here? *Seminars in Perinatology* 2005; **29**: 296–304.

Ong SS, Zamora J, Khan KS, Kilby MD. Prognosis for the co-twin following single-twin death: a systematic review. *BJOG: an International Journal of Obstetrics and Gynaecology* 2006; **113**: 992–8.

Taylor MJ. The management of multiple pregnancy. *Early Human Development* 2006; **82**: 365–70.

Multiple Pregnancy at a Glance

Incidence	Twins 1.3%, triplets 0.1%; incidence of twins increasing because of fertility treatment and older mothers	
Terms	Dizygotic (DZ):	Different oocytes fertilized by different sperm
	Monozygotic (MZ):	Division of zygote after fertilization
	Dichorionic:	Two placentas
	Monochorionic (MC):	Shared placenta
Twin types	DC: (approx 70%)	Can be identical (MZ) or not (DZ); do not share placenta or sac
	MCDA: (approx 30%)	Identical (MZ), share placenta (MC) but not amniotic sac (DA)
	MCMA: (approx 1%)	Identical (MZ), share placenta (MC) and amniotic sac (MA)
Aetiology	Ovulation induction, genetic factors, increasing age and parity	
Diagnosis	Usually at ultrasound scan. Vomiting, 'large for dates', 3+ fetal poles	
Complications	Maternal:	Pre-eclampsia, anaemia, gestational diabetes, operative delivery
	All twins:	Increased morbidity and mortality due to most obstetric complications partic.: miscarriage, preterm labour, placental insufficiency/intrauterine growth restriction (IUGR), antepartum and postpartum haemorrhage and malpresentations
	MC twins:	Congenital abnormalities, twin–twin transfusion (TTTS), IUGR even more common
Management	All twins:	Early diagnosis, identification of chorionicity. Consultant care. Iron and folic acid supplements. Anomaly scan Increased surveillance for pre-eclampsia, diabetes, anaemia Serial ultrasound at 28, 32 and 36 weeks
	MC twins:	Ultrasound fortnightly from 12 weeks for TTTS and IUGR. Laser treatment if TTTS
	Delivery:	38 weeks if DC; 36–37 weeks if MC
	Labour:	Caesarean section if first twin not cephalic and usual indications as for singletons. Cardiotocography. After first twin, lie of second twin checked: external cephalic version (ECV) to longitudinal lie if necessary. Amniotomy when presenting part engaged, then maternal pushing. Ventouse or breech extraction if fetal distress

Twin–Twin Transfusion Syndrome (TTTS) at a Glance

Incidence	15% of all MC twins
Pathology	Unequal blood distribution in shared placenta leading to discordant blood volumes, liquor and often growth
Diagnosis	Discordant liquor volumes. Recipient twin larger, polyhydramnios, fluid overload, heart failure Donor twin smaller, 'stuck' with oligohydramnios
Complications	Late miscarriage and severe preterm delivery, *in utero* death, neurological damage
Management	Ultrasound surveillance from 12 weeks. Laser therapy if TTTS diagnosed
Prognosis	Very poor untreated. With laser, approx. 60% both twins survive; 85% one twin survives

28 Labour 1: Mechanism—anatomy and physiology

Labour is the process whereby the fetus and placenta are expelled from the uterus, which normally occurs between 37 and 42 weeks' gestation. The diagnosis is made *when painful uterine contractions accompany dilatation and effacement of the cervix*. It is divided into stages. In the *first stage*, the cervix opens to 'full dilatation' to allow the head to pass through. The *second stage* is from full dilatation to delivery of the fetus. The *third stage* lasts from delivery of the fetus to delivery of the placenta.

Labour	
Diagnosis:	Painful contractions lead to dilatation of the cervix
First stage:	Initiation to full cervical dilatation
Second stage:	Full cervical dilatation to delivery of fetus
Third stage:	Delivery of fetus to delivery of placenta

Mechanical factors of labour

Three mechanical factors determine progress during labour:
1 The degree of force expelling the fetus (the powers).
2 The dimensions of the pelvis and the resistance of soft tissues (the passage).
3 The diameters of the fetal head (the passenger).

The powers (Fig. 28.1)

Once labour is established, the uterus contracts for 45–60 s about every 2–3 minutes. This pulls the cervix up (effacement) and causes dilatation, aided by the pressure of the head as the uterus pushes the head down into the

Obstetrics and Gynaecology, 3rd edition. By Lawrence Impey and Tim Child. Published 2008 by Blackwell Publishing, ISBN: 978-1-4051-6095-7.

pelvis. Poor uterine activity is a common feature of the nulliparous woman and in induced labour [→ p.251], but is rare in multiparous women.

The passage

The bony pelvis

This has three principal planes. At its *inlet*, the transverse diameter is about 13 cm, wider than the 11-cm antero-posterior (AP) diameter (Fig. 28.2). The *mid-cavity* is almost round as the transverse and AP diameters are similar. At the *outlet*, the AP diameter (12.5 cm) is greater than the transverse diameter (11 cm). In the lateral wall of the round mid-pelvis, bony prominences called *ischial spines* are palpable vaginally. These are used as landmarks by which to assess the descent of the head on vaginal examination: the level of descent is called 'station' and is crudely measured in centimetres in relation to these 'spines'. Station 0 means the head is at the level of these spines; station +2 means it is 2 cm below and station −2 means it is 2 cm above (Fig. 28.3). A variety of pelvic shapes have been described, but diagnosis and therefore description of these is seldom useful in clinical practice.

The soft tissues

Cervical dilatation is a prerequisite for delivery and is dependent on contractions, the pressure of the fetal head on the cervix and the ability of the cervix to soften and allow distension. The soft tissues of the vagina and perineum need to be overcome in the second stage: the perineum often tears or is cut (episiotomy) to allow the head to deliver.

The passenger

The head is oblong in transverse section. Its bones are not yet fused and, on vaginal examination, spaces

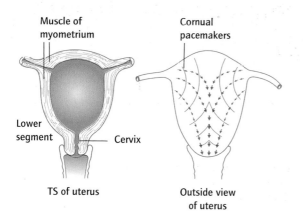

Fig. 28.1 The powers.

between them are palpable as sutures and fontanelles. The anterior fontanelle (bregma) lies above the forehead. The posterior fontanelle (occiput) lies on the back of the top of the head. Between these two is the area called the vertex. In front of the bregma is the brow (Fig. 28.4). Because the head is not round, several factors determine how easily it fits through the pelvic diameters.

Attitude

The attitude is the degree of flexion of the head on the neck (Fig. 28.5). The ideal attitude is maximal flexion, keeping the head bowed. This is called *vertex presentation*, and the presenting diameter is 9.5 cm, running from the anterior fontanelle to below the occiput at the back of the head. A small degree of extension results in a larger diameter. Extension of 90° causes a *brow*

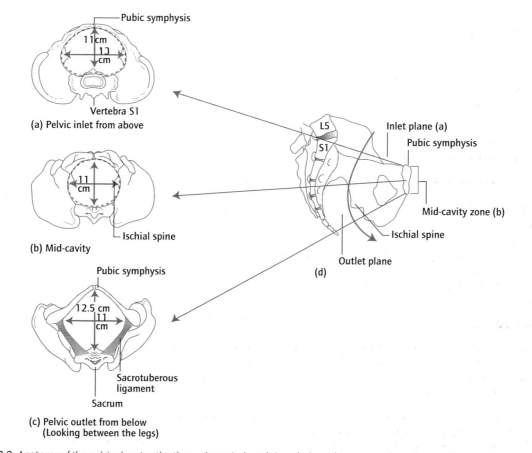

Fig. 28.2 Anatomy of the pelvis showing the three planes (a, b and c), and where they are on a lateral view of the pelvis (d).

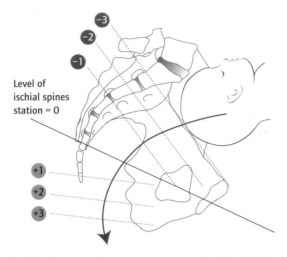

Level of
ischial spines
station = 0

Fig. 28.3 Descent of the head in labour in relation to the ischial spines.

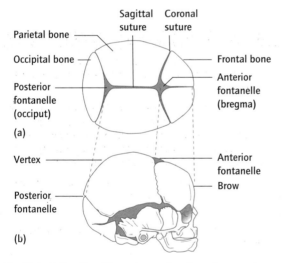

Parietal bone

Sagittal suture Coronal suture

Occipital bone

Frontal bone

Posterior fontanelle (occiput)

Anterior fontanelle (bregma)

(a)

Vertex

Anterior fontanelle

Posterior fontanelle

Brow

(b)

Fig. 28.4 (a) Fetal head from above, showing sutures and fontanelles. (b) Fetal head from the side.

presentation, and a much larger diameter of 13 cm. A further 30° of extension (with the face looking parallel and away from the body) is a *face presentation*. Extension of the head can mean that the fetal diameters are too large to deliver vaginally.

Attitude of the head

What is palpable

Well flexed (vertex)

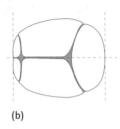

(a)

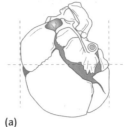

(b)

Deflexed

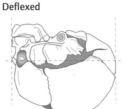

(a)

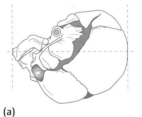

(b)

Extended (brow)

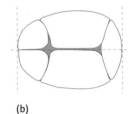

(a)

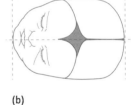

(b)

Hyperextended (face)

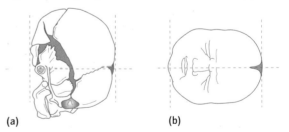

(a)

(b)

Fig. 28.5 Attitude of the fetal head showing how extension of the head changes the presenting diameter and what is palpable on vaginal examination.

Position

The position is the degree of rotation of the head on the neck (Fig. 28.6). If the sagittal suture is transverse, the oblong head will fit the pelvic inlet best. But at the outlet

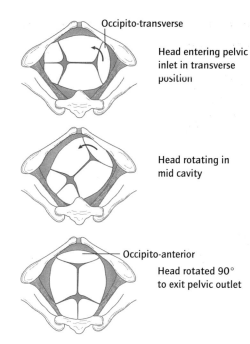

Occipito-transverse

Head entering pelvic inlet in transverse position

Head rotating in mid cavity

Occipito-anterior

Head rotated 90° to exit pelvic outlet

Fig. 28.6 View from below showing rotation of the head (position) according to the three planes of the pelvis.

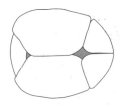

Fig. 28.7 Diagram of moulding showing compression and overlap of sutures.

larger head may cause a longer and more difficult labour.

the sagittal suture must be vertical for the head to fit. The head must therefore normally rotate 90° during labour. It is usually delivered with the *occiput anterior* (occipito-anterior [OA]). In 5% of deliveries it is occipito-posterior (OP) and more difficulty may be encountered. Persistence of the occipito-transverse (OT) position implies non-rotation and delivery without assistance is impossible.

Size of the head

The head can be compressed in the pelvis because the sutures allow the bones to come together and even overlap slightly. This slightly reduces the diameters of the head and is called *moulding* (Fig. 28.7). Pressure of the scalp on the cervix or pelvic inlet can cause localized swelling or *caput*. It is relatively unusual for a normally formed head to be simply too big to pass through the bony pelvis (cephalopelvic disproportion), although a

---

Terms describing the fetal head

Presentation is the part of the fetus that occupies the lower segment or pelvis: i.e. head (cephalic) or buttocks (breech)

Presenting part is the lowest part of the fetus palpable on vaginal examination: the lowest part of the head or breech. For a cephalic presentation, this can be the vertex, the brow or the face, depending on the attitude. For simplicity, these are often described as separate 'presentations'

Position of the head describes its rotation: occipito-transverse (OT), occipito-posterior (OP) or occipito-anterior (OA)

Attitude of the head describes the degree of flexion: vertex, brow or face

---

Movements of the head (Fig. 28.8)

Engagement in occipito-transverse (OT)
Descent and flexion
Rotation 90° to occipito-anterior (OA)
Descent
Extension to deliver
Restitution and delivery of shoulders

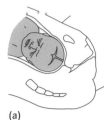

Engagement: The oblong-shaped head normally enters the pelvis in the occipito-transverse (OT) position, because the transverse diameter of the inlet is greater than the antero-posterior diameter.

(a)

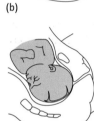

Descent and flexion: The head descends into the round mid-cavity and flexes as the cervix dilates. Descent is measured by comparison with the level of the ischial spines (see Fig. 28.3) and is called station.

(b)

Rotation: In the mid-cavity, the head rotates 90°(internal rotation) so that the face is facing the sacrum and the occiput is anterior, below the symphisis pubis (occipito-anterior, OA). This enables it to pass through the pelvic outlet which has a wider antero-posterior than transverse diameter. In 5% of cases, the head rotates to occipito-posterior (OP).

(c)

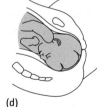

Rotation completed, further descent: The perineum distends.

(d)

Extension and delivery.

(e)

Restitution: The head then rotates 90° (external rotation) to the same position in which it entered the inlet, facing either right or left, to enable delivery of the shoulders.

(f)

Cervical dilatation: the 'stages' of labour

Initiation and diagnosis of labour

Involuntary contractions of uterine smooth muscle occur throughout the third trimester and are often felt as Braxton Hicks contractions. How this leads to labour is not fully understood, but the fetus has a role, and prostaglandin production has a crucial role both in reducing cervical resistance and increasing release of the hormone oxytocin from the posterior pituitary gland. This aids stimulation of contractions, which arise in one of the pacemakers situated at each cornu of the uterus.

Painful regular contractions lead to effacement and dilatation of the cervix. Effacement is when the normally tubular cervix is drawn up into the lower segment until it is flat (Fig. 28.9). This is commonly accompanied by a 'show' or pink/white mucus plug from the cervix and/or rupture of the membranes, causing release of liquor.

The first stage

This lasts from the diagnosis of labour until the cervix is dilated by 10 cm (fully dilated). The descent, flexion and internal rotation described occur to varying degree. If the membranes have not already ruptured, they normally do so.
The latent phase is where the cervix usually dilates slowly for the first 3 cm and may take several hours.
The active phase follows: Average cervical dilatation is at the rate of 1 cm/h in nulliparous women and about 2 cm/h in multiparous women. The first stage should not normally last longer than 16 h.

The second stage

This lasts from full dilatation of the cervix to delivery. Descent, flexion and rotation are completed and followed by extension as the head delivers.
The passive stage lasts from full dilatation until the head reaches the pelvic floor and the woman experiences the desire to push. Rotation and flexion are commonly completed. This stage may last a few minutes, but can be much longer.

Fig. 28.8 (a–f) Movement of the head in labour.

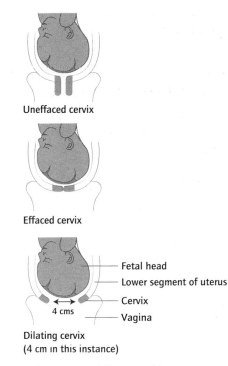

Uneffaced cervix

Effaced cervix

Fetal head
Lower segment of uterus
Cervix
4 cms
Vagina

Dilating cervix
(4 cm in this instance)

Fig. 28.9 Effacement and dilatation of the cervix.

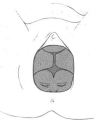

Fig. 28.10 Head delivery over the perineum by extension.

The active stage is when the mother is pushing. The pressure of the head on the pelvic floor produces an irresistible desire to bear down, although epidural analgesia may prevent this. The woman gets in the most comfortable position for her, but not supine, and pushes with contractions. The fetus is delivered, on average, after 40 minutes (nulliparous) or 20 minutes (multiparous). This stage can be much quicker, but if it takes >1 h spontaneous delivery becomes decreasingly likely.

Delivery

As the head reaches the perineum, it extends to come up out of the pelvis (Fig. 28.10). The perineum begins to stretch and often tears, but can be cut (episiotomy) usually only if progress is slow or fetal distress [→ p.237] is present. The head then restitutes, rotating 90° to adopt the transverse position in which it entered the pelvis. With the next contraction, the shoulders deliver: the anterior shoulder comes under the symphysis pubis first,

usually aided by lateral body flexion in a posterior direction; the posterior shoulder is aided by lateral body flexion in an anterior direction. The rest of the body follows.

The third stage

This is the time from delivery of the fetus to delivery of the placenta. It normally lasts about 15 minutes and normal blood loss is up to 500 mL. Uterine muscle fibres contract to compress the blood vessels formerly supplying the placenta, which shears away from the uterine wall.

Perineal trauma

The perineum is intact in about one-third of nulliparous women and in half of multiparous women. A *first degree tear* involves minor damage to the fourchette. *Second degree tears* and *episiotomies* involve perineal muscle. *Third degree tears* involve the anal sphincter also and occur in 1% of deliveries. They are subclassified according to the degree of damage [→ p.246]. *Fourth degree* tears also involve the anal mucosa.

Further reading

Bernal AL. Overview of current research in parturition. *Experimental Physiology* 2001; **86**: 213–22.

Jaffe RB. Role of the human fetal adrenal gland in the initiation of parturition. *Frontiers of Hormone Research* 2001; **27**: 75–85.

Mechanism of Normal Labour at a Glance

When	37–42 weeks
Diagnosis	Contractions with effacement and dilatation of the cervix
First stage	Average duration 10 h, nulliparous; 6 h, multiparous Uterus contracts every 2–3 min Latent (<3 cm) and active (4–10 cm) phases Cervix dilates until the widest diameter of head passes through Head descends remaining flexed to maintain the smallest diameter (Variable descent occurs before labour: 'engagement') 90° rotation from occipito-transverse (OT) to occipito-anterior (OA) (or occipito-posterior [OP]) begins Amniotic membranes usually rupture or are ruptured artificially
Second stage	Contractions continue Head descends and flexes further, rotation usually completed Pushing starts when head reaches pelvic floor (active second stage)
Delivery	Head now extends as it is delivered over perineum Head restitutes, rotating back to the transverse before the shoulders deliver
Third stage	Placenta is delivered. Average duration 15 min

29 Labour 2: Management

The word 'management' for labour is misleading: supervision is more appropriate. Labour is a normal physiological process and most women will deliver safely without any management. Nevertheless, advances in obstetric care have contributed to its safety. The principal difficulty is that, in attempting to prevent rare but serious bad outcomes whilst not knowing who is at most risk, we cannot target intervention accurately enough. An example is induction of labour for post dates: this will prevent approximately 1 stillbirth for every 300 women induced at 41–42 weeks [→ p.210], and is usually advised, because we cannot predict the stillbirth. But such 'medicalization' of a natural process can initiate a cascade of intervention. For instance, induction of labour means epidural analgesia is more likely to be used. Epidural analgesia means cardiotocography [→ p.239] is used, and increases the chances of an instrumental delivery [→ p.256]. Obstetricians therefore spend much of their time sorting out problems that they have themselves created.

Many women also fear labour, for its pain, for interventions such as instrumental deliveries and because it is a time of risk to the fetus. Such fear can be reduced by information, reassurance, accommodating reasonable wishes and, most importantly, by not treating labour as a disease. Such support, particularly in labour, improves outcomes and reduces the need for intervention (*Cochrane* 2007: CD003766) (Fig. 29.1). This is not surprising because, albeit simplistically, fear leads to adrenaline secretion, and adrenaline is a potent inhibitor of uterine contractions.

Because of these problems, increasing numbers of women, at opposite ends of a spectrum, request elective Caesarean section or wish to deliver outside hospital.

Obstetrics and Gynaecology, 3rd edition. By Lawrence Impey and Tim Child. Published 2008 by Blackwell Publishing, ISBN: 978-1-4051-6095-7.

General care of the woman in labour

Physical health in labour

Observations: The temperature, pulse and blood pressure should be monitored. If abnormal, or the circumstances predispose to abnormalities (e.g. epidural), measurement should be more frequent. Hypotension associated with epidural analgesia will respond to intravenous fluids ± ephedrine; hypertension should be treated as antenatally.

Mobility and delivery positions: Freedom of movement is encouraged. Most women deliver semi recumbent: squatting, kneeling or the left-lateral position all increase the dimensions of the pelvic outlet. Pregnant women should not lie flat on their back: the gravid uterus compresses the main blood vessels, reducing cardiac output and causing hypotension, and often fetal distress. This is called aortocaval compression (Fig. 29.2) and in the supine position it is prevented by maintaining at least 15° of left lateral tilt.

Hydration: Dehydration in labour is common and women should be encouraged to drink water. Intravenous fluid is also necessary if an epidural is used or if labour is prolonged.

Stomach and food: Eating is often discouraged because stomach contents can be aspirated (Mendelson's syndrome) if a general anaesthetic is required. Ranitidine is often given to reduce the stomach acidity. However, general anaesthesia should rarely be used in obstetric practice, and routine starvation of women in labour is inhumane.

Pyrexia in labour: This is best defined as >37.5°C. This is associated with an increased risk of neonatal illness and is not always a result of chorioamnionitis (*BJOG* 2001; **108**: 594). It is more common with epidural analgesia and prolonged labour. Cultures of the vagina, urine and blood are taken. Antipyretics are normally administered

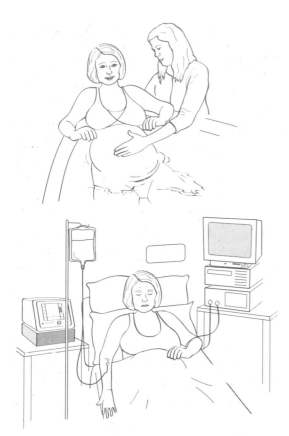

Fig. 29.1 Maternal anxiety is bad for labour.

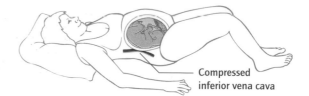

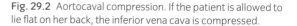

Fig. 29.2 Aortocaval compression. If the patient is allowed to lie flat on her back, the inferior vena cava is compressed.

although it is not known if these are beneficial for the baby; intravenous antibiotics are warranted if the fever reaches 38°C or there are other risk factors for sepsis [→ p.161].

The urinary tract: Neglected retention of urine can irreversibly damage the detrusor muscle [→ p.64]. An epidural usually removes bladder sensation. The woman must be encouraged to micturate frequently in labour; if she has an epidural, catheterization may be needed. Routine catheterization of all, however, is unnecessary.

Mental health in labour

The importance of psychological well-being in labour is crucial. The impact of this is seldom remembered but fear and anxiety cause adrenaline secretion and adrenaline slows labour.

Environment: This need not be too clinical. Resuscitation equipment can be hidden. Music and privacy may help. More women now choose to deliver at home [→ p.247], or in less clinical atmospheres such as birthing centres.

The birth attendant: The continuous presence of a 'caregiver' is reassuring. This reduces the length of labour, the use of analgesia, and the augmentation and obstetric intervention (*Cochrane* 2003: CD003766). Continuous support, explanation and encouragement are needed. This should be from the midwife as well as partner, or from non-medical supporters or 'doulas'.

The partner or accompanying person is an important potential source of support for the woman. He/she may need support too.

Control: Women have differing expectations of labour. Some want labour to be safe, quick and reasonably painless. Others have definite views, either because they view labour as a positive experience rather than a means to an end or because they have preconceptions based on previous or other people's experiences. They should be encouraged to write their views on a 'birth plan', which can be discussed so that expectations are realistic and the woman does not regard deviation from the plan as failure. Most requests in uncomplicated labour can then be safely accommodated as most labours need little or no intervention. If an unwanted intervention becomes necessary, adequate explanation is important.

Progress in labour: problems and their treatment

Monitoring progress: the partogram

Progress in labour is dependent on the powers, the passage and the passenger. A partogram (Fig. 29.3) is used to record progress in dilatation of the cervix (±

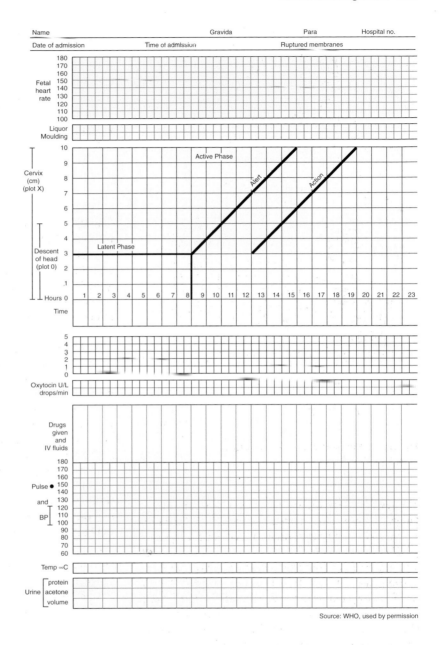

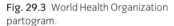

Fig. 29.3 World Health Organization partogram.

Source: WHO, used by permission

descent of the head). This is assessed on vaginal examination and plotted against time. After the latent phase (i.e. at about 3 cm dilated) the usual minimum rate of dilatation is 1 cm/h: 'alert' and 'action' lines on the partogram indicate slow progress, although debate remains as to exactly where they should be placed. This visual record therefore aids identification of abnormal progress and also forms a record of maternal vital signs, fetal heart rate (FHR) and liquor colour.

The power

'Inefficient uterine action' is the most common cause of slow progress in labour. Classifications are meaningless. It is common in nulliparous women and in induced labour, but is rare in multiparous women. Continuous support during labour is associated with a reduction in the length of labour (*Cochrane* 2003: CD003766). This probably increases contractions by reducing anxiety.

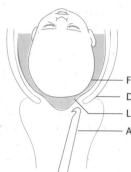

Fetal head
Dilating cervix
Liquor in the amniotic sac
Amnihook

Fig. 29.4 Amniotomy.

Mobility should also be encouraged. Persistently slow progress is treated by augmentation, initially with amniotomy (Fig. 29.4) and then oxytocin (Fig. 29.5).

Hyperactive uterine action occurs with excessively strong or frequent or prolonged contractions. FHR may be abnormal as placental blood flow is diminished and labour may be very rapid. It is associated with the use of too much oxytocin, or as a side effect of prostaglandin administration to induce labour, and with placental abruption. Treatment depends on the cause: if there is no evidence of an abruption, a tocolytic such as salbutamol can be given intravenously or subcutaneously, but Caesarean section is often indicated because of fetal distress.

Nulliparous labour

The first stage: Slow progress in the nulliparous woman is usually due to inefficient uterine action, even if contractions are frequent or feel strong. Strengthening the powers artificially is called augmentation, and this can even sometimes correct passenger problems of attitude or position. This is performed by artificially rupturing the membranes (ARM or amniotomy); if this fails to further cervical dilatation in 1–2 h, artificial oxytocin is administered intravenously as a dilute solution and the dose is gradually increased (*Cochrane* 2000: CD000015). Provided electronic fetal monitoring is used, this approach is safe because of the relative immunity of the nulliparous uterus to rupture. Oxytocin will usually increase cervical dilatation within 4 h if it is going to be effective. If full dilatation is not imminent within 12–16 h, the diagnosis is reconsidered and Caesarean section is performed: problems with the passage or passenger are more likely and the immunity of the uterus to rupture is diminished.

The passive second stage: If descent is poor, an oxytocin infusion should be started and pushing delayed by up to 2 h. If an epidural has been used, the urge to push that is characteristic of the active second stage is diminished.

The active second stage: Pushing need not be directed unless an epidural is present. If the stage lasts longer than 1 h, spontaneous delivery becomes less likely because of maternal exhaustion; fetal hypoxia and maternal trauma are also more common. If the head is distending the perineum, an episiotomy can be performed; if not, traction is often applied to the fetal head with a ventouse or forceps [→ p.256].

Multiparous labour

The first stage: Slow progress in the multiparous woman is unusual. The multiparous uterus is seldom 'inefficient' and the pelvic capacity has been 'proven' in the previous labour unless delivery has previously been by Caesarean section [→ p.252]. The cause is therefore more likely to be the fetal head: its attitude or position, or because it is much bigger than before. In addition, the multiparous uterus is more prone to rupture than the nulliparous uterus. Augmentation of labour with oxytocin must therefore be preceded by careful exclusion of a malpresentation.

The second stage: Instrumental delivery, although rarely needed, requires similar caution.

Augmentation and induction

Augmentation is the artificial strengthening of contractions in established labour
Induction is the artificial initiation of labour

The passenger

The fetus can contribute to a poor progress in labour.

Occipito-posterior (OP) position

This disorder of rotation [→ p.226] is often combined with varying degrees of extension and causes a larger

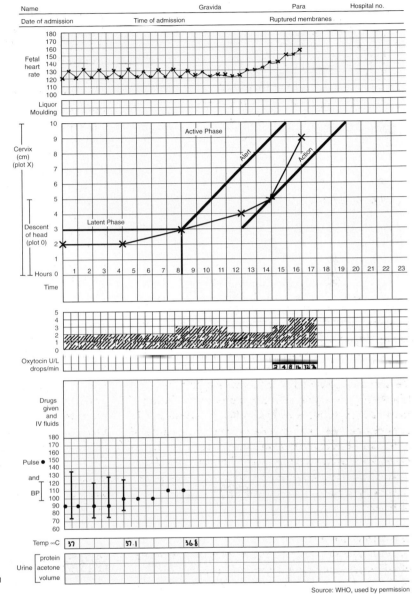

Fig. 29.5 A partogram showing delay in first stage managed with oxytocin.

diameter to negotiate the pelvic outlet. Labour is often longer and more painful, with backache and an early desire to push. The occiput is palpated posteriorly near the sacrum on vaginal examination (Fig. 29.6). If progress in labour is normal, no action is needed: many fetuses rotate to occipito-anterior (OA) spontaneously or deliver OP. If labour is slow, augmentation is used. If the position is persistent (5% of deliveries), delivery will be 'face to pubis' and completed by flexion rather than extension over the perineum. A few do not progress to full dilatation and Caesarean section is required. If associated with a prolonged active second stage, instrumental delivery can usually be achieved with rotation to OA position using a ventouse or with manual rotation. Kielland's forceps [→ p.258], requiring particular expertise, are associated with most success in these circumstances.

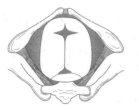

Fig. 29.6 The occipito-posterior (OP) position associated with extension of the head.

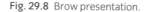

Fig. 29.8 Brow presentation.

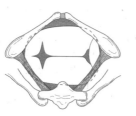

Fig. 29.7 The occipito-transverse (OT) position: delivery is impossible without rotation.

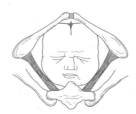

Fig. 29.9 Face presentation (chin is posterior).

Occipito-transverse (OT) position

This occurs when normal rotation has been incomplete. The occiput lies on the left or the right, and this is palpated on vaginal examination (Fig. 29.7). This is the position in which the head normally enters the pelvis and is a normal finding in the first stage. Only if vaginal delivery has not been achieved after 1 h of pushing in second stage is the position significant. This is usually associated with poor 'powers'. Rotation with traction is required for delivery to occur: this is usually achieved with the ventouse.

Brow presentation

Extension of the fetal head on the neck [→ p.225] results in a large (13 cm) presenting diameter that will not normally deliver vaginally (Fig. 29.8). It occurs in 1 in 1000 labours. The anterior fontanelle, supraorbital ridges and the nose are palpable vaginally. Caesarean section is required.

Face presentation

Complete extension of the head results in the face being the presenting part. It occurs in 1 in 400 labours. Fetal compromise in labour is more common. The mouth, nose and eyes are palpable vaginally. The presenting diameter is 9.5 cm, allowing vaginal delivery in most cases so long as the chin is anterior (mento-anterior position): delivery is completed by flexion over the perineum. If the chin is posterior (mento-posterior position; Fig. 29.9), extension of the head over the perineum is impossible, as it is already maximally extended and Caesarean section is indicated.

Fetal abnormality

Rarely, abnormalities such as fetal hydrocephalus may obstruct delivery.

Breech presentation and transverse or oblique lie in labour are discussed in Chapter 26.

Common causes of failure to progress in labour	
Powers:	Inefficient uterine action
Passenger:	Fetal size Disorder of rotation, e.g. occipito-transverse (OT), occipito-posterior (OP) Disorder of flexion, e.g. brow
Passage:	Cephalo-pelvic disproportion Possible role of cervix

The passage

Cephalo-pelvic disproportion

This implies that the pelvis is simply too small to allow the head to pass through, but it can almost never be diagnosed with accuracy. It depends on fetal as well as pelvic size: therefore, although commonly used to describe a person, it is more applicable to a pregnancy. In the absence of a gross pelvic deformity, which is extremely rare in healthy Caucasian women, it is a *retrospective* diagnosis best defined as the inability to deliver a particular fetus despite: (i) the presence of adequate uterine activity and (ii) the absence of a malposition or presentation. The word 'retrospective' means that it can normally only be diagnosed after labour has failed to progress and not with any accuracy before labour. Measuring the pelvis clinically or with X-rays or computed tomography (CT) scanning is unhelpful as the pelvis is not completely rigid and the scalp bones can overlap. Cephalo-pelvic disproportion is slightly more likely with large babies, with very short women or where the head in a nulliparous woman remains high at term. Elective Caesarean section is still generally inappropriate in such women, but the term 'trial of labour' is sometimes thoughtlessly used.

Pelvic variants and deformities

Normal variants in pelvic shape have been extensively classified but this is virtually never useful in modern practice. The 'gynaecoid' or ideal pelvis is found in 50–80% of Caucasian women. The 'anthropoid' pelvis (20%) has a narrower inlet, with a transverse diameter often less than the antero-posterior (AP) diameter. The android pelvis (5%) has a heart-shaped inlet and a funnelling shape to the mid-pelvis. In the platypelloid pelvis (10%) the oval shape of the inlet persists within the mid-pelvis.

Abnormal pelvic architecture is usually confined to developing countries where health and nutrition are poor.

Rickets and osteomalacia, poorly healed pelvic fractures, spinal abnormalities (such as major degrees of kyphosis or scoliosis), poliomyelitis and congenital malformations are very rare in the West.

Other pelvic abnormalities

Rarely, a pelvic mass such as an ovarian tumour or uterine fibroid blocks engagement and descent of the head. This will be palpable vaginally and Caesarean section is indicated.

The cervix

The role of the cervix is to prevent the fetus from literally dropping out before term: the rare cervical 'incompetence' [→ p.190] causes painless preterm delivery. During normal labour, it is not simply the strength of contractions that removes this natural obstruction but a complex mechanism involving hydration of the cervical collagen. The cervix itself, in addition to the contractions, may determine the course of labour, but the clinical relevance of this remains poorly understood.

Care of the fetus

Permanent fetal damage attributable to labour is uncommon: only about 10% of cases of cerebral palsy are attributed solely to intrapartum problems. Nevertheless, fetal death or damage, usually neurological, has devastating effects. There are several causes of damage:

1 Fetal hypoxia, commonly described as 'distress', is the best known.
2 Infection/inflammation in labour, e.g. group B streptococcus [→ p.161].
3 Meconium aspiration leading to chemical pneumonitis.
4 Trauma is rarely spontaneous and more commonly due to obstetric intervention, e.g. forceps.
5 Fetal blood loss [→ p.200].

Fetal distress

Definition

The term 'fetal distress' is a clinical diagnosis made by indirect methods. It should be defined as *hypoxia that might result in fetal damage or death if not reversed or the fetus delivered urgently*, but the term is widely abused. In reality hypoxia is simply the best known cause of intrapartum fetal damage and its effects are unpredictable and vary considerably. The convention is that a pH of <7.20 in the fetal scalp (capillary) blood (see below) indicates significant hypoxia.

In reality, the mean cord arterial pH at birth is about 7.20, so a capillary pH of <7.20 will not be uncommon in labour, and conventional practice overdiagnoses fetal distress. Indeed, it is only below 7.00 (*Obstet Gynecol* 1991; **78**: 1103) that neurological damage is considerably more common. Even at this level, most babies have no sequelae; further, most babies with neurological damage had a normal pH at birth. This reflects the influences of other factors, antepartum (e.g. intrauterine growth restriction [IUGR] [→ p.203]) or intrapartum (e.g. maternal fever [→ p.241]) on neonatal outcome.

Aetiology

Why hypoxia occurs is poorly understood. Contractions temporarily reduce placental perfusion and may compress the umbilical cord, so longer labours and those with excessive time (>1 h) spent pushing are more likely to produce hypoxia. Acute hypoxia in labour can be due to placental abruption, hypertonic uterine states and the use of oxytocin, prolapse of the umbilical cord and maternal hypotension.

Epidemiology

Prediction of the 'at-risk' fetus is imprecise. Intrapartum risk factors include long labour, meconium, the use of epidurals and oxytocin; antepartum factors include the high-risk pregnancy and IUGR fetuses are more vulnerable. Fetuses with these risk factors are usually monitored in labour with cardiotocography (CTG) [→ p.239].

Diagnosing fetal distress

As hypoxia is a relatively rare cause of handicap, the effects of attempts to prevent it will be limited. The diagnosis of fetal distress is usually made from the finding of significant fetal acidosis (scalp pH <7.20) or ominous FHR abnormalities. The following are methods employed in the detection of fetal distress.

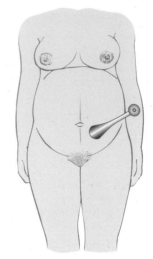

Fig. 29.10 Pinard's stethoscope for intermittent auscultation (IA) in labour.

Colour of the liquor: meconium

Meconium is the bowel contents of the fetus that stains the amniotic fluid. It is rare in preterm fetuses but common (30%) after 42 weeks. Meconium very diluted in amniotic fluid is seldom significant, but with undiluted meconium ('pea-soup') perinatal mortality is increased fourfold. Nevertheless, the presence or absence of meconium is not a reliable indicator of fetal well-being (*Obstet Gynecol* 2003; **102**: 89). It is an indication for caution (and hence closer surveillance with a CTG) because: (i) the fetus may aspirate it, causing meconium aspiration syndrome; and (ii) because hypoxia is more likely.

Fetal heart rate (FHR) auscultation

The heart is auscultated every 15 minutes during the first stage, and every 5 minutes in the second, with a Pinard's stethoscope (Fig. 29.10) or a hand-held Doppler for 60 s after a contraction. The distressed or potentially distressed fetus normally exhibits abnormal heart rate patterns, which can be heard. This method of intrapartum fetal surveillance is appropriate for low-risk pregnancies, and if abnormalities are detected, a CTG is indicated.

Cardiotocography (CTG)

This records the FHR on paper, either from a transducer placed on the abdomen or from a clip or probe in the vagina attached to the fetal scalp. Another transducer synchronously records the uterine contractions. Interpretation is complex and difficult, requiring experience. A combination of abnormal patterns increases the likelihood of fetal distress. There are several important features:

Baseline rate: This should be 110–160 beats/minute. *Tachycardias* are associated with fever, fetal infection and, if in conjunction with other abnormalities, fetal hypoxia. *A steep, sustained deterioration in rate* suggests acute fetal distress (Fig. 29.11a).

Variability: The short-term variation in FHR should be >5 beats/minute (Fig. 29.11b), except during episodes of fetal sleep, which usually last less than 45 minutes. Prolonged reduced variability, particularly with other abnormal features, *suggests* hypoxia (Fig. 29.11d).

Response to contractions: *Accelerations* of the fetal heart with movements or contractions are reassuring (Fig. 29.11b).

'*Early decelerations*' are synchronous with a contraction as a normal response to head compression and therefore are usually benign (Fig. 29.11c).

'*Variable decelerations*' vary in timing and classically reflect cord compression, which can ultimately cause hypoxia.

'*Late decelerations*' persist after the contraction is completed and are *suggestive* of fetal hypoxia (Fig. 29.11d). The depth of the deceleration is usually unimportant.

A normal CTG is reassuring, but the false positive rate of abnormal patterns is high: confirmation of hypoxia should be made by fetal scalp pH sampling to avoid unnecessary intervention, except in acute situations (e.g. prolonged fetal bradycardia) or if access to the fetal scalp is not possible. The use of CTG is widespread: in high-risk situations its use is logical but is poorly evaluated. In low-risk labour, it does reduce the incidence of neonatal seizures but does not improve long-term neonatal outcome (*Cochrane* 2006: CD006066), while increasing the rates of Caesarean section and other obstetric interventions.

Fetal electrocardiogram monitoring

Limited evidence suggests that if used in conjunction with a CTG, this improves neonatal outcomes whilst preventing some of the associated increase in operative delivery (*Cochrane* 2006: CD000116).

Fetal blood (scalp) sampling

A metal tube called an amnioscope is inserted vaginally through the cervix. The scalp is cleaned and a small cut is made, from which blood is collected in a microtube (Fig. 29.12). The pH and base excess are immediately analysed. If the pH is <7.20, delivery, unless imminent, is expedited by the fastest route possible. As discussed above, as most acidotic babies have no problems, this conventional threshold for intervention leads to an over diagnosis of fetal distress but less so than if CTG monitoring is used without it.

Fetal distress: simplified scheme for screening and diagnosis	
Level 1:	Intermittent auscultation of fetal heart. If abnormal, or meconium, or long, or high-risk labour, *proceed to*
Level 2:	Continuous cardiotocography (CTG). If sustained bradycardia, deliver. If other abnormalities, simple measures to correct. If fail, *proceed to*
Level 3:	Fetal blood sampling (FBS). If abnormal *proceed to*
Level 4:	Delivery by quickest route

Role of CTG in obstetric practice

Despite the disadvantages outlined, many of the problems with CTG are associated with poor interpretation, inappropriate timing, or a failure to use fetal blood sampling in conjunction. A computer-based package (K2) should be available on all delivery wards and provides excellent tuition in CTG interpretation. In many units a 20-minute CTG on admission is performed for all women in labour, but this has no neonatal benefits and may increase operative delivery rates (*Lancet* 2003; **361**: 465). Intermittent auscultation (IA) remains appropriate for low-risk pregnancy, with subsequent continuous CTG only if it is abnormal, if labour is prolonged, or if there is meconium, or a maternal fever.

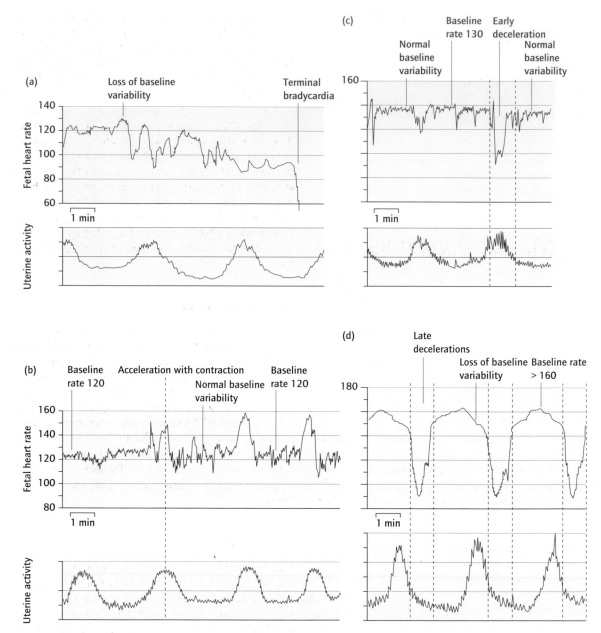

Fig. 29.11 (a) Acute fetal distress; the fetus is dying. (b) Normal cardiotocography (CTG); acceleration of the fetal heart with contractions. (c) Early decelerations are synchronous with a contraction. (d) Late decelerations, tachycardia, reduced variability suggestive of fetal distress.

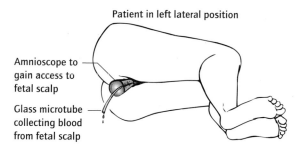

Patient in left lateral position

Amnioscope to gain access to fetal scalp

Glass microtube collecting blood from fetal scalp

Fig. 29.12 Fetal blood sampling (FBS) in labour.

The pros and cons of cardiotocography (CTG)	
Advantages:	Visual record that includes variability
	High sensitivity for fetal distress/hypoxia
	Reduction in short-term neurological morbidity
Disadvantages:	Cumbersome; reduces maternal mobility
	Increased rate of obstetric intervention
	No proven reduction in mortality or long-term handicap
	More puerperal sepsis

Management of fetal distress

Fetal distress is not always progressive and resuscitative measures are taken before fetal blood sampling (FBS) or delivery. The woman is placed in the left lateral position to avoid aortocaval compression [→ p.232]; oxygen and intravenous fluid are administered. Any oxytocin infusion is stopped; tocolytics [→ p.234] can even be given. A vaginal examination is also made to exclude cord prolapse or very rapid progress. If simple measures fail, FBS is performed: delivery is expedited if the pH is <7.20. If pH is >7.20 but the abnormal FHR pattern continues or deteriorates, a second scalp sample will be needed in about 30 minutes. If fetal scalp sampling is impossible, or the fetal heart shows a sustained bradycardia, delivery is undertaken anyway.

Other causes of fetal damage and their treatment

Fetal infection and the inflammatory response

Severe fetal infection due to group B streptococcus [→

p.160] affects about 1.7 per 1000 live births where strategies to prevent it are not used. Treatment encompasses screening for the organism and treatment of high-risk groups, which in labour comprise women with a maternal fever or prolonged rupture of the membranes.

There is increasing evidence that even a low-grade maternal fever is a strong risk factor for seizures, fetal death and cerebral palsy, even in the *absence* of evidence of infection (*BJOG* 2001; **108**: 594). It is still unknown whether this is due to causes of the fever (in addition to infection) or to the fever itself (i.e. overheating), so that the therapeutic role for antibiotics or antipyretics is unknown. Nevertheless this appears to be independent of fetal hypoxia and is probably much more important than is currently thought (*AmJOG* 2008; **49**: e1–6).

Meconium aspiration

Meconium is aspirated by the fetus into its lungs, where it causes a severe pneumonitis. This is more common in the presence of fetal hypoxia, but it can occur without it. Where the meconium is thick, amniofusion of saline into the uterus to dilute the meconium reduces the incidence of meconium aspiration (*Cochrane* 2000: CD00014). Maternal safety, however, remains unproven and this is seldom performed. When meconium is present at delivery, it is sucked out from the baby's airways before the body is delivered, to prevent the first gasp from aspirating it into the lungs.

Fetal trauma

Fetal trauma may be iatrogenic, principally from instrumental vaginal delivery or breech delivery. An uncontrolled vaginal delivery with rapid decompression of the head can also cause damage. Shoulder dystocia [→ p.262] often results in trauma, but prediction and therefore prevention is imprecise.

Fetal blood loss

This is very rare and is due to vasa praevia [→ p.200], feto-maternal haemorrhage or, on occasion, placental abruption.

Care of the mother

Pain relief in labour

Labour is normally extremely painful, but analgesia is a mother's choice: tolerance of pain and attitudes to childbirth differ widely. At opposite ends of a spectrum, some women prefer maximal analgesia while others prefer a more natural approach. There are also instances where analgesia, particularly epidural analgesia, is medically advisable. The methods employed can modify either pain or the emotional response to pain.

Non-medical

Preparation at antenatal classes, the presence of a birth attendant as well as the partner and the maintenance of mobility all help women cope with labour pain. Back-rubbing or transcutaneous electrical nerve stimulation (TENS) are beneficial for some in early labour. Immersion in water at body temperature is effective and should be distinguished from water birth [→ p.247], where the baby is actually delivered under water. A variety of other methods have not been adequately scientifically tested but are helpful to some women: these include hypno-therapy, acupuncture, localized pressure on the back, the application of superficial heat or cold, massage and aromatherapy (*Cochrane* 2006; CD003521).

Inhalational agents

Entonox is an equal mix of nitrous oxide and oxygen. It has a rapid onset and is a mild analgesic. However, it is insufficient for all but the most 'motivated' mothers and can cause light-headedness, nausea and hyperventilation as women attempt to obtain the maximum effect.

Systemic opiates

Pethidine or Meptid (occasionally diamorphine) are widely used as intramuscular injections. Advantages include easy administration (which can be patient-controlled: patient-controlled analgesia [PCA]). Most women become less concerned about their pain. However, the analgesic effect is small and many patients become sedated, confused or feel out of control. Anti-emetics are usually needed. They also cause respiratory depression in the newborn, which requires reversal with naloxone.

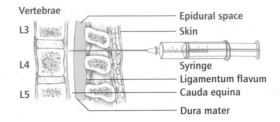

Fig. 29.13 Spinal analgesia, transverse section of the spinal column.

Anaesthesia for obstetric procedures

Spinal anaesthesia

Local anaesthetic is injected through the dura mater into the cerebrospinal fluid (CSF) (Fig. 29.13). This rapidly produces a short-lasting but effective analgesia that is the method of choice (if an epidural is not *in situ*) for Caesarean section or mid-cavity instrumental vaginal delivery [→ p.257]. The principal complications are hypotension and 'total spinal' analgesia: the latter is very rare.

Pudendal nerve block

Local anaesthetic is injected bilaterally around the pudendal nerve where it passes by the ischial spine. This is suitable for low-cavity instrumental vaginal deliveries.

Epidural analgesia

This is the injection of local anaesthetic, with or without opiates, via an 'epidural catheter' into the epidural space, between the vertebrae L3 and L4. Local anaesthetic is either infused continuously or used to 'top up' intermittently (Fig. 29.14). Complete sensory (except pressure) and partial motor blockade from the upper abdomen downwards is the norm. It is therefore suitable both for the entire labour as well as obstetric procedures.

Advantages
This is the only method in labour that can make women pain-free and is very popular. It can also be advised on purely medical grounds, if labour is long, to help reduce blood pressure in hypertensive women, to abolish a premature urge to push, and as analgesia for instrumental delivery or Caesarean section.

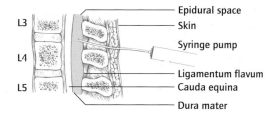

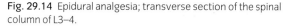

L3

L4

L5

Epidural space
Skin
Syringe pump
Ligamentum flavum
Cauda equina
Dura mater

Fig. 29.14 Epidural analgesia; transverse section of the spinal column of L3–4.

Contraindications to epidural analgesia

Sepsis
Coagulopathy or anticoagulant therapy (unless low-dose heparin)
Active neurological disease
Spinal abnormalities
Hypovolaemia

Disadvantages

Increased midwifery supervision is needed to check the blood pressure and pulse regularly. The woman is bed-bound, and pressure sores may occur without careful nursing, although low-dose regimes in combination with spinal blockade allow some mobility. Reduced bladder sensation causes urinary retention. Maternal fever is more common. The Caesarean section rate is not increased, although instrumental delivery is more common (*Cochrane* 2005: CD000331), particularly if the passive second stage is not modified [→ p.244]. Transient hypotension (*BJOG* 2002; **109**: 274) is minimized if intravenous fluid is given first. Transient fetal bradycardias are also common, but seldom precipitate fetal distress. There is little evidence for an association between epidural analgesia and back pain after delivery.

Major complications of technique

'Spinal tap' (0.5%) is inadvertent puncture of the dura mater causing leakage of CSF and often a severe headache. Characteristically the pain is worse when sitting up and alleviated by lying down. It is treated with analgesics and if persistent for >48 h, with the administration of a 'blood patch' to seal the leak. Very rarely, inadvertent intravenous injection produces convulsions and cardiac arrest. Or inadvertent injection of local anaesthetic into the CSF combined with progression up the spinal cord causes 'total spinal analgesia' and respiratory paralysis.

Epidural analgesia is very safe in expert hands but needs increased midwifery care and modification of the second stage of labour.

Problems with epidurals

Spinal tap
Total spinal analgesia
Hypotension
Local anaesthetic toxicity
Higher instrumental delivery rate
Poor mobility
Urinary retention
Maternal fever

Conduct of labour

Initiation of labour

The woman is advised to admit herself or to call the midwife if painful contractions are regular and at 5–10 minute intervals, or if the membranes have ruptured. A brief history of the pregnancy and past obstetric history is taken, and temperature, blood pressure, pulse and urinalysis are recorded. The presentation is checked and a vaginal examination is performed to check for cervical effacement and dilatation to confirm the diagnosis of labour. The degree of descent is also assessed. The colour of any leaking liquor is noted. Every 15 minutes, the fetal heart is listened to for 1 minute following a contraction; if the pregnancy is high risk or meconium is seen or there is maternal fever, a CTG [→ p.239] is started. Routine shaving or the administration of an enema are obsolete.

Account must at this stage be taken of the woman's wishes for labour, and the birth plan should be read. These wishes should be respected as far as possible: and the care that she is given should be adjusted accordingly (see different approaches to delivery [→ p.247]). Described below is the basic care that should be given to all labouring women.

The diagnosis of labour

Painful contractions with effacement and dilatation of cervix
Painful contractions with show and/or ruptured membranes suggestive

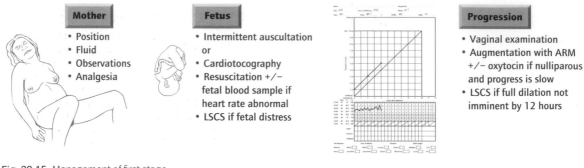

Fig. 29.15 Management of first stage.

First stage of labour (Fig. 29.15)

The mother

The mother is made comfortable and encouraged to remain mobile. The supine position is avoided. Continuous support, attention and explanation are needed. Pain is better tolerated when progress is made. If analgesia is requested, nitrous oxide provides short-term relief but commonly an epidural is used. The vital signs and fluid balance are monitored; catheterization is often needed if an epidural is used, but it should not be routine.

The fetus

The colour of the liquor is observed. The fetal heart is auscultated for 60 s after a contraction every 15 minutes; or it is monitored with CTG if the pregnancy is 'high risk', a heart rate abnormality is detected or if labour is longer than about 5 h. If the heart rate pattern is abnormal, the fetus may be hypoxic. Oxygen, intravenous fluid and the left lateral position (to avoid aortocaval compression) are used. Any oxytocin is usually stopped. If the abnormal heart rate pattern persists, a fetal scalp blood sample is taken. If there is fetal distress (i.e. scalp blood pH <7.20), expedition of delivery in the first stage can only be accomplished by Caesarean section.

Progress

Progress is assessed by 2–4-hourly vaginal examination. Dilatation is estimated digitally in centimetres; descent of the head is measured by its relationship to the ischial spines: these measurements are recorded on the partogram. Slow dilatation after the latent phase (<1 cm/h) can be treated with ARM (or amniotomy). If progress continues to be slow, oxytocin is used in a nulliparous woman, but in a multiparous woman a malpresentation or malposition must be carefully excluded first. If the cervix is not fully dilated by 12–16 h, Caesarean delivery is usually appropriate unless delivery can be anticipated in the next hour or two.

Second stage of labour (Fig. 29.16)

If there is no epidural, 'non-directed' pushing is encouraged only when the mother has the desire to push or the head is visible. If an epidural is *in situ*, it is normal to wait at least an hour before pushing, and oxytocin is administered if the woman is nulliparous and descent is poor. If numb from an epidural, she is encouraged to push about three times for about 10 s during each contraction. During this time, considerable support and encouragement are required.

If delivery is not imminent after 1 h of pushing, instrumental vaginal delivery is normally indicated. Fetal distress is normally diagnosed in the same manner as for the first stage, but expedition of delivery is usually possible with the ventouse or forceps. Careful assessment is required to ensure that all the prerequisites [→ p.258] for this are met.

Normal delivery

As the head approaches the perineum, the attendant's hands are scrubbed and gloved. The mother should be however she feels most comfortable, but *not* flat on her

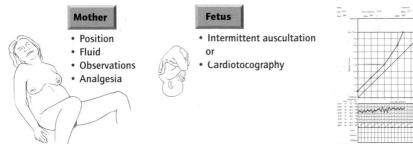

Fig. 29.16 Management of second stage.

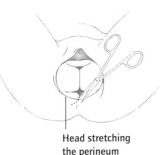

Head stretching
the perineum

Fig. 29.17 Episiotomy.

back. The routine use of an episiotomy has no benefit (*Cochrane* 2000: CD000081): episiotomy should be reserved for where there is fetal distress, where the head is not passing over the perineum despite maternal effort, or a large tear is likely. If it is to be performed, the perineum is infiltrated with local anesthetic and a 3–5 cm cut is made with scissors from the centre of the fourchette to the (mother's) right side of the perineum (Fig. 29.17).

A swab is pushed against ('guarding') the perineum as the head distends it, and she is asked to stop pushing and to pant slowly. This enables a controlled and slow delivery of the head and reduces perineal damage. Once all the head is delivered, the airways are sucked out if meconium is present. The head then restitutes. With the next contraction, maternal pushing and gentle downward traction on the head lead to delivery of the anterior shoulder; traction is then directed upwards to deliver the posterior shoulder, once again guarding the perineum. Unless requiring resuscitation, the baby is delivered onto the mother's (preferably bare) abdomen and wrapped to keep warm; the umbilical cord need not be clamped and cut immediately (Fig. 29.18).

Third stage of labour (Fig. 29.19)

Oxytocin is administered intramuscularly to help the uterus contract once the shoulders are delivered (*BJOG* 1996; **103**: 1068) (not until after the last fetus if it is a multiple pregnancy). A combination of ergometrine and oxytocin (Syntometrine) is often used but frequently leads to maternal vomiting. Once placental separation is evident from lengthening of the cord and the passage of blood, continuous gentle traction on the cord allows delivery of the placenta (controlled cord traction). At the same time, the left hand pushes down suprapubically to prevent uterine inversion [→ p.264].

The placenta is checked for missing cotyledons and the vagina and perineum for tears. Once these are sutured, a swab and needle count is performed, blood loss is recorded, the mother is cleaned, made comfortable and encouraged to breastfeed if she wishes. Maternal observation should continue for at least 2 h.

Retained placenta

This is defined as a third stage longer than 30 minutes, and occurs after 2.5% of deliveries. Partial separation may cause considerable blood loss into the uterus

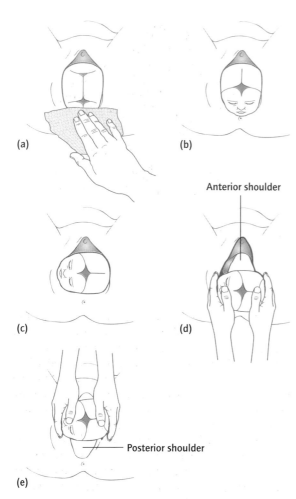

Fig. 29.18 Normal delivery. (a) 'Guarding' the perineum as the head distends it. (b) The head delivers. (c) The head restitutes. (d) The anterior shoulder is delivered by gentle downward traction until the next contraction. (e) The posterior shoulder is delivered by gentle upward traction.

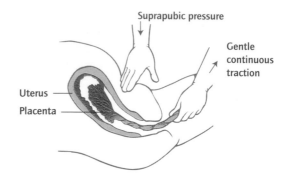

Fig. 29.19 Management of third stage. Delivery of the placenta.

Classification of perineal trauma	
First degree:	Injury to skin only
Second degree:	Involving perineal muscles but not anal spincter
Episiotomy:	Equivalent to second degree but may extend to third/fourth
Third degree:	Involving anal sphincter complex 3a: <50% of external anal sphincter torn 3b: >50% of external anal sphincter torn 3c: internal anal spincter also involved
Fourth degree:	Involving anal sphincter and anal epithelium

without any external signs. An oxytocin infusion is started and 10 units can be injected into the vein of the cord and 'milked' up it. In the absence of bleeding, an hour is left for natural separation, after which the placenta is 'manually removed'. A hand in the uterus, under general or spinal anaesthesia, gently separates the placenta from the uterus, with the second hand on the abdomen preventing the uterus from being pushed up. Blood is usually cross-matched and intravenous antibiotics are given.

Perineal repair (Fig. 29.20)

First and second degree tears and uncomplicated episiotomies without anal sphincter damage are sutured under local anesthetic. Failure to suture reduces healing and may cause more pain. Absorbable synthetic material is used (e.g. Dexon or Vicryl). continuous rather than separate sutures for the muscle and a subcuticular layer for the skin. A rectal and vaginal examination excludes sutures that are too deep and retained swabs, respectively.

Third and fourth degree tears occur in about 1% of deliveries. Risk factors include forceps delivery, large babies, nulliparity and the (now obsolete) use of midline episiotomy. The sphincter is repaired under epidural or spinal anaesthetic with the visualization and asepsis afforded by an operating theatre. The torn ends of the external sphincter are mobilized and sutured, usually overlapping, with the internal sphincter sutured sepa-

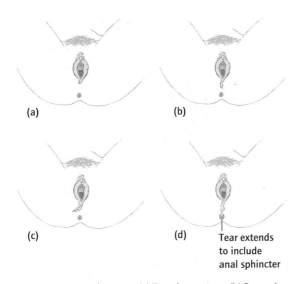

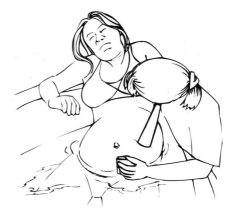

Fig. 29.21 Water birth.

(a)   (b)

(c)   (d)   Tear extends
to include
anal sphincter

Fig. 29.20 Perineal trauma. (a) First degree tear. (b) Second degree tear. (c) Mediolateral episiotomy. (d) Third degree tear.

rately if damaged. Adequate repair requires experience. Antibiotics and laxatives are given, as well as analgesia. Physiotherapy assessment, sometimes with anal manometry [→ p.271], is usual. Long term, about 30% of women have sequelae, usually incontinence of flatus or urgency, but occasionally frank incontinence.

Different approaches to delivery

Natural approaches to labour

Childbirth is a major life event. Whilst safety is the most important factor, it is usually taken for granted. The experience can be 'negative' for other reasons, particularly if the woman is immobile and attached to monitors or 'drips'. Whilst the safety of childbirth has increased, this cannot all be attributed to the increased 'medicalization' that has occurred in the last few years, much of which has been without scientific basis. There is increasing pressure among women to be allowed more choice and participation in decisions about their labours: now that labour is safer, we should try to make it more rewarding.

Home birth: Progress and fetal condition are monitored in the normal way and non-epidural analgesia may be administered. Intervention for slow progress may be delayed but if required, the woman is transferred to hospital. It is suitable for low-risk, preferably multiparous women, and in those with a planned, rather than inadvertent home birth, safety does not appear to be compromised. Indeed, the environment may lead to better psychological well-being and a reduced incidence of complications: it is just more difficult to manage them if they occur. Suitable plans for transport into hospital are therefore important, should this become necessary.

Water birth (Fig. 29.21): The labour and delivery are conducted in a large bath of water maintained at 37°C. Water is relaxing and analgesic. The baby is delivered under water and does not breathe until brought rapidly to the surface. It is used for motivated low-risk women, provided that trained personnel are available. Intermittent auscultation and vaginal examinations are easily performed under water. Despite its widespread usage, there is still incomplete evidence regarding the safety of this method.

Fast labour: 'active management'

Some women prefer labour to be quick and painless. For these, the early use of an epidural and 'active management of labour' may help this. The policy was developed to reduce the length of labour. The principles apply to nulliparous women and are: (i) early diagnosis of labour;

(ii) 2-hourly vaginal examinations; (iii) early correction of slow progress with amniotomy and oxytocin (augmentation); and (iv) Caesarean section by 12 h if delivery is not imminent. In addition, there is one-to-one midwifery care, a comprehensive antenatal education programme and continuous audit. Early augmentation minimizes the effect of inefficient uterine action. This shortens labour and the 'latent phase' [→ p.228] so long as it is only used once the cervix is fully effaced. Prolonged labour is rare and Caesarean and vaginal operative delivery rates are low. This policy has been criticized because suggestions that the chance of Caesarean section was reduced were not proven in clinical trials (*NEJM* 1995; **333**: 745).

Avoiding labour: Caesarean section for maternal request

For discussion see p. 260.

Criteria for home birth
Woman's request
'Low risk' on basis of antenatal or past obstetric and medical complications
37–41 weeks
Cephalic presentation
Clear liquor
Normal fetal heart rate (FHR)
All maternal observations normal

Further reading

Alfirevic Z, Devane D, Gyte GM. Continuous cardiotocography (CTG) as a form of electronic fetal monitoring (EFM) for fetal assessment during labour. *Cochrane Database of Systematic Reviews* 2006: CD006066.

Anim-Somuah M, Smyth R, Howell C. Epidural versus non-epidural or no analgesia in labour. *Cochrane Database of Systematic Reviews* 2005: CD000331.

Cluett ER, Pickering RM, Getliffe K, St George Saunders NJ. Randomised controlled trial of labouring in water compared with standard of augmentation for management of dystocia in first stage of labour. *British Medical Journal* 2004; **328**: 314.

Consensus Statement from the maternity care working party. 2007. *Making normal birth a reality*. RCM, RCOG, NCT. http://www.rcog.org.uk/resources/public/pdf/normal_birth_consensus.pdf

Friedman EA. Primigravid labor: a graphicostatistical analysis. *Obstetrics and Gynecology* 1955; **6**: 567–89.

Hodnett E, Gates S, Hofmeyr G, Sakala C. Continuous support for women during childbirth. *Cochrane Database of Systematic Reviews* 2007: CD003766.

Impey L, Boylan P. Active management of labour revisited. *BJOG: an International Journal of Obstetrics and Gynaecology* 1999; **106**: 183–7.

Murphy DJ. Failure to progress in the second stage of labour. *Current Opinion in Obstetrics and Gynecology* 2001; **13**: 557–61.

National Institute of Clinical Excellence (NICE). The use of electronic fetal monitoring. *Inherited Guideline C*. 2001. http://www.nice.org.uk

Nelson KB. Infection, inflammation and the risk of cerebral palsy. *Current Opinion in Neurology* 2000; **13**: 133–9.

Smith CA, Collins CT, Cyna AM, Crowther CA. Complementary and alternative therapies for pain management in labour. *Cochrane Database of Systematic Reviews* 2006: CD003521.

World Health Organization. Partograph in management of labour. World Health Organization Maternal Health and Safe Motherhood Programme. *Lancet* 1994; **343**: 1399–404.

Slow Progress in Labour at a Glance

Definitions		'Slow labour' is progress slower than 1 cm/h after latent phase
		'Prolonged labour' is >16 h duration after latent phase
Epidemiology		Common in nulliparous women; rare in multiparous
Aetiology	Powers:	Inefficient uterine action
	Passenger:	Fetal size, disorder of rotation, e.g. occipito-transverse (OT), occipito-posterior (OP)
		Disorder of flexion, e.g. brow
	Passage:	Cephalo-pelvic disproportion, rarely cervical resistance (if induction)
Management	General:	Wait if natural labour wanted, mobilize, improve support
	Nulliparous:	Amniotomy; oxytocin
	Multiparous:	Amniotomy; oxytocin if malpresentation/malposition excluded
	If this fails:	Caesarean section if first stage
		Instrumental delivery if second stage (if prerequisites met)

Occipito-posterior (OP) Position at a Glance

Definition	Abnormality of rotation, with face upwards. Some extension common
Epidemiology	5% of deliveries, more common in early labour
Aetiology	Idiopathic, inefficient uterine action, pelvic variants
Features	Slow labour. Back pain, early desire to push. Occiput posterior on vaginal examination
Management	Nil required if progress normal
	If slow progress, amniotomy and oxytocin
	If these fail in first stage, Caesarean section
	If second stage, >1 h of pushing, instrumental delivery if criteria met

Fetal Monitoring in Labour at a Glance

Modes of fetal injury	Hypoxia, meconium aspiration, trauma, infection/?inflammation, blood loss
Fetal distress	Hypoxia that may result in fetal damage or death if not reversed or the fetus delivered urgently
High-risk situations	Fetal conditions, e.g. intrauterine growth restriction (IUGR), prolonged pregnancy Medical complications, e.g. diabetes and pre-eclampsia Intrapartum factors: long labours, presence of meconium, maternal fever

Monitoring methods	Intermittent auscultation (IA), inspection for meconium:
	If IA abnormal or high-risk situation: cardiotocography (CTG)
	    Normal features: rate 110–160, accelerations, variability >5 beats/minute
	    Abnormal features: tachy- or bradycardias, decelerations, reduced variability
	If CTG abnormal: resuscitate, fetal blood sample

Intervention	If fetal blood sample abnormal, delivery by quickest route:
	    Caesarean section if first stage
	    Instrumental vaginal delivery if second stage and criteria met

Pain Relief in Labour at a Glance

Types	Non-medical:	Support, transcutaneous electrical nerve stimulation (TENS), water
	Medical:	Entonox, opiates, epidural
Epidural	Injection of local anaesthetic into epidural space:	
	Advantages:	Best pain relief. Prevents premature pushing
	Disadvantages:	Increased supervision, maternal fever, reduced mobility, increased instrumental delivery rate, hypotension, urinary retention
	Complications:	Spinal tap, 'total spinal analgesia', local anaesthetic toxicity
	Contraindications:	Sepsis, coagulopathy, active neurological disease, hypovolaemia, spinal abnormalities, cardiac outflow obstruction

30 Labour 3: Special circumstances

Induction of labour

Labour that is started artificially is induced. It is different from augmentation [→ p.234], when the contractions of established labour are strengthened. Theoretically, induction is performed in situations where allowing the pregnancy to continue would expose the fetus and/or mother to risk greater than that of induction. In practice, there are many instances when labour is induced and quantification of risk is virtually impossible.

Methods of induction

Whether induction is successful depends on the state, or 'favourability', of the cervix. This is related to 'consistency', the degree of effacement or early dilatation, how low in the pelvis the head is (station) and the cervical position (anterior or posterior within the vagina). These are often scored out of 10, as the 'Bishop's score': the lower the score, the more unfavourable the cervix (Fig. 30.1). Transvaginal assessment of cervical length may also be used (*Ultrasound Obstet Gynecol* 2001; **18**: 623).

Induction with prostaglandins

Prostaglandin E$_2$ (PGE$_2$) gel (normally 2 mg) is inserted into the posterior vaginal fornix. Misoprostol is cheaper and slightly more effective but, as hyperstimulation is more common (*Cochrane* 2003: CD000941), concerns regarding safety remain. Medical induction is the best method in most nulliparous women, and in multiparous women when the cervix is very unfavorable. It either starts labour, or the 'ripeness' of the cervix is improved to allow amniotomy. If one dose does not increase the

cervical ripeness, another may be given a minimum of 6 h later, providing there is no uterine activity; more than two doses are not helpful. Prostaglandins may be more effective if first administered in the evening.

Induction with amniotomy ± oxytocin

The forewaters are ruptured with an instrument called an amnihook (artificial rupture of the membranes [ARM]). An oxytocin infusion is then usually started within 2 h if labour has not ensued (*Cochrane* 2001: CD003250). Oxytocin is often used alone if spontaneous rupture of the membranes has already occurred [→ p.254], although prostaglandins are as effective.

Methods of induction	
Medical:	Prostaglandins/misoprostol
	Oxytocin (after amniotomy/membrane rupture)
Surgical:	Amniotomy

Natural induction

Cervical sweeping involves passing a finger through the cervix and 'stripping' between the membranes and the lower segment of the uterus (Fig. 30.2). At 40 weeks, this reduces the chance of induction and postdates pregnancy (*Cochrane* 2001: CD000451). However, it can be uncomfortable.

Indications for induction

In practice the decision to induce, and the choice of method and timing, are dependent on each individual case.
Fetal indications include high-risk situations such as prolonged pregnancy [→ p.210], suspected intrauterine growth restriction (IUGR) or compromise [→ p.203],

Obstetrics and Gynaecology, 3rd edition. By Lawrence Impey and Tim Child. Published 2008 by Blackwell Publishing, ISBN: 978-1-4051-6095-7.

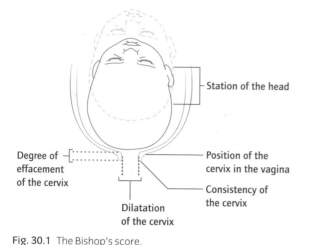

Fig. 30.1 The Bishop's score.

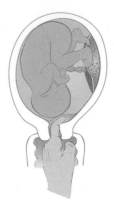

Fig. 30.2 Sweeping the membranes. A finger is inserted through the cervix and rotated: the membranes are peeled off the lower segment.

antepartum hemorrhage, poor obstetric history and prelabour term rupture of the membranes [→ p.254]. *Materno-fetal indications*, where both mother and fetus should benefit, include pre-eclampsia and maternal disease such as diabetes. *Maternal indications* are social reasons and *in utero* death.

Common indications for induction
Prolonged pregnancy
Suspected growth restriction
Prelabour term rupture of the membranes
Pre-eclampsia
Medical disease: hypertension and diabetes

Contraindications

Absolute contraindications include acute fetal compromise, abnormal lie, placenta praevia or pelvic obstruction such as a pelvic mass or pelvic deformity causing cephalo-pelvic disproportion. It is usually considered inappropriate after more than one Caesarean section. *Relative contraindications* include one previous Caesarean section and prematurity.

Management of induced labour

Because of both the indication for induction and the use of drugs, the fetus is at increased risk in labour. Cardiotocography (CTG) should be used for an hour, 1 h after the use of prostaglandins or when they stimulate uterine activity. Oxytocin is commonly required in labour, and also warrants CTG monitoring. Induction commonly increases the time spent in 'early labour', and the woman should be warned of this.

Complications

Labour may fail to start or be slow due to inefficient uterine activity. The risk of instrumental delivery or Caesarean section is probably higher, even allowing for the higher-risk pregnancies. Paradoxically, overactivity of the uterus can occur. This hyperstimulation is rare but can result in fetal distress and even uterine rupture. The umbilical cord can prolapse [→ p.262] at amniotomy. Postpartum hemorrhage (PPH) is more likely, as is intrapartum and postpartum infection. Iatrogenic prematurity can follow, by accident (incorrect gestation) or design.

Labour/vaginal delivery after a previous Caesarean section

Repeat, elective Caesarean sections account for more than one-quarter of all Caesarean sections performed, yet vaginal delivery after Caesarean (VBAC) can often be safely achieved.

Factors influencing vaginal delivery after one Caesarean section

Contraindications to vaginal delivery include the usual absolute indications for Caesarean section [→ p.259], a vertical uterine scar and multiple previous Caesareans. After two Caesareans, vaginal delivery is in practice seldom attempted in the UK.

Prediction of success: If a vaginal delivery is attempted, some 60–80% of women will deliver vaginally; the others will require an emergency Caesarean section in labour. Prediction of success is not reliable (*Obstet Gynecol* 2007; **109**: 800); factors associated with increased success include spontaneous labour, inter-pregnancy interval less than 2 years, low age and body mass index, Caucasian race, a previous vaginal delivery (chance of vaginal delivery 90%) and when the previous Caesarean section had been performed elec-tively (e.g. for breech presentation) or for fetal distress, as opposed to dystocia. Further, a smaller subsequent fetus and engagement of the head are good prognostic features.

Safety of vaginal delivery after Caesarean section

Unfortunately, no randomized controlled trials have been performed to compare VBAC with elective Caesar-ean. Women should be fully appraised of risks. In the absence of robust evidence, it is usual for them to decide on the mode of delivery.

Maternal: Maternal safety is related to the success rate of VBAC: the safest is a vaginal delivery, the least safe is emergency Caesarean section, with elective Caesarean between. Therefore, when attempting a VBAC, the maternal safety depends on the chance of such an emergency delivery. Overall, the risk of blood transfusion or uterine infection is about 1% higher with an attempt at VBAC. Serious maternal morbidity, however, is greater with increasing number of prior Cae-sarean deliveries: a particular risk is of placenta accreta [→ p.196].

Fetal: These are increased (3- to 10-fold) with VBAC (*JAMA* 2002; **287**: 2684). This is largely because elective Caesarean section, performed at 39 weeks, eliminates the risk of antepartum stillbirth beyond that time. The risk of VBAC itself is small: the usual, rare risks of labour, and rupture of the old uterine scar (Fig. 30.3) [→ p.264]. This occurs in 0.7% of

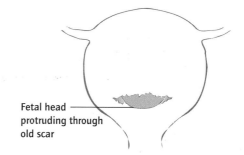

Fig. 30.3 Rupture of scar from previous Caesarean section.

Fetal head protruding through old scar

VBAC attempts overall, and has an approximately 10% perinatal mortality. The risk is higher with an un-successful VBAC (i.e. emergency Caesarean) and if labour is induced. It is related to the thickness of the lower uterine segment (*Lancet* 1996; **347**: 281). Nevertheless, the risk of stillbirth related to VBAC is low: approximately the same risk as found in a first labour. In contrast, transient tachypnoea of the newborn (TTN) is more common where elective Caesarean has been performed. Importantly, fetal morbidity is increased with increasing number of prior Caesarean deliveries.

Management of labour after a Caesarean section

Delivery in hospital and CTG are advised because of the risk of scar rupture. Induction, particularly with prostaglandins, is usually avoided as it is associated with a risk of rupture up to three times higher than with spontaneous labour. Caesarean is preferable unless induction is performed with amniotomy and the cervix is ripe or the fetal head is engaged. Augmentation also increases the risk of scar rupture and is performed with caution. Epidural analge-sia is safe, but labour should not be prolonged. Scar rupture usually presents as fetal distress, sometimes accompanied by scar pain, cessation of contractions, vaginal bleeding and even maternal collapse. Immediate laparotomy and Caesarean is indicated if rupture is suspected.

Prelabour term rupture of the membranes

In 10% of women after 37 weeks, the membranes rupture before the onset of labour. The reason is unknown in the majority of patients. This is to be distinguished from prelabour *preterm* rupture of the membranes [→ p.194], when the fetus is not mature.

Diagnosis of prelabour term rupture of the membranes

Typically, there is a gush of clear fluid, which is followed by an uncontrollable intermittent trickle. This is occasionally initially confused with urinary incontinence. The diagnosis, however, is seldom in doubt, although the finding of reduced liquor volume on ultrasound may help. A few have only a 'hindwater' rupture: that is, liquor is definitely leaking, but membranes remain present in front of the fetal head.

Risks of prelabour term rupture of the membranes

Cord prolapse is rare and usually a complication of transverse lie or breech presentation. There is a small but definite risk of neonatal infection: this is increased by vaginal examination (Fig. 30.4), the presence of group B streptococcus (GBS) [→ p.160] and increased duration of membrane rupture (*AmJOG* 1998; **179**: 635).

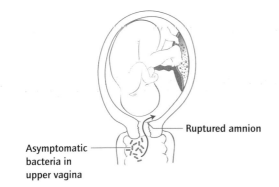

Fig. 30.4 Ascending infection can complicate prelabour rupture of the membranes.

Labels: Ruptured amnion; Asymptomatic bacteria in upper vagina

Management

Confirmation is made by identification of liquor. The lie and presentation are checked. Digital vaginal examination is usually avoided, but may be performed in a sterile manner if there is a risk of cord prolapse (abnormal lie or fetal distress); a vaginal swab is used to screen for infection. Fetal auscultation or CTG is performed. Management options are to await the spontaneous onset of labour, or to induce labour.

Induction of labour does not increase the risk of Caesarean section, and is associated with a lower chance of maternal infection. It is also associated with a lower risk of the baby being admitted to the neonatal unit. This policy is therefore slightly safer (*Cochrane* 2006; CD005302), particularly if the mother is a GBS carrier.

Waiting for spontaneous labour is common practice. Only 20% of women do not labour spontaneously within 24 h. The maternal pulse, temperature and fetal heart rate are measured every 4 h. The presence of meconium or evidence of infection warrants immediate induction. After 18–24 h, it is usual to prescribe antibiotics as a prophylaxis against GBS unless the presence of this bacterium in the vagina and rectum has recently been excluded using swabs, and to induce labour.

Further reading

Royal College of Obstetricians and Gynaecologists. Birth after previous Caesarean section. Green Top Guidelines. 2007. http://www.rcog.org.uk/resources/Public/pdf/green_top45_birthafter.pdf

Dare MR, Middleton P, Crowther CA, Flenady VJ, Varatharaju B. Planned early birth versus expectant management (waiting) for prelabour rupture of membranes at term (37 weeks or more). *Cochrane Database of Systematic Reviews* 2006; CD005302.

Kayani SI, Alfirevic Z. Induction of labour with previous caesarean delivery: where do we stand? *Current Opinion in Obstetrics and Gynecology* 2006; **18**: 636–41.

Landon MB, Hauth JC, Leveno KJ, *et al*. Maternal and perinatal outcomes associated with a trial of labor after prior cesarean delivery. *New England Journal of Medicine* 2004; **351**: 2581–9.

Mackenzie IZ. Induction of labour at the start of the new millennium. *Reproduction* 2006; **131**: 989–98.

Delivery after Caesarean Section at a Glance

Incidence	Many still undergo elective Caesarean; usual practice if >1
Success	60–80% vaginal delivery rate if labour attempted
Contraindications	Vertical uterine scar; usual indications for Caesarean
Safety	Emergency Caesarean section risk 20–40% Fetal and maternal risks slightly higher with attempt at vaginal delivery, but elective Caesarean makes subsequent pregnancies higher risk for both Scar rupture rate 0.7%
Management	Cardiotocography (CTG), careful monitoring of progress

Induction of Labour at a Glance

Definition	Labour is started artificially	
Methods	Vaginal prostaglandin E_2 (PGE_2)/misoprostol; amniotomy and oxytocin	
Main indications	Fetal:	Prolonged pregnancy, prelabour term spontaneous rupture of membranes (SROM), Intrauterine growth restriction (IUGR)
	Materno-fetal.	Pre-eclampsia, diabetes
	Maternal:	Social
Contraindications	Absolute:	Acute fetal distress; where elective Caesarean indicated
	Relative:	Previous lower segment Caesarean section (LSCS)
Complications	LSCS, other interventions in labour, longer labour, hyperstimulation, postpartum hemorrhage (PPH)	

Prelabour Term Rupture of the Membranes at a Glance

Definition	Membranes rupture after 37 weeks before the onset of labour
Incidence	10%: 80% start labour in <24 h
Features	Gush of fluid. Check temperature, lie/presentation. Avoid vaginal examination
Investigations	Cardiotocography (CTG), high vaginal swab (HVS)
Management	Antibiotics if >18 h duration. Consider immediate induction as risks lower, or wait 24 h

31 Instrumental and operative delivery

Forceps or ventouse delivery

These allow the use of traction if delivery needs to be expedited in the second stage of labour. The shape of the pelvis will only allow delivery if the occiput is anterior [→ p.227], or occasionally posterior. Rotation is therefore sometimes also needed. In the absence of rotation, instrumental delivery simply adds power. No instrument can drag a fetus that is too large through the pelvis, and technique and judgement are required. The aim is to prevent fetal and maternal morbidity associated with a prolonged second stage or expedite delivery where the fetus is compromised.

Ventouse

Also known as the vacuum extractor, this consists of a rubber or metal cap, connected to a handle; the cap is fixed near the fetal occiput by suction (Fig. 31.1). Traction during maternal pushing will deliver the occipito-anterior (OA) positioned head, but also usually allows the shape of the pelvis to simultaneously rotate a malpositioned head to the OA position. The ventouse can be used for most instrumental deliveries, the metal ventouse being most suitable for more difficult deliveries.

Obstetric forceps

These come in pairs that fit together for use. Each has a 'blade', shank, lock and handle. When assembled, the blades fit around the fetal head and the handles fit together (Fig. 31.2). The lock prevents them from slipping apart. *Non-rotational forceps* (e.g. Simpson's,

Neville–Barnes) grip the head in whatever position it is and allow traction. They are therefore only suitable when the occiput is anterior. These forceps have a 'cephalic' curve for the head and a 'pelvic curve' which follows the sacral curve. *Rotational forceps* (e.g. Kielland's) have no pelvic curve and enable a malpositioned head to be rotated by the operator to the OA position, before traction is applied.

Safety of ventouse and forceps

Failure: Both methods of delivery can fail: this is more common with the ventouse, particularly if the cup is placed inaccurately.

Maternal complications and the need for analgesia are greater with forceps (*Cochrane* 2000: CD000224), but use of either instrument can cause vaginal laceration, blood loss or third degree tears [→ p.246] (*BJOG* 1996; **103**: 845). Cervical and uterine tears are very rare.

Fetal complications are slightly worse with the ventouse. An unsightly 'chignon', a swelling of the area of scalp that was drawn into the cup by suction is usual. It diminishes over a period of hours, but a mark may be visible for days. Scalp lacerations, cephalhaematomata and neonatal jaundice are more common with the ventouse. Facial bruising, facial nerve damage and even skull and neck fractures occasionally occur with injudicious use of forceps, and prolonged traction by either instrument is dangerous.

Changing instrument: This is associated with increased fetal trauma, and is usually only appropriate if a ventouse has achieved descent to the pelvic outlet, but then comes off the head and is replaced by a low cavity forceps delivery (see below).

Indications for instrumental vaginal delivery

Prolonged second stage is the most common indication. Instrumental vaginal delivery is usual if 1 h of pushing

Obstetrics and Gynaecology, 3rd edition. By Lawrence Impey and Tim Child. Published 2008 by Blackwell Publishing, ISBN: 978-1-4051-6095-7.

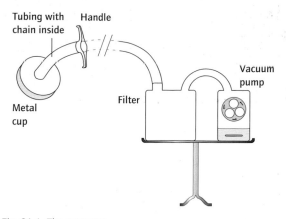

Fig. 31.1 The ventouse.

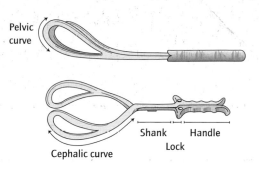

Fig. 31.2 Forceps (non-rotational).

(active second stage) has failed to deliver the baby. If the mother is exhausted it may be performed earlier. The length of passive second stage is less important.

Fetal distress: This is more common in the second stage: delivery can be expedited.

Prophylactic use of instrumental vaginal delivery is indicated to prevent pushing in some women with medical problems such as severe cardiac disease or hypertension.

In a breech delivery [→ p.215], forceps are often applied to the after-coming head to control the delivery.

Prevention of instrumental vaginal delivery

Whilst the ventouse and forceps have clear benefits, e.g. delayed second stage, avoidance of such circumstances is preferable.

All labours: Continuous support from the midwife [→ p.232] is essential, and delivery should be in the most comfortable maternal position possible.

Where epidural analgesia is used: In spite of the excellent analgesia and consequent popularity, epidural analgesia increases the risk of instrumental delivery (*AmJOG* 2002; **186**: S69): if used, maternal pushing should be delayed at least an hour after the diagnosis of second stage unless the head is visible, oxytocin should be considered if descent of the head is poor (only in nulliparous women), and pushing should be directed.

Types of instrumental vaginal delivery

The type of delivery and choice of instrument is determined by the *position* and *descent* of the head: no instrument should be regarded as 'first choice' for all situations, but an overall comparison of forceps and ventouse is shown on p. 259. With either instrument, if moderate traction does not produce immediate and progressive descent, Caesarean section is indicated. 'High' forceps deliveries (the head is not engaged) are dangerous and obsolete. Caesarean section at full cervical dilatation is increasingly used as an alternative to instrumental delivery. However, it is often difficult surgically and is associated with increased maternal trauma and neonatal unit admission (*Lancet* 2001; **358**: 1203).

Low-cavity delivery

The head is well below the level of the ischial spines, bony prominences palpable vaginally on the lateral wall of the mid-pelvis [→ p.224] and is usually occipito-anterior (OA) (Fig. 31.3a). Forceps or a ventouse are appropriate (see box below), the former being better if maternal effort is poor. A pudendal block [→ p.242] with perineal infiltration is usually sufficient analgesia.

Mid-cavity delivery

The head is still not palpable abdominally, but is at or just below the level of the ischial spines (Fig. 31.3a). Epidural or spinal anaesthesia are usual. If there is any doubt that delivery will be successful, it is attempted in the operating theatre, with full preparations for a Caesarean section. This is called a 'trial' of forceps or ventouse. The

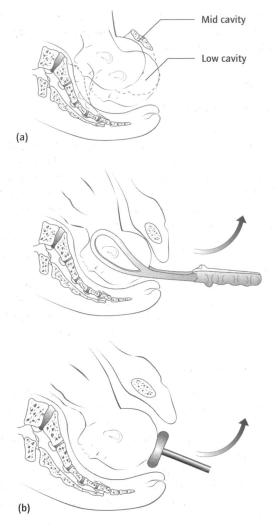

Fig. 31.3 (a) Side view of pelvis showing level of head for mid-cavity and low-cavity forceps delivery. (b) Forceps and ventouse in position on the fetal head showing direction of traction.

position may be OA, occipito-transverse (OT) or occipito-posterior (OP).

Occipito-anterior position: Forceps or a ventouse can be used.

Occipito-transverse position: Usually this is a result of insufficient descent of the head to make it rotate. Therefore, descent is achieved with the ventouse, with rotation resulting. Non-rotational forceps are contraindicated.

Rotation *in situ* followed by descent can also sometimes be achieved by manual rotation or with Kielland's rotational forceps (see below).

Occipito-posterior position: This is often accompanied by extension of the fetal head [→ p.226] making the presenting diameter too large for the pelvis. One-fifth of the head may still be palpable abdominally. The need for instrumental delivery is unusual in multiparous women and if required, this position should be suspected. Simply dragging out a baby in this position may fail or cause severe perineal damage. Rotation of 180° can be achieved manually, or with the ventouse, but is most successful with Kielland's forceps. Some regard these forceps as dangerous, but in trained, skilled hands, they are extremely effective.

Common indications for ventouse or forceps delivery
Prolonged active second stage
Maternal exhaustion
Fetal distress in second stage

Prerequisites for instrumental vaginal delivery

Both forceps and the ventouse are potentially dangerous instruments and their use is subject to stringent conditions. *The head must not be palpable abdominally* (therefore deeply engaged); on vaginal examination the head must be *at or below the level of the ischial spines*. *The cervix must be fully dilated*: the second stage must have been reached (occasional exceptions are made by experts delivering with the ventouse for fetal distress). *The position of the head must be known*: incorrect placement of forceps or ventouse may cause fetal and maternal trauma as well as result in failure. There must be *adequate analgesia*. The *bladder should be empty*: catheterization is normally required. The operator must be skilled and delivering for a *valid reason*.

Prerequisites for ventouse or forceps delivery
Head not palpable abdominally
Head at/below ischial spines on vaginal examination
Cervix fully dilated
Position of head known
Adequate analgesia
Valid indication for delivery
Bladder empty

> **Forceps or ventouse?**
>
> *Ventouse causes:*
> Higher failure rate
> (but lower segment Caesarean section [LSCS] not more
> common if forceps then used)
> More fetal trauma
> No difference in Apgar scores
> Less maternal trauma

Instrumental delivery rates

A 'normal' vaginal delivery usually produces less blood loss, requires less analgesia and is safer and more pleasant for mother and baby unless a valid indication for intervention is present. In the UK, approximately 20% of nulliparous and 2% of multiparous women are delivered by forceps or ventouse.

Caesarean section

Delivery by Caesarean section occurs for 20–30% of babies in the developed world. The usual operation is the lower segment operation (lower segment Caesarean section [LSCS]), in which the abdominal wall is opened with a suprapubic transverse incision and the lower segment of the uterus is also incised transversely to deliver the baby (Fig. 31.4). Very occasionally, such as with extreme prematurity, multiple fibroids or where the fetus is transverse, the uterus may be incised vertically: this is called a classic Caesarean section. After

delivery of the placenta, the uterus and abdomen are sutured. A trial (CAESAR) examining different surgical techniques is in progress.

Indications

Emergency Caesarean section

This is performed in labour.
Prolonged first stage of labour is diagnosed when full dilatation is not imminent by 12 h, or earlier if labour was initially rapid. Occasionally, full dilatation is achieved but not all the criteria for instrumental delivery are met. Most commonly, it is due to abnormalities of the 'powers': inefficient uterine action. The 'passenger' (malposition or malpresentation) or 'passage' (pelvic abnormalities and cephalo-pelvic disproportion) can also contribute [→ p.237].
Fetal distress is diagnosed from abnormalities of the fetal heart rate, normally in conjunction with fetal blood sampling [→ p.239]. A Caesarean section is performed if it is the quickest route of delivery for the baby.

Elective Caesarean section

This is performed to avoid labour. It is normally performed at 39 weeks' gestation to reduce the risk of neonatal lung immaturity (*BJOG* 1995; **102**: 101). If earlier, administration of steroids [→ p.194] should be considered (*BMJ* 2005; **331**: 662).
Absolute indications are placenta praevia, severe antenatal fetal compromise, uncorrectable abnormal lie, previous vertical Caesarean section and gross pelvic deformity.

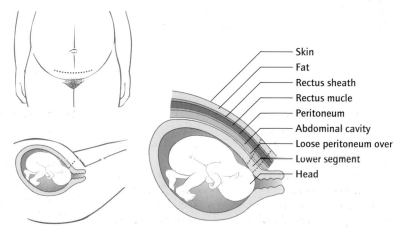

Skin
Fat
Rectus sheath
Rectus mucle
Peritoneum
Abdominal cavity
Loose peritoneum over
Lower segment
Head

Fig. 31.4   Layers of the abdominal wall for delivery of fetus by Caesarean section.

Relative indications include: breech presentation, twin pregnancy, diabetes mellitus and other medical diseases, previous Caesarean section and older nulliparous patients.

When delivery is needed before 34 weeks, it is usual to perform a Caesarean section rather than induce labour. The most common indications are severe pre-eclampsia and severe intrauterine growth restriction.

Elective Caesarean for maternal request

This is becoming increasingly common. The ethics surrounding this are complex (*BJOG* 2002; **109**: 593). As emergency Caesarean sections in labour have become commonplace it is not surprising that some women would rather have the Caesarean without several hours of labour first. In most cases, if the obstetrician understands and addresses the reasons for the request, both conflict and a Caesarean section can be avoided: Caesarean section is commonly perceived to be the answer to many concerns, but in reality such problems and anxieties can be addressed within the context of a normal birth. If this is not possible, most obstetricians now agree to the procedure.

Common reasons for Caesarean section	
Emergency:	Failure to progress in labour
	Fetal distress
Elective:	Previous Caesarean section(s)
	Breech presentation

Definition of type/urgency of Caesarean section	
Emergency	Immediate threat to mother or fetus, e.g. severe fetal distress
Urgent	Maternal/fetal compromise not immediately life-threatening, e.g. dystocia
Scheduled	Needing early delivery but no compromise
Elective	At time to suit mother and team
Peri-/postmortem	For fetus and mother during maternal arrest/for fetus after maternal death

Safety and complications of Caesarean section

Maternal

Although serious complications are rare, these are greater than with a normal vaginal delivery. They are more common where the procedure is an emergency, in labour, than when it is elective. Complications may also be related to the indication for the Caesarean: as it is frequently used for complicated pregnancies. Complications include *haemorrhage* and the need for *blood transfusion, infection of the uterus or wound* (up to 20%), rare *visceral*, e.g. bladder or bowel damage, postoperative pain and immobility, and *venous thromboembolism*. Prophylactic antibiotics, which reduce the incidence of infection (*Cochrane* 2002: CD000933), and thromboprophylactic measures [→p.181] are routine. Overall, approximately 1 in 5000 women will die after a Caesarean.

Fetal

An elective procedure increases the risk of *fetal respiratory morbidity* at any given gestation, and in an uncomplicated pregnancy should not be performed before 39 weeks. Although usually minor, this occurs in up to 4% even at this stage. *Fetal lacerations* are rare and usually minor. *Bonding and breastfeeding* are particularly affected by emergency procedures. Controversial evidence suggests that neonatal morbidity and mortality is increased with elective Caesarean section (*BMJ* 2007; **335**: 1025). This is surprising given the small but clear risks of labour and may result from confounding variables in the data.

Subsequent pregnancies

Caesarean sections become increasingly difficult although in practice of course no 'limit' can be set. A small increase in stillbirth in subsequent pregnancies is debated (*BJOG* 2008; **115**: 726). Importantly, the incidence of placenta praevia is more common in pregnancies after a Caesarean. Further, the placenta may implant more deeply than normal, in the myometrium (accreta) or through into surrounding structures (percreta) [→ p.196]. For a third Caesarean section, the overall risk of placenta accreta is 0.57%, and 40% if the placenta is praevia (*Obstet Gynecol* 2006; **107**: 1226). This placental invasion can be diagnosed with ultrasound scanning or MRI with reasonable accuracy. Surgery should be performed by the most senior person available, with full anaesthetic and urological back up. Blood must be cross matched. For percreta, facilities ready for internal iliac artery embolisation are advised; for accreta, leaving the uterus *in situ* or compression of the placental site, after piecemeal removal of the placenta, with a Rusch balloon may alleviate or reduce haemorrhage. Ultimately, hysterectomy may be required: delay in performing this can be lethal. This problem is a good argument against the widespread use of Caesarean section.

Caesarean section rates

Discussion of Caesarean section rates is on p. 277.

Further reading

Murphy DJ. Failure to progress in the second stage of labour. *Current Opinions in Obstetrics and Gynecology* 2001; **13**: 557–61.

Royal College of Obstetricians and Gynaecologists. Operative vaginal delivery. Green Top Guideline No 26. 2005. http://www.rcog.org.uk/resources/Public/pdf/operative_vaginal_delivery.pdf

Royal College of Obstetricians and Gynaecologists. Placenta praevia and placenta praevia accreta: diagnosis and management. Green Top Guideline No 27. 2005. http://www.rcog.org.uk/resources/Public/pdf/placenta_praevia_accreta.pdf

Royal College of Obstetricians and Gynaecologists. *The National Sentinel Caesarean Section Audit*. The Royal College of Obstetricians and Gynaecologists Press, London, 2001.

Villar J, Carroli G, Zavaleta N, *et al*. World Health Organization, 2005. Global Survey on Maternal and Perinatal Health Research Group. Maternal and neonatal individual risks and benefits associated with caesarean delivery: multicentre prospective study. *British Medical Journal* 2007; **335**: 1025. Epub 2007; Oct 30.

Forceps and Ventouse at a Glance	
Descriptions	Ventouse attaches by suction, allowing traction with rotation Non-rotational forceps grip and allow traction Rotational forceps grip, allow rotation and then traction
Rates	20%, nulliparous; 2%, multiparous
Indications	Prolonged second stage, fetal distress in second stage, when maternal pushing contraindicated
Prerequisites	Cervix fully dilated, position of head known, head deeply engaged and mid-cavity or below, adequate analgesia, empty bladder, valid indication
Complications	Maternal trauma: Lacerations, haemorrhage, third degree tears Fetal trauma: Lacerations, bruising, facial nerve injury, hypoxia if prolonged delivery

Caesarean Section at a Glance	
Descriptions	Lower segment (>99%); classical (vertical) rare
Rates	20–30%
Common indications	Elective: Breech presentation, previous lower segment Caesarean section (LSCS), placenta praevia Emergency: Failure to advance, fetal distress
Complications	Haemorrhage, uterine/wound sepsis, thromboembolism, anaesthetic

32   Obstetric emergencies

Shoulder dystocia

Definition and consequences

This is when additional manoeuvres are required after normal downward traction has failed to deliver the shoulders after the head has delivered. Occurring in approximately 1 in 200 deliveries, it requires urgent and skilled help. Excessive traction on the neck damages the brachial plexus, resulting in Erb's (waiter's tip) palsy, which is permanent in about 50% of cases (Fig. 32.1). The delay, and possibly unskilled attempts at delivery, can be lethal: the mean time from delivery of the head to delivery of the shoulders in a series of lethal cases was only 5 minutes (*BJOG* 1998; **105**: 1256).

Risk factors and prevention

The principal risk is the large baby, but only about half of all cases occur in babies over 4 kg. Further, antenatal prediction of fetal size, even with ultrasound, is poor. Other reported factors include previous shoulder dystocia, increased maternal body mass index (BMI), labour induction, low height, maternal diabetes and instrumental delivery. Antenatal prediction (*AmJOG* 2006; **195**: 1544) is limited by the poor sensitivity even of integration [→ p.149] of these risk factors, coupled with the rarity of a serious outcome and the fact that prevention involves Caesarean section. Most cases are therefore considered unpreventable.

Management

This requires rapid and skilled intervention: teaching of this rather than attempted prevention is current prac-

Obstetrics and Gynaecology, 3rd edition. By Lawrence Impey and Tim Child. Published 2008 by Blackwell Publishing, ISBN: 978-1-4051-6095-7.

262

tice. A sequence of actions is recommended. Because the obstruction is at the pelvic inlet, excessive traction is useless, and will cause Erb's palsy: gentle downward traction is used. Initially, senior help is requested, and the legs are hyperextended onto the abdomen (McRoberts' manoeuvre); suprapubic pressure is also applied. These methods work in about 90% of cases. If they fail, internal manoeuvres are required, necessitating episiotomy. If the shoulders are transverse, pressure behind the anterior shoulder will rotate it to the widest diameter; this can be combined with pressure on the anterior part of the posterior shoulder (Wood's screw manoeuvre). If this fails, the posterior arm is grasped and, by extension at the elbow, the hand is brought down. The trunk will either follow, or rotation of the body using the arm is performed, causing the anterior shoulder to enter the pelvis. Last resorts include symphisiotomy, after lateral replacement of the urethra with a metal catheter, and the Zavanelli manoeuvre. This involves replacement of the head and Caesarean section, but by this time fetal damage is usually irreversible.

Cord prolapse

Definition and consequences

This occurs when, after the membranes have ruptured, the umbilical cord descends below the presenting part (Fig. 32.2). Untreated, the cord will be compressed or go into spasm and the baby will rapidly become hypoxic. It occurs in 1 in 500 deliveries.

Risk factors and prevention

Risks include preterm labour, breech presentation, polyhydramnios, abnormal lie and twin pregnancy. More than half occur at artificial amniotomy. The diagnosis is usually made when the fetal heart rate becomes abnor-

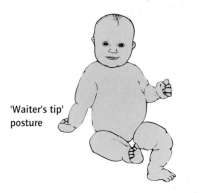

Fig. 32.1 Erb's palsy of right arm in characteristic 'waiter's tip' position.

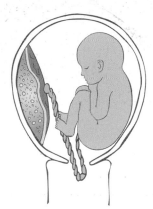

Fig. 32.2 Cord prolapse (here associated with flexed breech presentation).

mal and the cord is palpated vaginally, or if it appears at the introitus. The widespread practice of delivering breeches by Caesarean section has reduced the incidence.

Management

Initially, the presenting part must be prevented from compressing the cord: it is pushed up by the examining finger, or tocolytics such as terbutaline are given. If the cord is out of the introitus, it should be kept warm and moist but not forced back inside. The patient is asked to go on 'all fours', whilst preparations for delivery by the safest route are undertaken. Caesarean section, as fast as possible, is normally used, but instrumental vaginal delivery is appropriate if the cervix is fully dilated and the head is low. With prompt treatment, fetal mortality is rare.

Amniotic fluid embolism

Definition and consequences

This is when liquor enters the maternal circulation, causing sudden dyspnoea, hypoxia and hypotension, often accompanied by seizures and cardiac arrest. Acute heart failure is evident. It is extremely rare (approxi-

mately 1 in 50 000 pregnancies) but is an important cause of maternal mortality because 80% die: it accounted for 17 deaths in the UK in the 3 years 2002–05 (CEMACH 2007). If the woman survives for 30 minutes, she will rapidly develop disseminated intravascular coagulation (DIC), and often pulmonary oedema and adult respiratory distress syndrome (ARDS). In a few, haemorrhage from DIC is the first presentation.

Risk factors

It typically occurs when the membranes rupture, but may occur during labour, at Caesarean section and even at termination of pregnancy. There are multiple mild predisposing factors, particularly strong contractions in the presence of polyhydramnios, but prevention is impossible.

Management

The diagnosis is easily confused with other causes of collapse, and with eclampsia and is usually only made with certainty at postmortem. Resuscitation and supportive treatment as for any cause of collapse is key. Oxygen and fluid under central venous monitoring is used. Blood for clotting, full blood count, electrolytes and cross-match is taken. Blood and fresh frozen plasma (FFP) will be required. The patient is transferred to an intensive care unit.

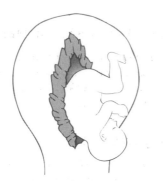

Fig. 32.3 Massive 'primary' rupture of the uterus with extrusion of the fetus.

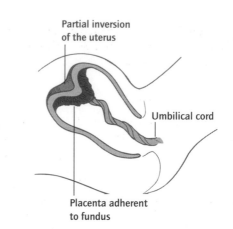

Fig. 32.4 Inverted uterus.

Uterine rupture

Definition and consequences

The uterus can tear *de novo* (Fig. 32.3) or an old scar (e.g. from a Caesarean section) can open. The fetus is extruded, the uterus contracts down and bleeds from the rupture site, causing acute fetal hypoxia and massive internal maternal haemorrhage. Rupture of a lower transverse Caesarean scar is usually less serious than a primary rupture or one from a classic Caesarean: the lower segment is not very vascular and heavy blood loss and extrusion of the fetus into the abdomen are less likely. Nevertheless, the neonatal mortality even from these is about 10%. Rupture occurs in 1 in 1500 pregnancies, and in 0.7% of women who attempt a vaginal delivery after a single previous lower section Caesarean section (LSCS). The diagnosis is suspected from fetal heart rate abnormalities or a constant lower abdominal pain; vaginal bleeding, cessation of contractions and maternal collapse may also occur.

Risk factors and prevention

Principal risk factors include *labours with a scarred uterus*: a classic Caesarean [→ p.259] or deep myomectomy [→ p.128] carry higher risks than that of previous LSCS. Rupture before labour of a scarred uterus is rare. *Neglected obstructed labour* is rare in the West but is a common obstetric emergency in developing countries. *Congenital uterine abnormalities* occasionally cause rupture before labour. Preventive measures include caution when using oxytocin in women with a previous Caesarean section, and elective Caesarean section in women with a uterine scar not in the lower segment.

Management

Maternal resuscitation with intravenous fluid and blood is required. Blood is taken for clotting, haemoglobin and cross-match is taken. Blood loss may be faster than can be replaced and urgent laparotomy for delivery of the fetus and cessation of maternal bleeding by repair or removal of the uterus is indicated. Uterine rupture has a high recurrence rate in subsequent pregnancies and early Caesarean delivery is required.

Other obstetric emergencies

Uterine inversion

This is when the fundus inverts into the uterine cavity (Fig. 32.4). It usually follows traction on the placenta and occurs in 1 in 20 000 deliveries. Haemorrhage, pain and profound shock are normal. A brief attempt is made immediately to push the fundus up via the vagina. If impossible, a general anaesthetic is given and replacement performed with hydrostatic pressure of several litres of warm saline, which is run past a clenched fist at the introitus into the vagina.

Epileptiform seizures

These are most commonly the result of maternal epilepsy or eclampsia [→ p.169], but can also be due to hypoxia from any cause. The airway is cleared with suction and oxygen administered. Cardiopulmonary resuscitation may be required. The patient is not restrained but is prevented from hurting herself. In the absence of cardiopulmonary collapse, diazepam will normally stop the fit in the first instance. However, it is wise to assume eclampsia is responsible, until this is excluded by the absence of suggestive examination and laboratory findings. Magnesium sulphate is not useful for non-eclamptic seizures and is therefore inappropriate where the diagnosis is uncertain, but it is superior to diazepam in the eclamptic woman (*Lancet* 1995; **345**: 1455).

Local anaesthetic toxicity

Excessive doses or inadvertent intravenous doses of local anaesthetic can cause transient cardiac, respiratory and neurological consequences, occasionally resulting in cardiac arrest. Prevention is most important; treatment involves resuscitation and even intubation until the effects have worn off.

Massive antepartum haemorrhage

This is discussed on p. 200 (and management section [→ p.304]). The key is to appreciate that blood loss may be internal, that replacement of normovolaemia and cessation of bleeding are required, and that, provided a coagulopathy (e.g. DIC) is treated, delivery of the fetus may save it and prevent further bleeding.

Massive postpartum haemorrhage

This is discussed on p. 267 (and management section [→ p.310]). The principles are the same. Surgical management is used only if medical management has failed, but procrastination is lethal.

Pulmonary embolus

This is discussed on p. 180 (and management section [→ p.309]). Most occur postpartum and can present with cardiac arrest. Thromboprophylaxis [→ p.181] is essential to prevent this common cause of maternal death.

Further reading

Dyachenko A, Ciampi A, Fahey J, Mighty H, Oppenheimer L, Hamilton EF. Prediction of risk for shoulder dystocia with neonatal injury. *American Journal of Obstetrics and Gynecology* 2006; **195**: 1544–9.

Kaczmarczyk M, Sparén P, Terry P, Cnattingius S. Risk factors for uterine rupture and neonatal consequences of uterine rupture: a population-based study of successive pregnancies in Sweden. *BJOG: an International Journal of Obstetrics and Gynaecology* 2007; **114**: 1208–14.

Moore J, Baldisseri MR. Amniotic fluid embolism. *Critical Care Medicine* 2005; **33**: S279–85.

Murphy D, MacKenzie I. The mortality and morbidity associated with umbilical cord prolapse. *British Journal of Obstetrics and Gynaecology* 1995; **102**: 826–30.

Murphy DJ. Uterine rupture. *Current Opinions in Obstetrics and Gynecology* 2006; **18**: 135–40.

Royal College of Obstetricians and Gynaecologists. Shoulder dystocia. Green Top Guideline No 42. 2005. http://www.rcog.org.uk/resources/Public/pdf/shoulder_dystocia_42.pdf

33 The puerperium

The puerperium is the 6-week period following delivery, when the body returns to its prepregnant state. Obstetric involvement is often lacking; midwives conduct most postpartum care. However, maternal morbidity and mortality associated with pregnancy is highest during this period. Many women continue to have problems after discharge, and the lack of medical interest means these problems often go untreated or even unrecognized.

Physiological changes in the puerperium

The genital tract: Immediately the placenta has separated, the uterus contracts and the criss-cross fibres of myometrium occlude the blood vessels that formerly supplied the placenta. Uterine size reduces over 6 weeks: within 10 days the uterus is no longer palpable abdominally (Fig. 33.1). Contractions or 'after pains' may be felt for 4 days. The internal os of the cervix is closed by 3 days. Lochia, a discharge from the uterus, may be blood-stained for at least 14 days, but thereafter is yellow or white. Menstruation is usually delayed by lactation, but occurs at about 6 weeks if the woman is not lactating.

The cardiovascular system: Cardiac output and plasma volume decrease to prepregnant levels within a week. Loss of oedema can take up to 6 weeks. If transiently elevated, blood pressure is usually normal within 6 weeks.

The urinary tract: The physiological dilatation of pregnancy reduces over 3 months and glomerular filtration rate (GFR) decreases.

The blood: Urea and electrolyte levels return to normal because of the reduction in GFR. In the absence of haemorrhage, haemoglobin and haematocrit rise with haemoconcentration. The white blood count falls. Platelets and clotting factors rise, predisposing to thrombosis.

General postnatal care

The mother and baby should not be separated, and privacy is important. Early mobilization is encouraged. Counselling and practical help with breastfeeding are often required. Uterine involution and the lochia, blood pressure, temperature, pulse and any perineal wound are checked daily. Careful fluid balance checks should prevent retention if a woman has had an epidural. Analgesics may be required for perineal pain, which is also helped by pelvic floor exercises. The full blood count may be checked before discharge, and iron is prescribed if appropriate, usually in conjunction with laxatives.

Ideally, the midwife or doctor who attended the delivery should visit the patient after delivery. The circumstances of the delivery should be discussed, particularly if there has been obstetric intervention, and the woman given the opportunity to ask questions about her labour. Discharge should be dependent on the mother's wishes: some like to leave hospital within 6 h of delivery; others will need a few days in hospital. The GP should be alerted of any complications. In the UK, a community midwife, preferably one who knows the woman, can visit daily for the next 10 days. Advice regarding contraception is given prior to discharge.

Psychiatric disease and suicide are now recognized as major contributors to maternal death. Most women have a psychiatric history but this is often not recorded. Psychiatric referral is recommended for women with such a history, and a postnatal plan including the GP is drawn up. Vigilance for evidence of depression is essential.

Obstetrics and Gynaecology, 3rd edition. By Lawrence Impey and Tim Child. Published 2008 by Blackwell Publishing, ISBN: 978-1-4051-6095-7.

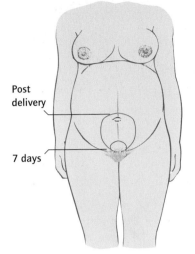

Post delivery

7 days

Fig. 33.1 Diagram of uterine involution.

Lactation

Physiology

Lactation is dependent on prolactin and oxytocin. Prolactin from the anterior pituitary gland stimulates milk secretion. Levels of prolactin are high at birth, but it is the rapid decline in oestrogen and progesterone levels after birth that causes milk to be secreted, because prolactin is antagonized by oestrogen and progesterone. Oxytocin from the posterior pituitary stimulates ejection in response to nipple suckling, which also stimulates prolactin release and therefore more milk secretion. As much as 1000+ mL of milk per day can be produced, dependent on demand. Since oxytocin release is controlled via the hypothalamus, lactation can be inhibited by emotional or physical stress. Colostrum, a yellow fluid containing fat-laden cells, proteins (including immunoglobulin A) and minerals, is passed for the first 3 days, before the milk 'comes in'.

Management

Women should be gently encouraged to breastfeed, when the baby is ready. Early feeding should be on demand. Correct positioning of the baby is vital: the baby's lower lip should be planted below the nipple at the time that the mouth opens in preparation for receiving milk, so that the entire nipple is drawn into the mouth. This could largely prevent the main problems of insufficient milk, engorgement, mastitis and nipple trauma. A restful, comfortable environment is important, not least because oxytocin secretion, and therefore milk ejection, can be reduced by stress. Supplementation is unnecessary, although vitamin K should be given (*BMJ* 1996; **313**: 199) to reduce the chances of haemorrhagic disease of the newborn.

Composition of human milk	
Protein	1.0%
Carbohydrate	7.0%
Fat	4.0%
Minerals	0.2%
Immunoglobulins	Mainly immunoglobulin A
Energy	70 kcal/100 mL

Advantages of breastfeeding
Protection against infection in neonate
Bonding
Protection against cancers (mother)
Cannot give too much
Cost saving

Postnatal contraception
Lactation not adequate alone, but important on global scale
Contraception is usually started 4–6 weeks after delivery
Combined contraceptive suppresses lactation and contraindicated if breastfeeding
Progesterone-only (pill or depot) safe with breastfeeding
Intrauterine device (IUD) safe: screen for infection first. Insert at end of third stage or at 6 weeks

Primary postpartum haemorrhage

Definition and epidemiology

Primary primary postpartum haemorrhage (PPH) is the loss of >500 mL blood <24 h of delivery. It occurs in

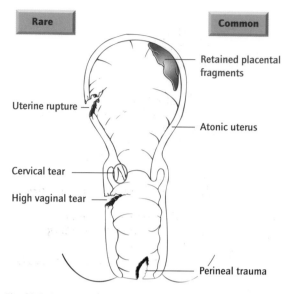

Rare

Common

Retained placental fragments

Uterine rupture

Atonic uterus

Cervical tear

High vaginal tear

Perineal trauma

Fig. 33.2 Causes and sites of postpartum haemorrhage (PPH).

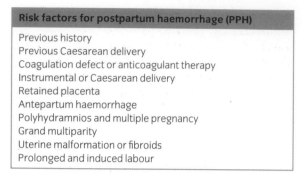

Risk factors for postpartum haemorrhage (PPH)

Previous history
Previous Caesarean delivery
Coagulation defect or anticoagulant therapy
Instrumental or Caesarean delivery
Retained placenta
Antepartum haemorrhage
Polyhydramnios and multiple pregnancy
Grand multiparity
Uterine malformation or fibroids
Prolonged and induced labour

about 10% of women and remains a major cause of maternal mortality.

Aetiology (Fig. 33.2)

Retained placenta occurs in 2.5% of deliveries. Partial separation can cause blood to accumulate in the uterus, which will rise. Collapse may occur in the absence of external loss.

Uterine causes account for 80%. The uterus fails to contract properly, either because it is 'atonic' or because there is a retained placenta, or part of the placenta. Atony is more common with prolonged labour, with grand multiparity and with overdistension of the uterus (polyhydramnios and multiple pregnancy) and fibroids. Blood loss exceeds 500 mL at many Caesarean sections.

Vaginal causes account for about 20%. Bleeding from a perineal tear or episiotomy is obvious, but a high vaginal tear must be considered, particularly after an instrumental vaginal delivery.

Cervical tears are rare, but associated with precipitate labour and instrumental delivery.

Coagulopathy is rare. Congenital disorders, anticoagulant therapy or disseminated intravascular coagulation (DIC) all cause PPH.

Prevention

Routine use of oxytocin in the third stage of labour reduces the incidence of PPH by 60%. Oxytocin is as effective as ergometrine (*Cochrane* 2001: CD001808) which often causes vomiting and is contraindicated in hypertensive women.

Clinical features

Blood loss should be minimal after delivery of the placenta. An enlarged uterus (above the level of the umbilicus) suggests a uterine cause. The vaginal walls and cervix are inspected for tears. Occasionally blood loss may be abdominal: there is collapse without overt bleeding.

Management

To resuscitate, the patient is nursed flat, intravenous access is obtained, blood is cross-matched and blood volume is restored. Anaesthetic, haematological and senior obstetric help are required in severe cases.

A retained placenta [→ p.245] should be removed manually if there is bleeding, or if it is not expelled by normal methods within 60 minutes of delivery.

To identify and treat the cause of bleeding, vaginal examination is performed to exclude the rare uterine inversion and the uterus is bimanually compressed. Vaginal lacerations are often palpable. Uterine causes are common and oxytocin and/or ergometrine is given intravenously to contract the uterus if trauma is not obvious. If this fails, an examination under anaesthetic (EUA) is performed: the cavity of the uterus is explored manually for retained placental fragments and the cervix and vagina inspected for tears, which should be sutured. If uterine atony persists, prostaglandin $F_{2\alpha}$ ($PGF_{2\alpha}$) is injected into the myometrium.

Persistent haemorrhage despite medical treatment requires surgery. Bleeding from a placental bed (well-contracted uterus with no trauma) may respond to placement of a Rusch balloon. Other methods to treat haemorrhage include a brace suture (*BJOG* 1997; **104**: 372) and uterine artery embolization. If these fail, hysterectomy should not be delayed.

Other problems of the puerperium

Secondary PPH

Secondary PPH is 'excessive' blood loss occurring between 24 h and 6 weeks after delivery. It is due to endometritis [→ p.74], with or without retained placental tissue, or, rarely, incidental gynaecological pathology or gestational trophoblastic disease [→ p.122]. The uterus is enlarged and tender with an open internal cervical os.

Vaginal swabs and a full blood count is taken, and cross-match in severe cases. Ultrasound is often used but differentiation between blood clot and retained placental tissue is poor. Antibiotics are given. If bleeding is heavy, evacuation of retained products of conception (ERPC [→ p.127]) is used. If the bleeding is more chronic, antibiotics are used initially alone: characteristically, endometritis due to retained tissue causes bleeding that slows, but does not stop, with antibiotics and gets worse again after the course is finished. Histological examination of the evacuated tissues will exclude gestational trophoblastic disease.

Postpartum pyrexia

This is a maternal fever of ≥38°C in the first 14 days. *Infection* is the most common cause. Genital tract sepsis (endometritis) is a major cause of maternal mortality, in addition to the long-term consequences of pelvic infection [→ p.76]. It is most common after Caesarean section: prophylactic antibiotics considerably reduce this. Group A streptococcus, staphylococcus and *Escherichia coli* are the most important pathogens in severe cases. The lochia may be offensive and the uterus is enlarged and tender. Urinary infection (10%), chest infection, mastitis, perineal infection and wound infection after Caesarean section are also common (Fig. 33.3). Careful examination of the

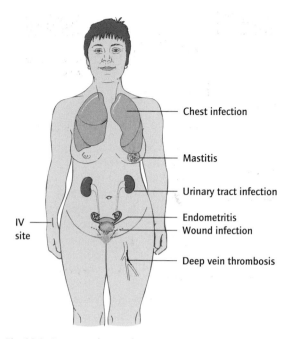

Fig. 33.3 Causes and sites of postpartum pyrexia.

Labels: Chest infection; Mastitis; Urinary tract infection; Endometritis; Wound infection; Deep vein thrombosis; IV site

abdomen, breasts, any intravenous access sites, chest and legs is required. Blood, urine, high vaginal and fetal cultures are taken. Broad-spectrum antibiotics are given. *Deep vein thrombosis* (DVT) often causes a low-grade pyrexia.

Thromboembolic disease

Deep vein thrombosis or pulmonary embolism is a leading cause of maternal mortality, although less than 0.5% of women are affected. Half the deaths are postnatal, usually after discharge from hospital. Early mobility and hydration is important for all women. Risk factors, prevention and treatment are discussed elsewhere [→ p.181].

Psychiatric problems of the puerperium

'Third day blues', consisting of temporary emotional lability, affects 50% of women. Support and reassurance are required.
Postnatal depression affects 10% of women but most do

not present and receive no help. Questionnaires, such as the Edinburgh Postnatal Depression Scale (EPDS) are helpful in identifying this extremely important problem, but screening is difficult (*Acta Psychiatr Scand* 2003; **107**: 10). Depression is more common in women who are socially or emotionally isolated, with a previous history, or after pregnancy complications. Postpartum thyroiditis [→ p.179] should be considered. The severity is variable, but symptoms include tiredness, guilt and feelings of worthlessness. Treatment involves social support and psychotherapy. Antidepressants (*Cochrane* 2001: CD002018) are used in conjunction with these. Postnatal depression frequently recurs in subsequent pregnancies and is associated (70% risk) with depression later in life.

Suicide is a major cause of death postpartum. Most women have a history of depressive or other psychiatric illness, particularly bipolar disorder. This must be recorded at the booking visit. In general, psychiatric drugs should be continued in pregnancy, but this decision should be made, preferably preconceptually, after assessment of the risks and benefits [→ p.182]. For depressive illness, selective serotonin reuptake inhibitors (SSRIs), such as fluoxetine, are preferred. Women with a history of mental illness should see a psychiatrist before delivery, and a multidisciplinary plan for postnatal discharge arranged.

Puerperal psychosis affects 0.2% of women and is characterized by abrupt onset of psychotic symptoms, usually around the fourth day. It is more common in primigravid women with a family history. Treatment involves psychiatric admission and major tranquillizers, after exclusion of organic illness. There is usually a full recovery, but some develop mental illness in later life and 10% relapse after a subsequent pregnancy.

Hypertensive complications

Pre-eclampsia and its complications [→ p.165] are a major cause of maternal mortality and most deaths occur postpartum. Although delivery is the only cure for pre-eclampsia, it often takes at least 24 h before the illness improves and the blood pressure, which usually peaks 4–5 days after delivery, may need treatment for weeks. In all pre-eclamptic patients, attention must be paid to the fluid balance, renal function and urine output, blood pressure and the possibility of hepatic or cardiac failure: discharge before 5 days may lead to complications being missed.

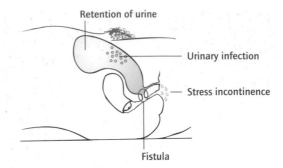

Fig. 33.4 Postpartum urinary problems.

The urinary tract (Fig. 33.4)

Retention of urine is common after delivery, and although it is usually painful it may not be after epidural analgesia. It may present with frequency, stress incontinence or severe abdominal pain, but the woman or staff may not notice the lack of voiding. Infection, overflow incontinence and permanent voiding difficulties [→ p.64] may follow. It can be identified by strict fluid charts and abdominal palpation. Post-micturition ultrasound can be used to assess the residual volume non-invasively. Treatment is with catheterization for at least 24 h.

Urinary infection occurs in 10% of women. It is usually asymptomatic but, as in pregnancy, often leads to symptomatic infection or pyelonephritis. Routine urine culture is advised.

Incontinence occurs in 20% of women. Overflow and infection should be excluded using post-micturition ultrasound or catheterization and a mid-stream urine (MSU) sample respectively. Obstetric fistulae are rare but can follow forceps or repeat Caesarean delivery. Symptoms of genuine stress incontinence [→ p.61] usually improve, particularly with formal pelvic floor exercises, but these have little preventive role.

Perineal trauma

Perineal trauma is repaired [→ p.246] after delivery of the placenta.

Pain occurs in 40% of all women after delivery and persists for more than 8 weeks in 10%. Superficial dyspareunia [→ p.294] is common, even years later. Pain is less

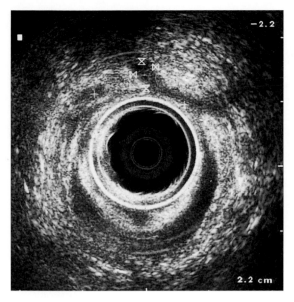

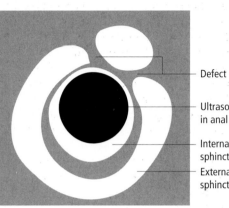

Defect

Ultrasound probe
in anal canal

Internal anal
sphincter

External anal
sphincter

Fig. 33.5 Ultrasound of disrupted anal sphincter.

when subcuticular Vicryl sutures have been used. The anti-inflammatory diclofenac is a highly effective anal geslc; ultrasound, salt baths and megapulse are of no benefit.

Paravaginal haematoma: Rarely, a woman experiences excruciating pain in the perineum a few hours after delivery. This is almost invariably due to a paravaginal haematoma, which is sometimes identifiable only on vaginal examination. This is drained under anaesthetic.

Bowel problems

Constipation and haemorrhoids both occur in 20% of women. Laxatives are helpful.

Incontinence of faeces or flatus is a distressing and an underreported symptom affecting 4% of women. Both pudendal nerve or anal sphincter damage [→ p.246] (Fig. 33.5) can be responsible and injury is often unrecognized. Forceps delivery, mid-line episiotomy, large babies, shoulder dystocia and persistent occipito-posterior positions are the main risk factors (*BMJ* 1994; **308**: 887). Affected women are evaluated using anal manometry and ultrasound, and managed according to symptoms. Formal repair may be required, after which deliveries should be by Caesarean section. The role of Caesarean section after an uncorrected anal sphincter injury or an asymptomatic one, however, is controversial.

Further reading

Glazener C, Abdalla M, Stroud P, *et al.* Postnatal maternal morbidity: extent, causes, prevention and treatment. *British Journal of Obstetrics and Gynaecology* 1995; **102**: 282–7.

National Institute for Health and Clinical Excellence (NICE). Antenatal and postnatal mental health. Clinical management and service guidance. NICE Clinical Guideline 45. 2007. http://www.nice.org.uk

Shevell T, Malone FD. Management of obstetric hemorrhage. *Seminars in Perinatology* 2003; **27**: 86–104.

Thakar R, Sultan AH. Management of obstetric anal sphincter injury. *The Obstetrician and Gynaecologist* 2003; **5**: 72–8.

Primary Postpartum Haemorrhage (PPH) at a Glance

Definitions	Primary: Blood loss >500 mL in first 24 h Secondary: Excessive blood loss between 24 h and 6 weeks
Epidemiology	10%; associated with Caesarean, forceps, prolonged labour, grand multiparity, antepartum haemorrhage (APH) and previous history
Aetiology	Uterine atony, retained placental parts; vaginal, uterine or cervical lacerations
Features	Look for poorly contracted uterus, bleeding perineum, vaginal or cervical lacerations
Investigations	Full blood count (FBC), clotting, cross-match; if severe, central venous pressure (CVP), cardiac monitor, oxygen saturation
Management	Bimanual uterine compression; suture cervical or vaginal tears Resuscitation with intravenous fluid, blood if necessary Ergometrine/oxytocin ± prostaglandin $F_{2\alpha}$ ($PGF_{2\alpha}$) Consider Rusch balloon, laparotomy, brace suture, embolization if these fail

Other Common Serious Problems of the Puerperium at a Glance

Secondary postpartum haemorrhage	Due to endometritis ± retained placental tissue. Give antibiotics, do evacuation of retained products of conception (ERPC) if no improvement
Pyrexia	Endometritis, wound, perineal, urine, breast, chest infection, thromboembolism Do cultures and give antibiotics
Urinary incontinence	20%. Exclude fistula and retention. Usually improves with time. Do urine culture and arrange physiotherapy
Urinary retention	Due to epidural or delivery, particularly forceps Catheterize for at least 24 h
Faecal incontinence	4%. Exclude rectovaginal fistula. Can be due to anal sphincter or pudendal nerve damage; associated with third-degree tears and forceps. Treat with physiotherapy ± sphincter repair
Postnatal depression	10%. Identification difficult and poor. Support, psychotherapy, drugs. Risk of suicide most with previous psychiatric illness
Thrombosis	0.5%. Major cause of mortality. Prophylaxis if high risk. Treat with subcutaneous low molecular weight heparin (LMWH)

34 Birth statistics and audit

Audit

This is the process whereby clinical care is systematically and critically analysed: comparing what *should be done* with what *is being done* allows changes to be made to what *will be done*. Practice can then be reanalysed, in a completion of the 'audit cycle'. The Confidential Enquiry into Maternal and Child Health (CEMACH) (www.cemach.org.uk) is an example of audit in obstetrics, which reports on maternal, perinatal and childhood mortality. This report, with lay and professional expert input, analyses, criticizes and makes recommendations; reports of later years examine their impact. On a local level, maternal and perinatal mortality are rare, and examination of 'near-miss maternal mortality', perinatal morbidity and intervention in pregnancy and labour are often more useful.

Perinatal mortality

Definitions and terms in the UK

Stillbirth occurs when a fetus is delivered after 24 completed weeks' gestation showing no signs of life.
Neonatal death is defined as death occurring within 28 days of delivery.
Early neonatal death occurs within 7 days of delivery.
Miscarriage occurs when a fetus is born with no signs of life before 24 weeks' gestation (however, if a fetus is delivered before 24 weeks, shows signs of life but subsequently dies, it is classified as a neonatal death).

Obstetrics and Gynaecology, 3rd edition. By Lawrence Impey and Tim Child. Published 2008 by Blackwell Publishing, ISBN: 978-1-4051-6095-7.

The perinatal mortality rate is the sum of stillbirths and early neonatal deaths per 1000 total births.
The 'corrected' perinatal mortality rate excludes those stillbirths and early neonatal deaths that are due to congenital malformations.

Different countries have different definitions concerning gestation and/or birthweight, so comparisons can be misleading. In 1992, in line with improvements in neonatal care, the earliest gestation defined as a stillbirth changed from 28 to the current 24 weeks in the UK. This is reflected in Fig. 34.1.

Perinatal mortality rate

In developed countries the perinatal mortality rate has been declining since the 1930s: in the UK it has declined from >50.0 to 8.2 per 1000 births in 2004 (not Scotland, where data is collected separately) (Fig. 34.1). The stillbirth rate in 2004 was 5.7 per 1000 births. The lowest rates are found in Scandinavian countries and the highest in Bangladesh and Central Africa.

Risk factors for perinatal mortality

Perinatal mortality is a reflection of obstetric care to only a limited extent and its decline has been more to do with better general health and nutrition, smaller families and improved neonatal care. The perinatal mortality rate is higher among lower socioeconomic groups, in those below 17 or above 40 years of age, in women who smoke, abuse drugs or have medical illnesses or poor nutrition. It is higher in highly parous women, in those of Asian or Afro-Carribean extraction and in those with multiple pregnancies.

Causes of perinatal mortality

Antepartum stillbirth is the principal contributor to perinatal mortality. The majority of cases are classified as 'unexplained' using traditional criteria. However,

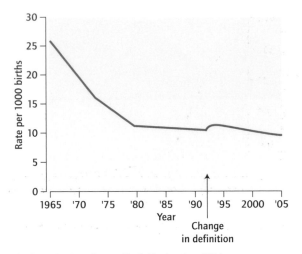

Fig. 34.1 Perinatal mortality in England and Wales.

intrauterine growth restriction (IUGR) is a frequent feature: if fetal growth is assessed according to individual maternal and pregnancy characteristics (customized growth charts) [→ p.206], then approximately 70% of hitherto unexplained antepartum stillbirths are actually small for dates (Fig. 34.2). This reflects the fact that absolute birthweight is less important than whether the birthweight is that expected from genetic characteristics.

Other common causes are pre-eclampsia [→ p.165], lethal congenital anomalies [→ p.148], preterm labour [→ p.190], antepartum haemorrhage [→ p.196] and intrapartum hypoxia [→ p.237].

Rarer causes of perinatal mortality include infection, birth trauma and fetal (e.g. vasa praevia) or feto-maternal haemorrhage.

Causes of death are classified by the Extended Wigglesworth and supplemented by the Obstetric Aberdeen classification system. However, many causes overlap: for instance, antepartum haemorrhage is associated with

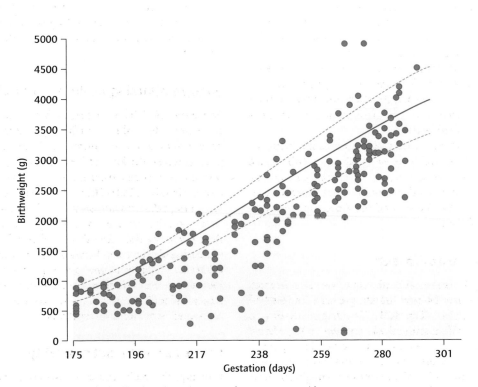

Fig. 34.2 Birthweight of 'unclassified stillbirths' after adjustment for constitutional factors.

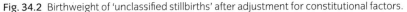

chronic compromise, pre-eclampsia, preterm labour and intrapartum hypoxia. Further, this classification takes little account of the issue of individual fetal growth.

Principal causes of perinatal mortality
Unexplained antepartum stillbirth
Intrauterine growth restriction (IUGR)
Prematurity
Congenital anomalies
Intrapartum hypoxia
Antepartum haemorrhage

Maternal mortality

Definitions

A maternal death is the death of a woman during pregnancy, or within 42 days of its cessation, from any cause related to or aggravated by the pregnancy or its management, but not from accidental or incidental causes.

A late maternal death is when a woman dies from similar causes but more than 42 days and less than a year after cessation of the pregnancy.

These are subdivided into '*direct' deaths*, which result from obstetric complications of the pregnancy, and '*indirect deaths*', which result from previous or new disease, which was not the result of pregnancy but nevertheless aggravated by it.

Recent new classifications are '*coincidental maternal deaths*', such as accidents or incidental death, which would have happened irrespective of the pregnancy, and '*pregnancy-related death*', including all 'maternal deaths' plus coincidental deaths, and therefore irrespective of the cause of death.

Maternal mortality rate

In the UK, the maternal death rate (direct and indirect, 2003–2005) was 14 per 100 000 pregnancies (0.01%) (CEMACH 2007) (Fig. 34.3). The rate in developed countries has fallen dramatically since the 1930s, when it was similar to that presently found in developing countries. In recent years this decline has 'bottomed out', although in up to 40% of cases the death might still have been avoided. Deaths in less developed countries are far

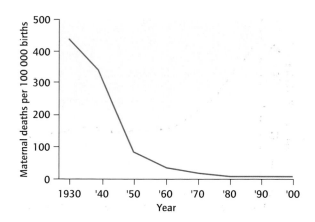

Fig. 34.3 Long-term changes in maternal mortality in the UK.

higher: rates of about 500 per 100 000 pregnancies (0.5%) are found in parts of Africa.

Maternal mortality has been reported triennially in England and Wales for over 50 years. This is now performed as part of CEMACH (www.cemach.org.uk). Of the 295 maternal deaths in the UK reported in 2007 for the period 2003–2005, 132 (6.24 per 100 000 maternities) were 'direct', 163 (7.71 per 100 000 maternities) indirect and 55 coincidental. Improved case ascertainment in the UK makes comparison with other countries difficult.

Factors affecting maternal mortality

Socioeconomic: The persisting high rates in developing countries reflect the contributory factors that have improved in developed countries. These factors include poor general nutrition and health, poverty, poor education and poor access to general and obstetric health care: in the triennium 2003–2005, of women who died from any cause, 14% admitted domestic abuse and 10% were from families known to child protection services. Recently, in the UK, increasing numbers of migrants and increasing obesity levels have also contributed.

Obstetric: Higher maternal age, high parity (mortality increases several-fold after four children), multiple pregnancy and multiple previous Caesarean deliveries are all associated with increased mortality.

Causes of maternal mortality

Globally, the main causes of maternal mortality are haemorrhage, obstructed labour, infection, severe

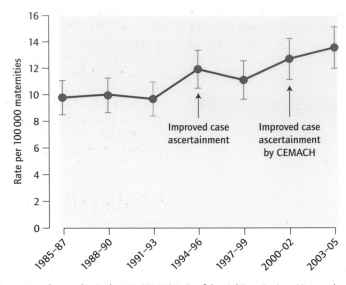

Fig. 34.4 Recent changes in maternal mortality in the UK. CEMACH, Confidential Enquiry into Maternal and Child Health.

pre-eclampsia and the consequences of illegal abortion. The causes are slightly different in developed countries: the latest figures from the UK are shown in Fig. 34.4 (CEMACH 2007).

Direct deaths (UK in 2003–2005)

Venous thromboembolic disease (41 deaths) is the most common direct cause. Deaths were from pulmonary embolism and cerebral venous thrombosis. Comments from CEMACH recommended better assessment of risk factors such as Caesarean section and a family history [› p.181], more prophylaxis and noted a failure to recognize clinical features in over half.

Haemorrhage (14 deaths): CEMACH has recommended protocols, fire drills, early and more senior intervention.

Hypertensive disease (18 deaths) were mostly as a result of intracranial haemorrhage associated with poorly controlled blood pressure. CEMACH has emphasized the importance of blood pressure control, fluid restriction and magnesium sulphate, and of recognition of pre-eclampsia.

Other causes include disorders of early pregnancy (mostly ectopic pregnancy), genital tract infection, amniotic fluid embolism, anaesthesia, acute fatty liver and genital tract trauma.

Indirect deaths (UK in 2003–2005)

Cardiac disease includes acquired and congenital cardiac disease, the incidence of which is rising among pregnant women. The importance of cardiological input has been emphasized by CEMACH.

Psychiatric disease is increasingly recognized, although most died after 42 days (i.e. late). Many were suicides, and although most had a psychiatric history, this was often not recorded or recognized. Nevertheless, suicide was less common than in the previous CEMACH report, possibly as a result of risks being highlighted.

Other indirect causes include drug/alcohol-related deaths, domestic violence, epilepsy and intracerebral haemorrhage.

Role of obstetric care

'Substandard care' has been assessed for many years in CEMACH reports. Recurrent features include a failure to recognize severe illness and poor communication and organization. In just over 50% of cases, substandard care was considered to be a major contributor. This, and consideration of organizational, demographic and socioeconomic features has led to a 'Top 10' list of recommendations in the recent report.

Principal causes of maternal death

Thromboembolism [→ p.180]
Hypertensive disorders [→ p.165]
Cardiac disease [→ p.177]
Ectopic pregnancy and abortion [→ pp.177, 119]
Haemorrhage [→ p.267]
Infection [→ p.269]
Neurological disease [→ p.178]
Psychiatric disease and suicide [→ p.182]

'Top Ten' Recommendations from CEMACH 2003–2005

1 Better preconception care, e.g. cardiac/psych. illness
2 Better access to care, e.g. early booking and . . .
3 See within 2 weeks of referral
4 Particular attention to health of migrant women
5 Adequate treatment of systolic hypertension
6 Caution re: Caesarean section rate
7 Improved skills: learning from events and . . .
8 Better training
9 Early warning systems for impending illness
10 More guidelines, e.g. obesity in pregnancy

Intervention in pregnancy and labour

The rate of obstetric intervention differs widely in different countries and hospitals or areas. Caesarean section is the most widely scrutinized, although induction rates, external cephalic version (ECV) [→ p.213] rates and instrumental delivery rates should also be audited. The Caesarean rate at different hospitals in the UK varies from <20% to >30%, and this cannot be entirely accounted for by population differences or 'case mix', be this medical or social differences, and is also dependent on the degree of supervision by, and interest from, senior staff and on institutional culture, midwifery skills and the percentage of home deliveries. A classification system called the Robson 'Ten Groups' examined 10 different groups of women, recording both the Caesarean section rate in that group, and the group's contribution to the

overall Caesarean section rate. This has been modified below (see box). It is clear that a previous Caesarean section is a major indication for another, whilst other multiparous women have a very low risk: this emphasizes the potential of avoiding the first Caesarean section. Likewise the use of induction is associated with an increase in Caesarean section (although care must be taken as it is usually 'higher risk' pregnancies that undergo induction). It is only by using such classifications that attempts can be made to alter practice.

Classification of Caesarean section

Indication*	Approx cs rate (%)	Approx % of total cs (%)[†]
Previous Caesarean section	70	20–25
Term breech presentation (if external cephalic version [ECV] available)	95	15
Nulliparous: cephalic, spontaneous labour	10	10
Nulliparous: cephalic, induced labour	20–25	10–15
Elective term Caesarean section (not breech or previous cs)	(100)	5
All multiparous women, cephalic, in labour	2	5
Preterm babies	40	5–10
Multiple pregnancies	60	5–8
Pure 'maternal request'	(100)	<5
Other	–	<5

cs, Caesarean section.
* Modified from Robson (2001).
[†] Individual units vary greatly.

Reasons why the Caesarean rate is high

Attempted reduction of perinatal and maternal risks. Most breech babies and the majority of women with one previous Caesarean section [→ p.252] undergo Caesarean section: these together account for the majority of elective Caesarean sections (not in labour). Cardiotography (CTG) in labour is widely used to try to avoid severe hypoxia [→ p.237], yet it is known to increase the risk of emergency Caesarean section. Clearly, as severe adverse outcomes become rarer, the 'net' is spread wider.
Obstetricians' lack of clinical skill. This undoubtedly contributes in the management of labour and interpreting

CTG, and skill at instrumental delivery and twin deliveries.

Fear of litigation. This is widely cited as contributory.

Maternal fear of labour [→p.231]. This contributes to prolonged labour an important factor that is seldom appreciated, but also to maternal request for Caesarean section: if a mother knows the chances of having a very long labour and *then* a Caesarean section are high, it is not surprising if she requests an elective one.

A belief that Caesarean section is the answer to most problems. Yet adverse perinatal outcomes and most adverse maternal ones are not related to labour.

Further reading

CMO's Annual Report 2007. 500 missed opportunities. http://www.dh.gov.uk/en/Publicationsandstatistics/Publications/AnnualReports/

Confidential Enquiry into Maternal and Child Health (CEMACH) *Saving Mothers' Lives: 2003–5.* London: RCOG Press, 2007. http://www.cemach.org.uk

Robson MS. Can we reduce the Caesarean section rate? *Best Practice & Research. Clinical Obstetrics & Gynaecology* 2001; **15**: 179–94.

Birth Statistics at a Glance	
Stillbirth	Fetus born dead at 24+ weeks
Neonatal death	Neonate dies <28 days after delivery (early is <7 days)
Perinatal mortality	Stillbirths plus early neonatal deaths; if 'corrected' excludes congenital anomalies Main causes: Unexplained antepartum, intrauterine growth restriction (IUGR), preterm labour, congenital anomalies, antepartum haemorrhage, intrapartum hypoxia, pre-eclampsia Rate: 7–9 per 1000 (1%) (UK)
Maternal mortality	Mother dies during or within 42 days of pregnancy from any cause related to (direct) or aggravated by (indirect) the pregnancy or its management, but not from accidental or incidental causes Main causes: Direct: venous thromboembolism, hypertensive disease, haemorrhage, sepsis, amniotic fluid embolism, ectopic pregnancy Indirect: cardiac disease, neurological and psychiatric disease Rate: 14 per 100 000 (approx 0.01%) (UK)

35 Legal issues in obstetrics and gynaecology

The UK's national annual insurance reserve estimate to cover the cost of clinical negligence litigation was £1 million in 1974–1975; for the year 2006–2007 £579.3 million was paid out for clinical negligence claims. Patients are more informed, they expect more, and they do not expect that pregnancy, as a normal life event, could go wrong. Funding options have also changed, with increased availability of legal expenses insurance and claimants' solicitors offering conditional fee agreements. In addition, the amount of compensation awarded has increased to keep track with inflation: in a successful clinical negligence claim the combined general and future damages awarded to look after the future care needs of a child with cerebral palsy can be several million pounds. There is no evidence, however, that more substandard practice is occurring.

Clinical negligence

In the UK, to establish that a doctor has been negligent, it must be established both that:

1 The doctor was in breach of his/her duty of care, either by act or omission; and that
2 This was on the balance of probabilities the most likely cause of harm.

The standard of care required is governed by the *Bolam* principle: 'A doctor is not guilty of negligence if he or she has acted in accordance with the practice accepted as proper by a responsible body of medical men skilled in that particular art' (Bolam vs. Friern Hospital 1957). This implies that imperfect medical care is not necessarily 'negligent'.

Establishing causation is particularly difficult in obstetrics. When an infant is born in poor condition and subsequently develops cerebral palsy, it is labour, as the most recent and apparently dangerous event, that is frequently blamed. Furthermore, patients frequently perceive labour-related events to be preventable. Hypoxia in labour, however, probably accounts for only 10% of cases of cerebral palsy [→ p. 203]. Guidelines to help establish whether hypoxia in labour is to blame have been drawn up (*BMJ* 1999; **319**: 1054), although they bear little relationship to whether cases are settled (*BJOG* 2003; **110**: 6).

Legal claims are funded in the UK by the Clinical Negligence Scheme for Trusts (CNST) insurance scheme, with Trusts paying insurance premiums to the National Health Service (NHS) Litigation Authority (www.nhsla.com), which is responsible for payments to claimants. There is a separate CNST standard for obstetrics in recognition of the fact that it is a high-risk area of clinical practice. The insurance premium is dependent on claims history and the fulfillment of a number of varied criteria, including risk management processes, minimum standards of clinical care, training guidelines and numbers of senior medical staff. Trusts can achieve three different standard 'levels' that influence the insurance premium they pay, and therefore act as financial incentives to make changes considered to be improvements to patient safety.

Clinical governance

The Chief Executive of a Trust now carries responsibility for the quality of medical care. Every Trust must have mechanisms to ensure the quality of care, identify faults and improve the service, and report annually on this. 'Clinical governance' has been developed, ostensibly to ensure the safety of patients and staff, and is described as 'a framework through which NHS organizations are accountable for continuously improving the quality of their services and safeguarding high standards of care by creating an environment in which excellence in clinical care will flourish'. Roughly translated, it means 'do a good job and prove it'.

Obstetrics and Gynaecology, 3rd edition. By Lawrence Impey and Tim Child. Published 2008 by Blackwell Publishing, ISBN: 978-1-4051-6095-7.

Clinical governance incorporates the implementation of evidence-based and 'effective' practice. Evidence-based guidelines for the management of common clinical situations have been drawn up, including guidance from the National Institute for Clinical Excellence (NICE; www.nice.org.uk), although they cannot entirely dictate the management of every clinical situation. It is easier to defend clinical practice if guidelines have been followed; equally, where a clear deviation has occurred, negligence is more likely to be alleged unless a clear reason for the deviation in practice is documented. Clinical governance also encompasses audit of clinical practice.

Risk management

Risk management aims to reduce risk of patient harm. Each NHS Trust has an incident reporting system to report adverse incidents: these range from third degree tears to maternal death. The organization has to routinely review, learn and, if necessary, change clinical practice or systems to try to prevent these from occurring again. CNST assessors audit NHS Trusts annually for evidence of working practices, protocols and guidelines that show good risk management systems (www.nhsla.com/RiskManagement/). In addition, the Healthcare Commission visits and assesses individual health care providers, providing scores on aspects such as use of resources, and 'quality of services'. The latter assesses a mass of criteria including cleanliness and sadly, in reality, is of minimal use for an individual in trying to decide where to be treated.

NHS complaints procedure

The NHS complaints procedure specifies time limits for the acknowledgement, investigation and resolution of a complaint. A complainant may obtain independent advice and representation for the Independent Complaints Advocacy Service (ICAS). If unsatisfied with a Trust's response, a complainant may request an independent assessment of their complaint with ultimate recourse to the Complaints Ombudsman. Many people seeking compensation cite a fear of other people experiencing the same situation or that communication after an adverse event was poor. Successful local resolution of a complaint can reduce the likelihood of litigation. If unhappy with the local response to the complaint, the complainant may take their case to the Healthcare Com-

mission (http://2007ratings.healthcarecommission.org.uk/homepage.cfm), and subsequently to the Health Service Ombudsman (www.ombudsman.org.uk/). They can also make an individual complaint about the healthcare professional to their regulatory body, e.g. the General Medical Council (GMC).

Consent

When negligent outcome is alleged it is common for patients to allege that they were not aware of the risks associated with the medical treatment. The Department of Health (DoH) consent forms now require discussion and documentation of the benefits, risks and side effects of treatment. It is considered preferable that the person performing the procedure takes the patient's consent, although this may often be impractical. Minor risks must be discussed if they are common; major risks must be discussed even if they are very rare.

Confidentiality

The doctor has a moral, professional, contractual and legal duty to maintain patient confidentiality. No details can be disclosed to a third party, including a relative, without the patient's consent. The Data Protection Act 1998 extends this duty to ensuring adequate protection and storage of information, such as patient records and communications. Confidentiality can be breached only in exceptional circumstances where the health and safety of others would otherwise be at serious risk.

Avoiding litigation
Communication
Consent
Clear documentation
Candour

Avoiding litigation

Besides ensuring you do your best medically, including referring to other more experienced colleagues if you are unsure, remembering the 4 'C's will help prevent allegations of negligence (Fig. 35.1). *Consent* must be thorough and this, and any discussion with or examination of a patient, must be *clearly documented*. Each entry in the notes must be legible, dated and signed, preferably with the doctor's name printed. *Communication* before and during treatment is essential, but even after an

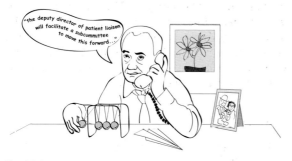

Fig. 35.1

adverse event has occurred, an adequate explanation, with *candour*, may be all that patients require.

Further reading

Clements RV. *Risk Management and Litigation in Obstetrics and Gynaecology*. London: RSM Press, 2001.
http://www.cgsupport.nhs.uk: for information on clinical governance
http://www.dh.gov.uk/en/Policyandguidance/Organisationpolicy/Complaintspolicy/index.htm
http://www.nhsla.com/Claims/Schemes/CNST/

Gynaecology management section

Management of bleeding or pain in early pregnancy

Fundamentals   Exclude ectopic pregnancy; ensure viability of intrauterine pregnancy

Causes	**Chapter reference**
Miscarriage	Chapter 14
Ectopic pregnancy	
Rarer: Molar pregnancy	**Where to see**
Gynaecological	Gynaecology 'on call'
	Gynaecology ward
	Theatre

Resuscitation   If collapse or heavy vaginal loss, intravenous (i.v.) access, give colloid and cross-match blood

History   Review of gynaecological history. Nature of pain and bleeding? Past pelvic operations? Ectopics? Pelvic inflammatory disease (PID)? Sexually transmitted infection (STI)? (i.e. ectopic risk factors)

Examination

General:	Anaemia, blood pressure (BP), pulse
Abdomen:	Tenderness, rebound tenderness
Pelvis:	Size of uterus, cervical excitation, adnexal mass/tenderness, cervical os open/closed (insert i.v. line first if ?ectopic), remove products in os if present

Investigations   Pregnancy test; ultrasound scan of pelvis (transvaginal sonography [TVS] if <7 weeks), full blood count (FBC), 'group and save' (G&S)

Management

If threatened:	Usually allow home if bleeding light
If missed:	Consider evacuation of retained products of conception (ERPC), medical or conservative management
If inevitable/incomplete:	Patient bleeding heavily: give ergometrine intramuscularly (i.m), confirm no products to be removed immediately from cervical os, do ERPC
	Patient not bleeding heavily: consider medical or conservative management
If complete:	(Empty uterus, history/examination) Allow home
If molar pregnancy:	Do ERPC, check histology and human chorionic gonadotrophin (hCG) and refer to centre
If certain ectopic:	Do laparoscopy or consider methotrexate if criteria met.

If unsure but possible ectopic (symptoms suggestive but uterus empty on ultrasound scan [USS] and no adnexal masses or pelvic free fluid [blood]):

Admit, i.v. access, do hCG:	If >1000 IU, do laparoscopy; if <1000 IU, repeat 48 h later
	If rise <66%, do laparoscopy. Repeat USS after 1 week if negative

After miscarriage or ectopic pregnancy:
Give anti-D if patient rhesus negative. Offer counselling or referral to support group

Management of heavy/irregular menstrual bleeding

Fundamentals	Treat bleeding according to severity of symptoms. Although rare, malignancy should be excluded

Causes

		Chapter references
Benign causes:	Idiopathic	Chapters 2–4, 9 & 13
	Anovulatory cycles, fibroids	
	Pelvic inflammatory disease (PID), polyps	**Where to see**
	Endometriosis, adenomyosis	Gynaecology ward
Malignant (rare):	Endometrial carcinoma (CA), cervical CA	Theatre
		Gynaecology clinic
Systemic:	Thyroid/clotting abnormalities	

History	Review of gynaecological history. Volume/timing/scale of blood loss? Effect on daily living? Intermenstrual/postcoital bleeding (PCB)? Dyspareunia/ dysmenorrhoea? Cervical smear history? Menopausal symptoms? When was last menstrual period (LMP)? Plans for fertility?

Examination

	General:	Weight, anaemia
	Abdominal:	Masses
	Pelvis:	Uterine size, consistency, mobility. Masses. Cervix

Investigations	Full blood count (FBC), consider thyroid function tests (TFTs) and pregnancy test. Do cervical smear if not up to date. Ultrasound scan (USS); biopsy if abnormal

Management

If <35 years:	Progestogen intrauterine system (IUS) if wants contraception Combined oral contraception (COC) to regulate/reduce volume if wants contraception Tranexamic acid, non-steroidal anti-inflammatory drugs (NSAIDs) if regular to reduce volume and if wanting to conceive Do hysteroscopy if this fails
If >35 years:	Do pelvic ultrasound ± hysteroscopy/endometrial biopsy first IUS if wants contraception COC to regulate/reduce volume if wants contraception and no contraindications Tranexamic acid, NSAIDs if regular to reduce volume Cyclical progestogens to regulate; hormone replacement therapy (HRT) if perimenopausal
If postmenopausal (PMB) only:	Urgent pelvic ultrasound; Pipelle biopsy or hysteroscopy if >4 mm endometrium or recurrent bleeding
If PCB only:	Do cervical smear ± colposcopy. If negative, consider cryotherapy
If malignancy:	Treat appropriately (Chapter 3–4)
If not:	With no response to medical treatment (including IUS), consider surgery: Hysteroscopic route (e.g. resection/ablation) If fibroids, consider myomectomy if patient wishes to conserve uterus
If treatment failure:	Hysterectomy, preferably vaginal if possible, or embolization

Management of the pelvic mass

Fundamentals   Exclude ovarian malignancy; remove persistent or enlarging masses unless asymptomatic fibroids or intrauterine pregnancy

Causes in postmenopausal women
Ovarian malignancy
Benign ovarian tumour
Fibroids
Rarer: Abscess, bladder, gastrointestinal tumour

Causes in premenopausal women
Pregnancy
Functional ovarian cyst
Benign ovarian tumour
Fibroids Ultrasound department
Rarer: Endometriosis, ectopic
         Abscess/hydrosalpinx
         Ovarian malignancy
         Bladder, pelvic kidney

Chapter references
Chapters 2, 3, 5, 8–10 & 14

Where to see
Gynaecology ward
Gynaecology clinic
Theatre

History   Review of gynaecological history. Menstruation? Pain? Weight loss?
Gastrointestinal/urinary symptoms? Investigate abnormal bleeding independently

---

Examination   General: Weight, anaemia, lymphadenopathy, breasts

Abdomen: Masses, ascites

Pelvis: Mobility, consistency of mass; separate from uterus?

Investigations   Ultrasound scan (USS). CA 125, urea and electrolytes (U&Es), full blood count (FBC), liver function tests (LFTs). Consider magnetic resonance imaging (MRI). Cross-match if for surgery

---

Management

Premenopausal women:
If fibroids: Manage according to symptoms and fertility plans [→ p.21]

If non-uterine mass <5 cm: If pain/possible abscess, laparoscopy
                              If not, reassess 2 months; if enlarged or solid/cystic, laparoscopy

If non-uterine mass >5 cm: Do laparoscopy ± laparotomy

Postmenopausal women:
Do laparoscopy. Proceed to laparotomy unless documented history of fibroids that are not enlarging

Management of urinary incontinence

Fundamentals	Incontinence is neither normal nor incurable, but treatment depends on the degree of inconvenience caused

Causes
Genuine stress incontinence (GSI)
Overactive bladder
Rarer: Chronic retention
            Fistula

Chapter reference
Chapter 8

Where to see
Gynaecology clinic
Urodynamics laboratory
Physiotherapy departments
Theatre

History	Review of gynaecological history. Incontinence with 'stress' or urgency? Daytime frequency? Nocturia? Enuresis? Haematuria? Dysuria? What is fluid/caffeine intake? How much is the patient's life affected? Smoker?

Examination	General:	Weight, chest problems (chronic cough)
	Abdomen:	Exclude masses, urinary retention
	Pelvis:	Exclude pelvic mass. Look for leak when coughing, prolapse, particularly of bladder neck (use Sims' speculum)

Investigations	Do mid-stream urine (MSU) and urinalysis
	Ultrasound or post-micturition catheterization if retention suspected
	Urinary diary: nocturia with small volumes suggests overactive bladder
	Consider methylene blue/intravenous pyelogram (IVP)/computed tomography (CT) urogram if possible fistula (continuous incontinence after recent pelvic surgery and/or irradiation)
	Cystometry if considering surgery for diagnosis of GSI or if failed medical treatment

Management

Optimize weight/fluid intake

If probable overactive bladder:	Bladder training and antimuscarinics. If no help then cystometry
If GSI likely:	Physiotherapy/Duloxetine ± surgery (only after cystometry) in form of tension-free vaginal tape/trans-obdurator tape (TVT/TOT)

Management of vaginal discharge

Fundamentals   Discharge is usually physiological or infective. Attention to detail prevents the diagnosis of 'intractable' discharge from being made

Causes
Candidiasis
Bacterial vaginosis (BV)
Atrophic vaginitis
Cervical eversion/ectropion
Trichomoniasis
Rarer: Malignancy
         Foreign body

Chapter references
Chapters 4 & 10

Where to see
Gynaecology clinic
Genitourinary medicine clinic
Microbiology laboratory

History   Review of gynaecological history. Ask about: Colour? Odour? Timing? Irritation?
Ask regarding: Pelvic pain? Sexual intercourse? Superficial dyspareunia?
Bloody discharge suggests malignancy of cervix or endometrium

Examination   Pelvis: Palpate for pelvic masses/tenderness

Speculum: Cervix: look for eversion/ectropion

Vaginal walls: Redness/irritation, atrophy, discharge

Investigations   Cervical smear, high vaginal swab (HVS) and cervical swab (including *Chlamydia*)
Take a slide and examine do whiff test, pH with litmus paper

Discharge and diagnosis

Cause	Itching	Discharge	pH	Redness	Odour	Treatment
Ectropion/eversion	No	Clear	Normal	No	Normal	Cryotherapy
Bacterial vaginosis	No	Grey/white	Raised	No	Fishy	Antibiotics
Candidiasis	Yes	'Cottage cheese'	Normal	Yes	Normal	Imidazole
Trichomonas	Yes	Grey/green	Raised	Yes	Yes	Antibiotics
Malignancy	No	Red/brown	Variable	No	Yes	Biopsy
Atrophic	No	Clear	Raised	Yes	No	Oestrogen

Management

If whiff test and swabs negative, infective cause unlikely:
Treat atrophic vaginitis with oestrogen cream (or consider hormone replacement therapy [HRT], if postmenopausal)
Treat cervical ectropion with cryotherapy or diathermy
Reassure if physiological

If infection present:
If candidiasis: Use clotrimazole pessary, and if recurrent, oral fluconazole
If BV: Use clindamycin cream or metronidazole
If sexually transmitted infection (STI):   Treat appropriately and arrange contact tracing

Management of the subfertile couple

Fundamentals	Consider basic criteria for fertility. Refer rapidly for assisted conception if failed treatment, especially if older woman

Common causes
Polycystic ovary syndrome (PCOS)
Pelvic inflammatory disease (PID)
Male factor
Endometriosis
Hyperprolactinaemia
Unexplained
Hypothalamic hypogonadism

Chapter references
Chapters 9, 10 & 11

Where to see
Gynaecology clinic
Fertility clinic or *in vitro* fertilization (IVF) unit
Andrology clinic
Theatre

Initial assessment

History	See the couple together. Offer counselling. Advise folic acid
	Review of gynaecological, medical and surgical history. Menstruation? Exercise? Smoking? Eating habits? Sexual intercourse frequency? (History from male if semen analysis abnormal)

Examination	General:	Health, blood pressure (BP), body mass index (BMI), hirsutism
	Pelvic:	Look for masses or reduced mobility

Investigations	Blood:	Check for ovulation: mid-luteal progesterone
		Cause for anovulation: follicle-stimulating hormone (FSH), luteinizing hormone (LH) (days 2–5), thyroid function (TFTs), prolactin, testosterone
		Check rubella immunity before pregnancy
	Semen analysis	
	Ultrasound:	Ovarian (polycystic ovary [PCO]) and uterine (fibroids/polyps) anatomy

Review

Results should be ready, and treatment can begin. Two or more causes may be found

If anovulation:	Reconsider weight gain or loss from history/examination
If prolactin raised:	Repeat and if persistent/high, do computed tomography (CT) of pituitary
	Start bromocriptine/cabergoline
If TFTs abnormal:	Treat appropriately
If PCOS:	Give clomifene days 2–6 and check mid-luteal progesterone in two subsequent cycles. Ultrasound monitoring. 10% multiple pregnancy rate
If FSH, LH low:	(Oestradiol low also) Start gonadotrophins
If FSH and LH high:	Recheck several times. If consistent, premature menopause: offer egg donation. Then pill/HRT for bone protection

If semen analysis abnormal, repeat:

If mild abnormalities:	Alteration in personal habits, testicular cooling. Try intrauterine insemination (IUI)
If marked abnormality:	Examine male, do FSH, LH, testosterone, prolactin, TFTs and refer to andrologist
If oligospermic:	Where no treatable cause found, consider IVF + intracytoplasmic sperm injection (ICSI)

(Continued)

Management of the subfertile couple (Continued)

If azoospermic:	Donor insemination or surgical sperm retrieval (SSR) followed by IVF + ICSI.
If all above normal:	Laparoscopy and dye test or hysterosalpingogram/HyCoSy
If fallopian tube damage:	
If both tubes blocked:	IVF
If peritubal adhesions:	Surgery (divide) at time of laparoscopy
If endometriosis:	Surgery (diathermy/laser) at time of laparoscopy

Subsequent management

General	Confirm ovulation with mid-luteal progesterone
If PCOS	If resistant to clomifene, try metformin, ovarian diathermy at laparoscopy, or gonadotrophins If still unsuccessful: consider IVF

Once situation optimized, e.g. previously anovulatory patient ovulating on treatment, wait 6 months. If pregnancy still not achieved or cause unexplained, consider IUI/IVF

Management of acute pelvic pain

Fundamentals   Alleviate pain; identify and treat cause; consider ectopic pregnancy

Common causes
Ectopic pregnancy
Septic/incomplete miscarriage
Ovarian cyst accident
Pelvic inflammatory disease, endometriosis
Renal tract infection/calculus
Appendicitis
Ovarian malignancy if older
None found

Chapter references
Chapters 5, 8–10 & 14

Where to see
Gynaecology 'on call'
Gynaecology clinic
Theatre

History   Review of gynaecological history. Timing? Nature/site of pain? Menstruation? Dyspareunia? Sexual/contraceptive history? Gastrointestinal symptoms/anorexia?

Examination   General: Appearance, shock, temperature, blood pressure (BP), pulse, anaemia

Abdomen: Site and degree of tenderness, bowel sounds

Pelvis: Masses, cervical excitation, adnexal tenderness, discharge

Investigations   Pregnancy test, swabs for culture if negative, ultrasound scan (USS), full blood count (FBC), mid-stream urine (MSU)

Differentiation between common causes of acute pelvic pain

	Ovarian cyst accident	Ectopic	Pelvic inflammatory disease (PID)	Appendicitis
Initial pain	Unilateral	Unilateral	Bilateral	Right-sided
Bleeding	Occasional	Usual	Often	Unusual
Discharge	Occasional	Bloody	Usual	No
Fever	Low grade	No	Often	Low grade
Peritonism	Often	Often	Often	Usual
Pregnancy test	Usually negative	Positive	Negative	Negative
Ultrasound	Usually shows cyst	Empty uterus	Normal	Normal pelvis

Management

Give analgesia, admit, nil by mouth

If probable ectopic: Laparoscopy
If ovarian cyst: Laparoscopy
If PID: Antibiotics
If unsure: Where pregnancy test negative, admit, observe, give antibiotics empirically, and do laparoscopy if no improvement

Management of chronic pelvic pain

Fundamentals	Exclude pathological causes with history and laparoscopy, offer support if apparently not pathological. Rare in postmenopausal women, so consider malignancy

Causes
Endometriosis
Adenomyosis
Chronic pelvic inflammatory disease (PID)
Irritable bowel syndrome (IBS)
Adhesions
Urinary tract: Interstitial cystitis
Pelvic pain syndrome

Chapter references
Chapters 9 & 10

Where to see
Gynaecology clinic
Pain clinics
Counselling sessions

History	Review of gynaecological history. Is pain cyclical? Dyspareunia? Bowel habit and effect of opening bowels on pain (bowel endometriosis or IBS)? Discuss effect on patient's life, and stress/life events
Ask about previous pelvic infection or surgery

Examination	General:	Health, weight, appearance; mental state
	Abdomen:	Tenderness, masses
	Pelvis:	Tenderness, masses, endometriosis on uterosacral ligaments

Investigations	Ultrasound scan (USS), mid-stream urine (MSU) sample, magnetic resonance imaging (MRI) if ?adenomyosis
Do high vaginal swab (HVS) and cervical swab
Laparoscopy

Management

If features of IBS:	Antispasmodics and refer to dietitian ± gastroenterologist
If other symptoms or signs (e.g. abnormal bleeding):	Investigate and treat appropriately
Initially:	Consider trial of ovarian suppression with combined oral contraceptive (COC) (or gonadotrophin-releasing hormone [GnRH] agonists). If improvement, can continue without further investigation. If no help, consider non-hormonal/gynaecological cause
Perform laparoscopy:	If wants firm diagnosis, declines drug treatment or if drugs fails. If wanting to conceive so cannot use ovarian suppression
If organic cause:	Treat appropriately [→ p.69]
If adhesions at laparoscopy:	Cut but ascribe pain to them with caution
If laparoscopy negative:	If intractable pain try ovarian suppression with COC or GnRH agonists
If successful:	Continue with ovarian suppression. If not possible then consider total hysterectomy and bilateral salpingo-oöphorectomy if family complete
If unsuccessful:	Pain management programmes, psychotherapy or counselling

Management of chronic dyspareunia

Fundamentals	Differentiate between deep and superficial dyspareunia, exclude organic, and consider pyschological factors

Causes

Deep causes:
Endometriosis
Chronic pelvic inflammatory disease (PID)
Pelvic mass
Irritable bowel
Ovarian cyst

Superficial causes:
Vagina/vulval infection
Surgery; childbirth
Psychological
Also: Vulval dysplasias; atrophic vaginitis

Chapter references
Chapters 6 & 9

Where to see
Gynaecology clinic

History	Review of gynaecological/obstetric history. Dyspareunia deep or superficial? Timing? Sexual history? Other symptoms? What is the patient's reaction to the problem?

Examination

General: Mental state

Abdominal: Masses, tenderness

Pelvic: If superficial, inspect vulva and vagina: pinpoint tender area
If deep, uterine mobility, adnexal and uterosacral tenderness/thickening (?endometriosis)

Investigations

Superficial: High vaginal swab (HVS) and cervical swab

Deep: Laparoscopy

Management

Superficial dyspareunia:

If painful ulceration:	Often herpes simplex	Swab, contact tracing, aciclovir
If discoloration:	Vulval condition intraepithelial neoplasia (VIN)	Biopsy, then treat
If vaginal discharge:	Trichomoniasis, candidiasis	Take swabs, treat [→ p.77]
If thin red epithelium:	Atrophic vaginitis	Topical oestrogen/hormone replacement therapy (HRT)
If mass:	Vaginal cyst, Bartholin's abscess	Surgery
If normal:	Psychological/vaginismus	Gradual dilatation; psychotherapy
If recent surgery/birth:	Perineal trauma	Unless obvious abnormality, wait 6 months before surgery (e.g. Fenton's repair)

Deep dyspareunia:

Do laparoscopy:	If organic cause found:	Treat (fibroids/retroverted uterus are rare as causes)
	If pelvis normal:	Treat as chronic pelvic pain [→ p.69]; consider psychotherapy

Management of the abnormal smear

Fundamentals   Cervical screening reduces the incidence of cervical carcinoma
Cervical intraepithelial neoplasia (CIN) is a histological diagnosis

Chapter reference
Chapter 4

Where to see
Gynaecology clinic
Colposcopy clinic
Pathology laboratory

History   Review of gynaecological history. Contraception and sexual intercourse? Menstruation? Cervical smear history? Vaginal discharge? Smoking?

Examination   To exclude coincidental disease or advanced carcinoma

Management

If smear is:

Mild dyskaryosis/borderline changes:	Repeat in 6 months, colposcopy if persistent
Moderate dyskaryosis:	Do colposcopy
Severe dyskaryosis:	Urgent colposcopy
Columnar atypia/cervical glandular intraepithelial neoplasia (CGIN):	Colposcopy; hysteroscopy if cause not found

If colposcopy suggests:

CIN I/human papilloma virus (HPV)	Do biopsy, repeat smear in 6 months
CIN II–III:	Large loop excision of transformation zone (LLETZ)
Invasion:	Diagnostic cone biopsy

If histology shows:

CIN II–III	Repeat smear in 6 months
Invasion <3 mm (Stage 1 a(i) CA):	Do cone biopsy
Deeper/lymph invasion:	Treat as cervical carcinoma

Obstetric management section

Management of common problems in the antenatal clinic

Fundamentals   Listen to the patient. Beware of unexplained proteinuria or reduced fetal movements

Chapter references
Chapters 20, 21 & 24–26

Where to see
Antenatal clinic
Antenatal ward
Ultrasound department

Management

If reduced fetal movements:
Check fetal size, consider ultrasound scan (USS) for growth. Do cardiotocography (CTG). Warn about continuing surveillance of movements [→ p.206]

Possible ruptured membranes (spontaneous rupture of membranes [SROM]):
Ask regarding contractions. If history suggestive of SROM, admit to hospital for confirmation. Check presentation. Do sterile speculum examination of posterior vaginal fornix to look for fluid. Avoid digital examination unless contractions or CTG abnormal

Hypertension, but blood pressure (BP) <170/110 mmHg, no proteinuria:
Possible early/mild pre-eclampsia. Recheck BP and urinalysis twice a week and refer for USS. Do a full blood count (FBC), urea and electrolytes (U&E), liver function tests (LFTs), uric acid

Hypertension, BP ≥170/110 mmHg ± 1+ proteinuria:
Admit to hospital and manage as pre-eclampsia

No hypertension, >/=2+ (new) proteinuria:
Admit to hospital to exclude or confirm pre-eclampsia

Symphysis–fundal height >2 cm below number of weeks at 24 weeks or more:
Arrange USS for size, and umbilical artery Doppler if small size confirmed

Antepartum haemorrhage:
Admit to hospital. Do CTG

Abnormal lie:
If <37 weeks: review at 37 weeks
If ≥37 weeks: admit to hospital and do USS

Breech at/after 37 weeks:
Refer for USS and consider external cephalic version (ECV)

Pregnancy at or beyond 41 weeks:
Recheck gestation. Offer cervical sweep. Offer induction by T+10 days. If not, daily CTG

Suspected polyhydramnios:
Do USS: if confirmed, look for fetal anomaly on ultrasound and check glucose levels [→ p.175]

Management of the small for dates fetus

Fundamentals   Perinatal mortality is higher with lower birthweight, but most mortality is of apparently normally grown fetuses

Common causes
Constitutional factors
Idiopathic
Maternal disease, e.g. pre-eclampsia
Smoking
Multiple pregnancy

Chapter references
Chapters 20, 21 & 25

Where to see
Antenatal clinic
Ultrasound department

History   Review of obstetric and medical history. Previous birthweight? Smoking? Complications (e.g. pre-eclampsia)? Vaginal bleeding? Fetal movements?

Examination   General: Blood pressure (BP) and urinalysis

Abdominal: Symphysis–fundal height

Investigations   Ultrasound scan (USS); umbilical artery (UA) Doppler, cardiotocography (CTG)

To identify the small for dates fetus
'Low-risk' pregnancy:
Measure symphysis–fundal height. If <2 cm less than gestation, refer for USS

'High-risk' pregnancy:
As above and serial USS measurement of fetal growth at 28, 32 and 36 weeks (frequency depends on risk)

Management

If ultrasound shows:
Size > 10th centile: Continue usual antenatal care
Size < 10th centile: Do UA Doppler. Look for fetal/maternal disease, e.g. pre-eclampsia

If <10th centile and Doppler shows:
Normal resistance: Repeat USS and UA Doppler every 2 weeks

High resistance: If >37 weeks, do CTG and induce
                   If <37 weeks, repeat twice weekly

Severe abnormality: If >34 weeks, CTG and deliver
                      If <34 weeks, fetal Doppler, steroids, daily CTG

If CTG shows: Normal: do daily
               Abnormal: deliver (usually lower segment Caesarean section [LSCS])

Management of hypertension in pregnancy

Fundamentals   Pre-eclampsia is common, is unpredictable and can kill the mother and the fetus. Monitor both

Causes		**Chapter references**
Pregnancy-induced:	Pre-eclampsia and transient	Chapters 17, 20 & 25
Underlying:	Essential and secondary	

Where to see
Antenatal ward
High-dependency ward
Antenatal clinic

History   Review of obstetric history. Did hypertension predate pregnancy/20 weeks? Risk factors for pre-eclampsia? Headache? Epigastric pain?

Examination   General: Recheck blood pressure (BP) and urinalysis. Look for epigastric tenderness, oedema, radio-femoral delay and renal bruits. Examine fundi

Abdominal: Symphisis–fundal height

Investigations   Do urea and electrolytes (U&E), full blood count (FBC), liver function tests (LFTs), uric acid, 24-h urine for protein (if >trace proteinuria) and vanillylmandelic acid (VMA). Ultrasound scan (USS) for growth, umbilical artery (UA) Doppler. Cardiotocography (CTG)

Management

As outpatient:
If BP < 170/110 mmHg and <0.3 g/24 h proteinuria
Do twice weekly BP and urinalysis, fortnightly USS for fetal growth, UA Doppler

Admission:
If BP ≥ 170/110 mmHg or >0.3 g/24 h proteinuria, or if symptoms or fetal compromise

Treat BP if:
BP ≥ 170/110 mmHg: Admit, give nifedipine, start methyldopa. If BP still ≥170/110 mmHg, repeat nifedipine

Delivery:
If eclampsia: Give magnesium sulphate, stabilize [→ p.170], fluid restrict, CTG. Deliver. Intensive monitoring

If other complications: Stabilize, fluid restrict. CTG. Deliver. Intensive monitoring

If no complications: If proteinuria and >34–36 weeks, admit, daily CTG, induction
If proteinuria and <34 weeks, steroids, monitor daily as in-patient including CTG, deliver (usually LSCS) if deterioration
If no proteinuria and BP < 170/110 mmHg, consider delivery at term

After delivery: Treat BP ≥ 170/110 mmHg, fluid balance; FBC, U&E, LFTs. Keep in hospital for 5 days

Management of abnormal or unstable lie at term

Fundamentals	Only abnormal after 37 weeks: exclude pathological cause, beware cord prolapse. Most spontaneously turn to cephalic and deliver normally

Common causes	**Chapter reference**
Lax multiparous uterus	Chapter 26
Abnormal uterus	
Pelvic obstruction, e.g. placenta praevia	**Where to see**
Polyhydramnios	Antenatal ward

History	Review of obstetric history. Diabetic? Multiparous?

Examination	Abdominal:	Palpation of lie, liquor volume, fetal size
	Vaginal:	(If not placenta praevia) Exclude pelvic mass

Investigations	Ultrasound scan (USS) for liquor volume, fetal/uterine abnormality, placental site

Management

If lie not longitudinal <37 weeks:	Recheck at 37 weeks
If lie not longitudinal >37 weeks:	Admit and stay unless cephalic for >48 h
If lie never longitudinal:	Lower segment Caesarean section (LSCS) at 39 weeks
If lie abnormal/unstable >41 weeks:	LSCS

Management of breech presentation

Fundamentals Breech presentation at term is associated with increased risk. External cephalic version reduces the incidence of breech delivery and Caesarean section

Causes	**Chapter reference**
Idiopathic	Chapter 26
Abnormal fetus	
Pelvic obstruction	**Where to see**
Twins	Antenatal clinic
Uterine anomaly	Ultrasound department
	Labour ward

History Review of obstetric history. Check gestation

Examination Abdominal: Confirm presentation

Vaginal: (If not placenta praevia)

Investigation Ultrasound scan (USS) to confirm, look for abnormalities, placenta praevia and suitability for external cephalic version (ECV)

Management

If <37 weeks:	Review at 37 weeks
If >37 weeks:	Counsel, and attempt ECV if no contraindication
If contraindication:	Lower segment Caesarean section (LSCS) at 39 weeks, check presentation first
If successful:	Manage as normal
If unsuccessful:	LSCS at 39 weeks, check presentation first

Management of antepartum haemorrhage

Fundamentals Resuscitate mother first, beware concealed haemorrhage, deliver baby if fetal distress or heavy maternal blood loss

Common causes
Placenta praevia
Placental abruption
Undiagnosed

Chapter reference
Chapter 24

Where to see
Antenatal ward
Theatre
Labour ward

Resuscitation If patient shocked, or heavy vaginal bleeding, or pain

Insert intravenous (i.v.) access, give colloid, cross-match blood and check full blood count (FBC), urea and electrolytes (U&E), clotting. Consider uncross-matched blood

Nurse in left lateral position, oxygen. Analgesia

History Review of obstetric history. Is placental site known? Pain (constant/contractions)? Volume and colour of blood loss?

Examination

General: Colour, pulse, BP

Abdomen: Tenderness, uterine activity, size and presentation, head engagement

Pelvis: Vaginal examination (VE) (if placenta praevia excluded)

Investigations Cardiotocography (CTG) (immediate), ultrasound scan (USS) to determine placental site/fetal viabilty
Catheterize if heavy bleed (hourly urine output), blood tests as above

Management

The shocked patient must receive full resuscitation

Placenta praevia:

Shock/heavy bleeding or >37 weeks: Lower segment Caesarean section (LSCS). Give blood. Risk of postpartum haemorrhage (PPH)

Blood loss stopped, <37 weeks: Give steroids if <34 weeks, anti-D if Rhesus negative
Keep in hospital; LSCS at 39 weeks

Placental abruption or undiagnosed bleed:

CTG abnormal: Emergency LSCS

Fetus dead: Anticipate coagulopathy and transfuse blood ±FFP
Induce labour. Intensive monitoring; consider CVP line

CTG normal, >37 weeks: Induce unless small painless bleed

CTG normal, <37 weeks: Steroids if <34 weeks, anti-D if Rhesus negative
Serial USS

Recurrent small painless bleeds without placenta praevia:
Inspect cervix, consider colposcopy. Serial USS

Management of prelabour rupture of the membranes

Fundamentals	Beware of infection; if present, deliver whatever gestation

Causes	**Chapter references**
Idiopathic	Chapters 23 & 30
Infection	
	Where to see
	Antenatal ward

History	Review of obstetric history. Known group B streptococcus (GBS) carrier? Gestation? Colour of fluid? Contractions?

Examination	General:	Temperature, pulse
	Abdomen:	Lie, presentation, engagement, tenderness
	Vaginal:	Only if abnormal lie or presentation. Can pass sterile speculum

Investigations	Cardiotocography (CTG), high vagina; swab (HVS). Ultrasound scan (USS) for growth, presentation, liquor volume if preterm

Management

If infection:	(Fever/tachycardia/abdominal tenderness/offensive liquor) Antibiotics and deliver whatever gestation
If <37 weeks:	Do 4-hourly pulse, temperature, and fetal heart rate. Give steroids if <34 weeks. Give erythromycin. Induce labour at 36 weeks
If >37 weeks:	Induction slightly safer but may prefer to wait. Give antibiotics if >18 h If meconium, induce immediately

Management of induction of labour

Fundamentals   Induction can fail. Easier to do in multiparous than nulliparous

Common indications Prolonged pregnancy Prelabour term spontaneous rupture of membranes (SROM) Medical conditions in pregnancy Intrauterine growth restriction (IUGR)	**Chapter reference** Chapter 30 **Where to see** Labour ward

History   Review of obstetric history. Check gestation, indication

Examination   Abdominal: Check longitudinal lie and cephalic presentation

Vaginal: To assess cervical 'ripeness'

Investigation   Cardiotocography (CTG)

Management

Cervix unripe: Give prostaglandin E_2 (PGE_2) usually in evening; reassess a.m. (>6 h later)
If cervix unchanged, repeat prostaglandin once
Otherwise, artificial rupture of membranes (ARM), oxytocin if no labour in 2 h

Cervix ripe: Do ARM and await labour. Oxytocin if no labour in 2 h

In labour: Anticipate slow progress initially and maintain encouragement. Treat as high risk

Management of slow progress in labour

Fundamentals	Oxytocin safe in nulliparous women, beware slow progress in multiparous/previous lower segment Caesarean section (LSCS)

Causes

		Chapter references
Powers:	Inefficient uterine action	Chapters 28 & 29
Passenger:	Occipito-posterior (OP) position, brow or face	**Where to see**
Passage:	Cephalo-pelvic disproportion	Labour ward

History   Review of obstetric history. Parity? Induction?

Look at partogram: length of labour, cervical dilatation

If slow progress in second stage, has passive stage been ignored? Oxytocin used?

Examination

General:	Temperature, pain relief, hydration, adequate support
Abdomen:	Note fetal size, degree of engagement
Vaginal:	Cervical dilatation, station of head, position and attitude, moulding

Investigations   Cardiotocography (CTG)

Management

First stage:
Consider mobilization if delay not extreme and mother willing

If nulliparous:	Do artificial rupture of membranes (ARM); start oxytocin if no further dilatation 2 h later
If multiparous:	Do ARM; start oxytocin 2 h later if no malposition
Both:	Do LSCS if no increase in rate of dilatation within 4 h of oxytocin

Second stage:

If nulliparous:	Anticipate if head high/epidural present: start oxytocin and delay pushing by 1 h
If multiparous:	No oxytocin: anticipate malposition or presentation
Both:	Push for 1 h; then instrumental delivery if prerequisites met; LSCS if not

Management of suspected fetal distress in labour

Fundamentals	Resuscitate first. Most suspected fetal distress cases are false alarms. Consider fetal blood sampling (FBS) unless bradycardia, when act quickly

Causes	Chapter reference
Unknown	Chapter 29
Chronic fetal compromise	
Prolonged labour; rapid labour	**Where to see**
Acute intrapartum events, e.g. cord prolapse	Labour ward

Resuscitation (of fetus)	Lie patient in left lateral, oxygen and stop any oxytocin infusion Intravenous (i.v.) fluid

History	Review of obstetric history and labour: Is it high risk, induced?
	Why is fetal distress suspected (i.e. abnormal cardiotogram [CTG], or pH of FBS). Flat on her back? Epidural or oxytocin?

Examination	General:	Take blood pressure, temperature
	Abdominal:	Uterine tenderness
	Vaginal:	Assess for cord prolapse and assess progress of labour

Management

If recent epidural insertion:	Increase i.v. fluid. Check BP.
If cord prolapse or bradycardia:	Urgent delivery (lower segment Caesarean section [LSCS] unless full dilatation)
If other CTG abnormality:	Do FBS and analyse pH
If pH <7.20:	Urgent delivery, LSCS unless full dilatation
If pH <7.25, ≥7.20:	Repeat FBS at 30 min
If CTG abnormality worsens/persists:	Repeat FBS at 30 min

Management of collapse on the labour ward

Fundamentals	Request senior help early and involve anaesthetic staff. Haemorrhage is the most common cause

Causes		**Chapter references**
Haemorrhage:	Intra-abdominal/revealed	Chapters 20, 21, 24, 32 & 33
Also:	Eclampsia or severe pre-eclampsia	
	Total spinal, local anaesthetic toxicity	**Where to see**
	Pulmonary or amniotic fluid embolus	Labour ward
	Maternal cardiac disease	High-dependency unit

Resuscitation	Clear airway, oxygen. Cardiopulmonary resuscitation (CPR) if necessary. Intravenous (i.v.) access
	If seizures, give diazepam; magnesium sulphate if eclampsia

History	Review of obstetric and medical history. Eye-witness account? Ante/postpartum? Vaginal bleeding? Pain? Seizures?

Examination	General:	Colour, pulse, temperature, blood pressure, sweating
		Lungs/heart
	Abdominal:	Uterine and abdominal tenderness; fetal lie
		If postpartum, uterine size

Investigations	Cross-match, clotting, full blood count (FBC), urea and electrolytes (U&E), liver function tests (LFTs). Cardiotocogram (CTG) if fetus undelivered

Management

Antepartum:

If bleeding heavy:	Placenta praevia or abruption [→ p.196] likely
If not but pale/tachycardic:	Abruption/uterine rupture [→ p.264] are likely

Postpartum:

If bleeding heavy:	Atonic uterus/retained placenta, or laceration [→ p.246] likely
If not, but pale/tachycardic:	Uterine rupture or atonic uterus full of blood

If sudden cardiorespiratory embarrassment:
Consider pulmonary embolus [→ p.181], amniotic fluid embolus [→ p.263], or cardiac decompensation in cardiac disease

If seizures:
Consider eclampsia [→ p.169], epilepsy or cardiorespiratory embarrassment

Management of massive postpartum haemorrhage

Fundamentals Blood loss may be faster than you can replace, so find cause. Call for senior and anaesthetic/haematological help early

Causes
Uterine atony
Retained placental parts
Perineal/vaginal trauma
Also: Cervical laceration
        Uterine rupture
        Coagulopathy

Chapter references
Chapters 32 & 33

Where to see
Labour ward
Theatre
Postnatal ward

Resuscitation Is placenta delivered? If not, do so. Lie patient flat, give oxygen; intravenous (i.v.) access, colloid or O-negative blood if *in extremis*. Compress uterus bimanually

History Review of obstetric history. Pain? Mode of delivery?

Examination	General:	Pallor, pulse, blood pressure
	Abdominal:	Size of uterus, abdominal tenderness
	Vaginal:	For bimanual compression. Exclude uterine inversion, palpate and inspect for vaginal tears

Investigations Check full blood count (FBC), urea and electrolytes (U&E), clotting, cross-match

Management

If perineal/vaginal trauma:	Suture
If uterus poorly contracted:	Give ergometrine and oxytocin infusion
If bleeding persistent:	Examination under anaesthetic (EUA): uterine cavity, cervix and vagina
	Remove placental tissue manually if present
If uterine atony confirmed:	Intra-myometrial prostaglandin $F_{2\alpha}$ ($PGF_{2\alpha}$) if oxytocics fail
If uterine bleeding persists:	Laparotomy, consider brace suture/tamponade with balloon/embolization/hysterectomy or ligation of the internal iliac arteries
After:	Check clotting, FBC. Watch fluid balance and oxygen saturation. Oxytocin infusion

Principles of blood volume replacement
Blood loss is often underestimated
Normovolaemia is the priority
Stop the source of bleeding
Use central venous pressure (CVP) monitoring to prevent fluid overload
Use fresh frozen plasma (FFP) if >5 U of blood are needed

Management of postpartum pyrexia

Fundamentals   Full investigation and treatment prevents mortality and morbidity

Causes	**Chapter references**
Uterine infection	Chapters 21 & 33
Wound infection	
Urine infection	**Where to see**
Also: Thromboembolism, mastitis	Postnatal ward
Chest infection	
Perineal infection	

History   Review of obstetric and medical history. Mode of delivery? Prolonged spontaneous rupture of membranes (SROM)? Pyrexia in labour? Pain? Cough? Shortness of breath? Dysuria?

Examination	General:	Temperature, pulse, blood pressure
	Abdomen:	Uterine or loin tenderness
	Vaginal:	Uterine tenderness, cervical os open?
	Other:	Breasts, legs, chest, perineum/wound, intravenous (i.v.) sites

Investigations	Routine:	FBC; blood, urine and high vaginal swab (HVS) cultures
	If appropriate:	Sputum, wound swab cultures; venogram

Management

If endometritis:	Antibiotics, review after culture sensitivity. Do evacuation of retained products of conception (ERPC) if not improving <24 h
If wound infection:	Keep clean and give antibiotics
If chest infection:	Antibiotics and arrange physiotherapy
If mastitis:	Antibiotics and consider possibility of breast abscess
If suspected deep vein thrombosis (DVT):	Low-molecular-weight heparin. Organize venogram/investigations for pulmonary embolus [→ p.181]

Management of preterm delivery

Epidemiology	8% of deliveries; 20% of mortality; 50% of childhood handicap
Aetiology	Infection: Vaginal e.g. BV, STDs, unknown UTI Cervix: 'Incompetence' usually idiopathic Fetal 'survival' response: PET, IUGR, placental abruption Multiple pregnancy: Higher risk with increasing number Uterine abnormalities: e.g. fibroids, congenital abnormalities Polyhydramnios: e.g. congenital abnormalities, diabetes Other associations: Male gender, low social class, extremes of age Iatrogenic delivery: Usually PET or IUGR
Screening	On history; TVS of cervical length
Prevention	Antibiotics if BV or UTI Cervical suture: either elective or ultrasound-indicated Reduction if high order multiple pregnancy (>2). Progesterone supplementation
Features	Abdominal pains, rupture of membranes, PV bleeding
Investigations	Ultrasound, CTG, swab (HVS) for infection
Management	Steroids if <34 weeks, tocolysis (e.g. nifedipine) to delay labour Antibiotics in labour LSCS for normal indications including breech Liaise with neonatologists

Appendix 1

Common drugs: safety and usage in pregnancy and breastfeeding

Drug	Risk*	Conclude	Alternatives	Breastfeeding
Antibiotics				
Metronidazole	Possible increased risk of preterm labour	Caution	Clindamycin	Safe
Penicillins	Nil known	Use if indicated	N/A	Safe
Erythromycin	Nil known	Use if indicated	N/A	Safe
Cephalopsorins	Nil known	Use if indicated	N/A	Safe
Augmentin	Possible increased neonatal risk if preterm birth	Caution	Penicillins	Safe
Tetracyclines	Discolour teeth if 2nd trimester	Avoid	Erythromycin	Safe
Trimethoprim	Folic acid antagonsist	Avoid	Cephalosporins	Safe
Fundamentals: bacterial infection in pregnancy requires treatment				
Analgesics				
Non-steroidals (normal dose)	Closure of fetal ductus arteriosus	Caution (avoid for analgesia)	Paracetomol	Safe
	Fetal oliguria			
	Possible cerebral haemorrhage	Monitor fetus with ultrasound		
Aspirin (low dose)	Nil known	Use if high risk of pre-clampsia	N/A	Safe
Paracetomol	Nil known	Safe	N/A	Safe
Opiates	Maternal/fetal dependency	Only if severe pain or drug dependency	(Methadone if opiate addict)	Beware accumulation
Fundamentals: best use paracteomol, plus codeine if more severe				
Anticoagulants				
Warfarin	Teratogenic	Only if artificial heart valves (seek advice)	LMWH	Safe
	Fetal haemorrhage			
LMWH (e.g. fragmin)	Maternal bleeding in OD	If indicated	N/A	Safe
	Safe for fetus			
Fundamentals: anticoagulation is probably under-used in pregnancy, warfarin only used in exceptional circumstances				
Antihypertensives				
ACE inhibitors	Fetal renal failure	Avoid	Methyldopa	Captopril safe
	Teratogenic (3% risk)		Nifedipine	
Methyldopa	Nil known	Best 1st line	N/A	Safe
Beta-blockers	Possible IUGR if early	Caution, 3rd line	Methyldopa	Safe
Ca antagonists	Nil known	Best 2nd line (e.g. nifedipine)	N/A	Safe
Thiazide diuretics	Maternal hypovolaemia	Avoid	Methyldopa	Safe
Fundamentals: severe hypertension in pregnancy is common and life-threatening and requires treatment				

(Continued)

Common drugs: safety and usage in pregnancy and breastfeeding (Continued)

Drug	Risk*	Conclude	Alternatives	Breastfeeding
Endocrine/hormone treatments				
Thyroid hormone	(Replacement therapy)	Use if indicated	N/A	Monitor thyoid
Propylthiouracil	Fetal hypothyroidism (rare)	Use, minimum dose	N/A	Monitor thyroid
Carbimazole	Fetal hypothyroidism (rare), aplasia cutis	Use, minimum dose	Propylthiouracil	Monitor thyroid
Insulin	(Replacement therapy) Maternal hypoglycaemia	Use with usual precautions	N/A	Safe
Metformin	Probably safe, few data	Caution	Insulin	Safe
Fundamentals: treatment of underlying disease greatly reduces maternal and fetal risks				
Immunosuppressants				
Ciclosporin	Nil known	Continue, monitor levels	N/A	Probably safe
Azathioprine	Minimal	Continue if indicated	N/A	Safe
Prednisolone	No fetal effects Maternal gestational diabetes, hypertension	Use minimum dose	N/A	Safe
Fundamentals: treatment of underlying disease (e.g. transplant) imperative and greatly reduces maternal and fetal risks				
Psychiatric medications				
Tricyclics	Largely safe	Use if high risk of relapse	Fluoxetine	Safe
SSRIs	Paroxetine teratogenic (3% risk) others probably safe	Use if high risk of relapse (avoid paroxetine, fluoxetine probably best)	Fluoxetine	Safe
Lithium	Teratogenic (cardiac) (10% risk)	Use only if high risk of relapse	Difficult	Watch for toxocity
Neuroleptics	Possible very mild teratogenicity largely unknown	Usually continue because of risk of relapse (avoid clozapine)	Difficult	Probably safe
Fundamentals: psychiatric disease is a major problem during/ after pregnancy so treatment may need to continue				
Antiepileptics				
Sodium valproate	Impaired childhood cognition teratogenic (4–9% risk)	Minimize combinations Consider change if <12 weeks	Carbamazepine N/A	Safe
Carbamazepine	Teratogenic (1–3% risk)	Usually continue	N/A	Safe
Lamotrigine	Teratogenic (1–5% risk)	Usually continue	N/A	Safe
Fundamentals: best sorted preconceptually. Seizure control imperative, but minimize combinations and doses. High-dose folic acid				
Other drugs				
Steroids (lung maturation: betamethasone and dexamethasone)	Nil known with single course	Use if high risk for preterm labour Betamethasone best	N/A	N/A
Beta-agonists	Nil known at anti-asthmatic doses	Use if indicated	N/A	Safe
Ursodeoxycholic acid	None known	For cholestasis	N/A	Not indicated

ACE, angiotensin-converting enzyme; IUGR, intrauterine growth restriction; LMWH, low-molecular-weight heparin; OD, overdose; SSRI, selective serotonin reuptake inhibitor.
* Note background risk of congenital malformations 1–2%.

Appendix 2

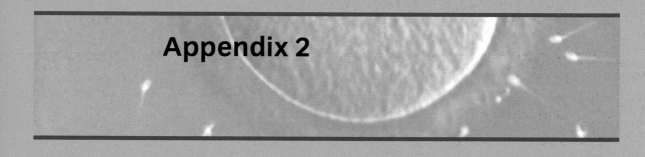

Normal maternal ranges in pregnancy

Full blood count

Hb	10.5–14.0 g/dL	Levels higher if routine supplementation given
WBC	5.0–11.0 g/dL	Levels unchanged in pregnancy, but rise in labour
Platelets	100–450 × 10⁹/L	Slight drop towards term

Note: High Hb associated with worse perinatal outcomes. Rapid drop in platelets suggestive of complications in PET

Thyroid function

Free T4	11–22 pmol/L	Slightly lower in early pregnancy
Free T3	43–5 pmol/L	Slightly lower in early pregnancy
TSH	0–4 mu/L	Aim for 1.5–2.0 if replacement therapy

Note: Undertreated and subclinical hypothyroidism associated with cognitive deficit in childhood

Renal function

Urea	2.8–3.8 mmol/L	Lowered in pregnancy
Creatinine	50–80 µmol/L	Lowered in pregnancy
Uric acid	0.14–0.2/0.35 µmol/L	×100 should be < gestation in weeks after 20 weeks
Na⁺	135–145 mmol/L	Unchanged in pregnancy
K⁺	3.5–4.5 mmol/L	Usually slightly low in pregnancy
Protein excr.	<0.3 g/24 h	Slightly raised

Note: Increased renal excretion in pregnancy. High creatinine/uric acid common with PET

Liver function

ALP	<500 IU/L	Raised in pregnancy
ALT	<30 IU/L	Slightly reduced in pregnancy
AST	<35 IU/L	Slightly reduced in pregnancy
Albumin	28–37 g/L	Slightly reduced in pregnancy

Note: Rapid rise in liver enzymes common with complications of PET

Other

ESR	>30	Elevated; no clinical use in pregnancy
CRP:	<8	Unchanged by pregnancy
Glucose:	<6.0 fasting	Slight fall in pregnancy
	<8.0 after food	

Note: Tight glucose control improves outcomes with maternal diabetes

Index

Note: Page numbers in *italic* refer to figures